Workbook for

Radiographic Image Analysis

Third Edition

Kathy McQuillen Martensen, MA, RT(R)
Director, Radiologic Technology Education
University of Iowa Hospitals and Clinics
Iowa City, Iowa

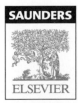

SAUNDERS

ELSEVIER

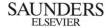

SAUNDERS
ELSEVIER

3251 Riverport Lane
St. Louis, Missouri 63043

Workbook for Radiographic Image Analysis, Third Edition   978-1-4377-0337-5

Notice

Knowledge and best practice in this field are constantly changing. As new research and experience broaden our understanding, changes in research methods, professional practices, or medical treatment may become necessary.

Practitioners and researchers must always rely on their own experience and knowledge in evaluating and using any information, methods, compounds, or experiments described herein. In using such information or methods they should be mindful of their own safety and the safety of others, including parties for whom they have a professional responsibility.

With respect to any drug or pharmaceutical products identified, readers are advised to check the most current information provided (i) on procedures featured or (ii) by the manufacturer of each product to be administered, to verify the recommended dose or formula, the method and duration of administration, and contraindications. It is the responsibility of practitioners, relying on their own experience and knowledge of their patients, to make diagnoses, to determine dosages and the best treatment for each individual patient, and to take all appropriate safety precautions.

To the fullest extent of the law, neither the Publisher nor the authors, contributors, or editors, assume any liability for any injury and/or damage to persons or property as a matter of products liability, negligence or otherwise, or from any use or operation of any methods, products, instructions, or ideas contained in the material herein.

The Publisher

ISBN: 978-1-4377-0337-5

Vice President and Publisher: Andrew Allen
Publisher: Jeanne Olson
Associate Developmental Editor: Luke Held
Publishing Services Manager: Patricia Tannian
Project Manager: Claire Kramer

Printed in the United States of America

Last digit is the print number: 9   8   7   6   5   4   3   2   1

Working together to grow
libraries in developing countries

www.elsevier.com | www.bookaid.org | www.sabre.org

ELSEVIER   BOOK AID
International   Sabre Foundation

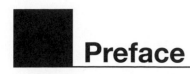

Preface

This workbook has been designed to provide students with a means of testing their understanding of the information covered in the *Radiographic Image Analysis* textbook. It follows the same format as the textbook with the first two chapters focusing on the technical and screen-film and digital imaging concepts that are considered when all procedures are evaluated. The workbook includes questions and images to evaluate for each of the technical and exposure concepts presented in the first two chapters of *Radiographic Image Analysis*. The remaining chapters guide the student through the image-analysis process of each body structure in a systematic fashion. The chapters can be followed as written, or the student may skip from chapter to chapter or procedure to procedure.

For these chapters the workbook provides the following features for each procedure presented:

- Study questions that focus on how the patient should be positioned to obtain an accurately positioned image and what criteria should be present when proper positioning is obtained. Also, there are questions that concentrate on improperly positioned images. The student is asked to state how the patient was mispositioned to obtain such an image.
- Poorly positioned images that separately focus on each topic and procedure. The images are different from those found in the textbook and sometimes present multiple positioning problems. Nonroutine scenarios and images are also presented.
- Answer keys to the study questions at the end of the workbook.

Student Guidelines

Prerequisite:	It is suggested that a course in anatomy and basic medical terminology be taken before studying radiographic procedures and analysis. For best understanding, it is effective to study the radiographic procedure in conjunction with the analysis.
Guideline 1	Read the learning objectives provided in the *Radiographic Image Analysis* textbook for the chapter being studied. These objectives outline key issues within the chapter and identify the knowledge you should understand after the chapter has been studied.
Guideline 2	Read the corresponding chapter in *Radiographic Image Analysis* and attend the procedure and analysis courses that focus on the subject matter.
Guideline 3	Fill in as many of the study question blanks as you can without referring to the textbook or the workbook answer key. Any blanks that you were unable to complete indicate the areas that require further study. If you left any questions unanswered or if you were uncertain of the correct answer, restudy the information that was covered in those questions.
Guideline 4	Check your study question answers with the answers provided at the end of the workbook. Restudy the information covered in any questions you answered incorrectly.
Guideline 5	Consult with your instructor about taking a final examination.

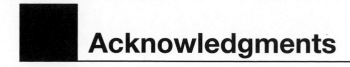Acknowledgments

I am pleased to acknowlege and recognize my friend and colleague Stephanie Harris, BS, RT(R)(CT)(M), for the help she provided in locating needed images, writing questions, reviewing the book, and providing support in areas too numerous to list. Stephanie is a dedicated educator with whom I am honored to work.

Contents

1 | Image Analysis Guidelines

STUDY QUESTIONS

1. An optimal radiographic image demonstrates what desired features?

A. _____

B. _____

C. _____

D. _____

E. _____

F. _____

G. _____

Using the Key Terms list at the beginning of Chapter 1 in the *Radiographic Image Analysis* textbook, complete the following.

2. Use the lateral chest drawing in Figure 1-1 to complete the following statements.

Figure 1-1

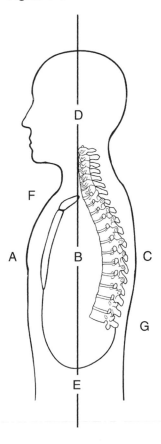

A. Letter B is situated on the _____ plane.

B. Letter A is placed _____ to letter B.

C. Letter C is placed _____ to letter B.

D. Letter D is placed _____ to letter B.

E. Letter E is placed _____ to letter B.

F. Letter F is placed _____ to letter B.

G. Letter G is placed _____ to letter B.

3. The inferior scapular angle moves toward the front and outer edge of the body when the humerus is abducted. What combination of the positioning terms is used to describe this movement? _____

4. When the humerus is brought from an abducted position to the patient's side, the inferior scapular angle moves toward the patient's back and closer to the midsagittal plane. What combination of the positioning terms is used to describe this movement? _____

5. What combination of the positioning terms is used to describe the portion of the scapula that is positioned closest to the patient's front and head? _____

6. If the IR was placed against the lateral aspect of the patient's leg and the central ray was centered to the medial aspect, what projection of the leg was taken? _____

7. Use the abdominal drawing in Figure 1-2 to complete the following statements.

Figure 1-2

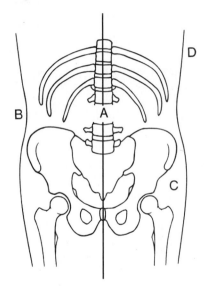

A. Letter A is situated on the _____ plane.

B. Letter B is placed _____ to letter A.

C. Letter A is placed _____ to letter B.

D. Letter C is placed _____ to letter A.

E. Letter D is placed _____ to letter A.

8. Use the drawing of the knee in Figure 1-3 to complete the following statements.

Figure 1-3

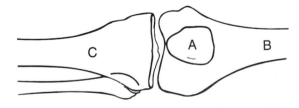

A. Letter B is placed _____ to letter A.

B. Letter C is placed _____ to letter A.

9. Use the following clues to complete the crossword puzzle shown in Figure 1-4.

Figure 1-4

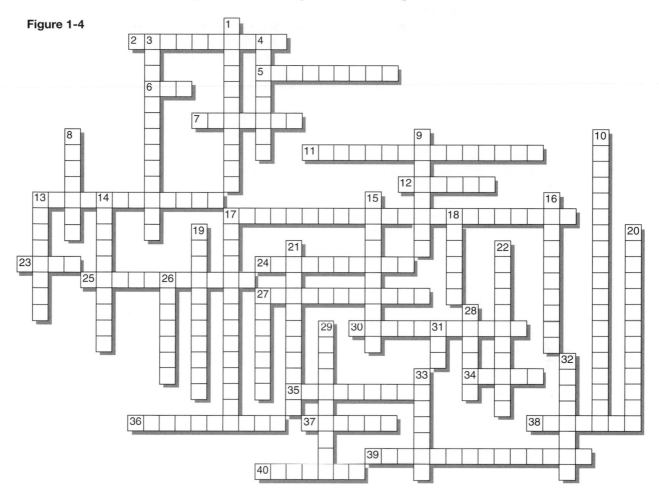

Across

2 Plane that divides the body into equal anterior and posterior halves
5 Position in which the patient lies on a cart and a horizontal beam is used
6 Absorbed dose to the most superficial layers of skin
7 Outline of an anatomic structure
11 Shortest exposure time to which the automatic exposure control (AEC) can respond
12 Situated far from the source or beginning
13 Filter used to remove photons from the beam to produce uniform density
17 How differently each tissue composition type will absorb photons
23 Device used to reduce amount of scatter radiation reaching the image receptor (IR)
24 Results of poor central ray and grid alignment
25 Determines maximum time that the AEC x-ray exposure will be allowed to continue
27 Diseases that cause the structure to be more radiolucent
30 Sthenic is example
34 Philosophy used to guide good radiation exposure practices
35 Absorption of radiation in heel of anode, causing less radiation intensity at anode end of IR
36 Ability to differentiate details from one another on an image
37 Foot end of patient
38 Radiation that has changed in direction from primary beam
39 Sharpness of structures
40 Contrast caused by x-ray attenuating characteristics of subject

Down

1 Decreased size of one axis of a structure
3 Law that states that radiation intensity is inversely proportional to square of its distance from x-ray source
4 Diseases that cause tissues to increase in mass density or thickness
8 Kilovoltage peak (kVp) that will provide adequate body part penetration and sufficient gray scale
9 Gown snap on an image
10 Biologic response of radiation exposure directly related to dose received
13 Number of gray shades used to represent different image structures
14 Results of using an angled central ray while part and IR remain parallel
15 Misrepresentation of size or shape of structure
16 Chamber in AEC system that collects radiation
17 Maximum permissible radiation dose limits
18 Law used to adjust milliampere-second (mAs) to maintain density when souce–image receptor distance (SID) is changed
19 Allowing passage of x-radiation
20 Device that receives radiation leaving patient
21 Plane that divides body into equal left and right halves
22 Motion that patient is unable to control
26 Act of throwing a structure
27 Degree of darkness on image
28 Technique whereby object–image receptor distance (OID) is increased to reduce amount of scatter radiation reaching IR
29 Preventing passage of x-radiation
31 System that automatically determines image density by stopping exposure
32 Head end of patient
33 Movement that bends a joint

10. State the distances indicated in Figure 1-5.

Figure 1-5

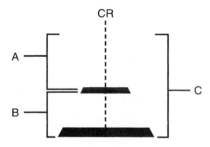

A. _____

B. _____

C. _____

11. Use the following (1 to 6) to define how radiographic images of the listed body parts are accurately displayed.
    1. Displayed as if the patient were standing upright
    2. Displayed as if hanging from the fingertips
    3. Displayed as if hanging from the shoulders
    4. Displayed as if hanging from the toes
    5. Displayed as if hanging from the hip
    6. Displayed as if hanging from the anterior surface

    A. _____ Chest

    B. _____ Wrist

    C. _____ Lumbar vertebrae

    D. _____ Humerus

    E. _____ Toes

    F. _____ Oblique foot

    G. _____ Lateral foot

    H. _____ Ankle

    I. _____ Lower leg

    J. _____ AP hip

    K. _____ Axiolateral shoulder

    L. _____ Cervical vertebrae

    M. _____ Abdomen

12. Evaluate the following projections for displaying accuracy.

Figure 1-6

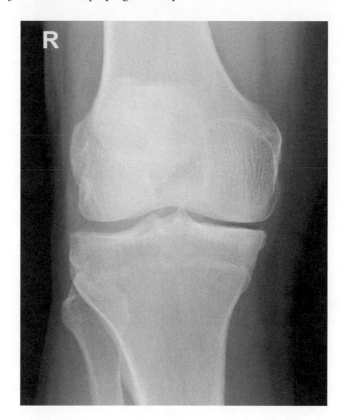

A. AP knee (Figure 1-6): _____

_____

Figure 1-7

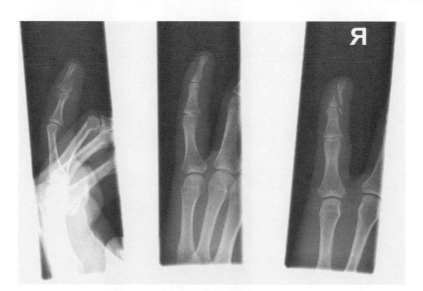

B. Left finger (Figure 1-7): _____

_____

Figure 1-8

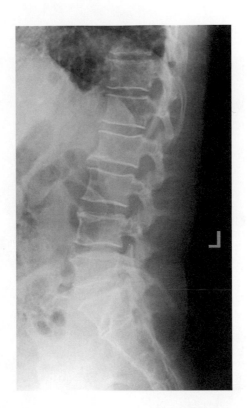

C. Left lateral lumbar vertebrae (Figure 1-8): _____

_____

Figure 1-9

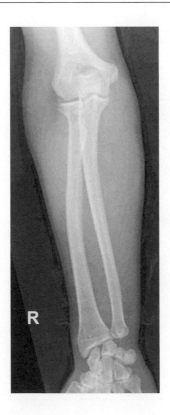

D. Right AP forearm (Figure 1-9): _____

_____

Figure 1-10

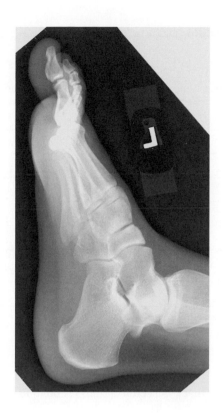

E. Left lateral foot (Figure 1-10): _____

_____

Figure 1-11

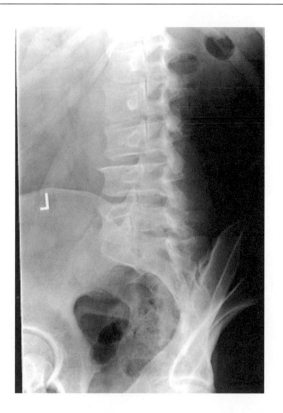

F. AP oblique (LPO) lumbar vertebrae (Figure 1-11): _____

_____

13. When an AP-PA projection or AP-PA oblique projection of the torso is accurately displayed, the patient's right side is on the viewer's _____ side.

14. List the demographic information that should be permanently photoflashed to the ID plate or displayed on the digital monitor.

    A. _____

    B. _____

    C. _____

    D. _____

    E. _____

    F. _____

15. State the guidelines that are followed when determining the best location to position the identification plate.

    A. _____

    B. _____

    C. _____

16. What marker is used for a patient that is placed in a right PA oblique projection (RAO position)?

    (A) _____

    Where is the marker placed on the IR in reference to the patient?

    (B) _____

17. A lateral vertebral projection is requested and the right side is placed closest to the IR.

    What marker is placed on the IR for this projection?

    (A) _____

    Where is the marker placed on the IR in reference to the patient?

    (B) _____

18. Evaluate the following projections for marker placement accuracy.

Figure 1-12

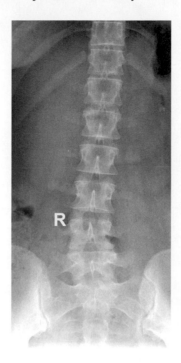

A. AP lumbar vertebrae (Figure 1-12): _____

_____

Figure 1-13

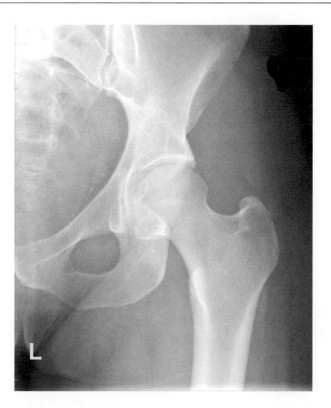

B. AP left hip (Figure 1-13): _____

_____

Figure 1-14

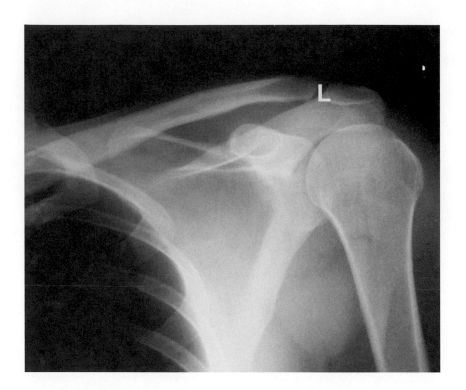

C. AP left shoulder (Figure 1-14): _____

_____

Figure 1-15

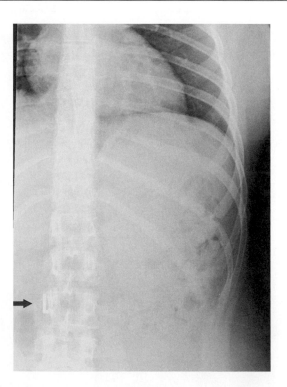

D. AP left lower ribs (Figure 1-15): _____

_____

Figure 1-16

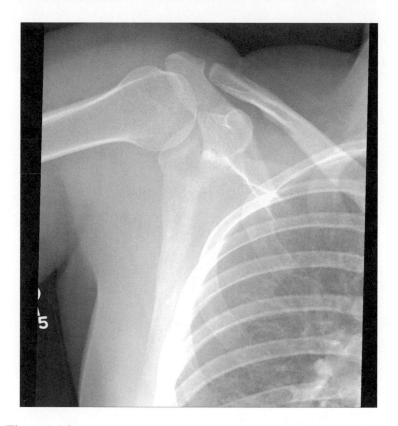

E. AP right scapula (Figure 1-16): _____

_____

19. The markers used in radiography are constructed of (A) _____ and are (B) _____ (radiolucent/radiopaque).

20. The marker placed on a lateral projection of the torso or skull represents the side of the patient that is positioned _____ (closer to/farther from) the IR.

21. Place an R where the marker should be positioned on the hip diagram in Figure 1-17.

Figure 1-17

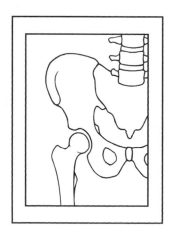

22. Place an L where the marker should be positioned on the lateral sacral diagram in Figure 1-18.

Figure 1-18

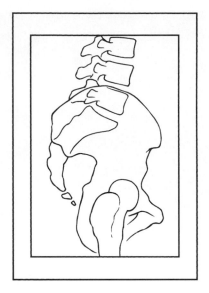

23. How is the image marked when a patient is placed in an AP oblique projection (LPO or RPO position)?

_____

_____

24. What procedure is followed when using a screen-film imaging system and the marker has not been demonstrated within the collimated field but is only faintly seen along its border?

_____

_____

_____

25. Use the following (1 to 4) to complete the following body habitus statements.
    1. Hypersthenic
    2. Sthenic
    3. Hyposthenic
    4. Asthenic

   A. The _____ body habitus demonstrates the longest thoracic cavity.

   B. The _____ body habitus demonstrates the broadest diaphragm.

   C. The _____ body habitus requires a crosswise IR to be used when imaging the thoracic cavity.

   D. The _____ body habitus demonstrates the widest and shortest thoracic cavity.

   E. The _____ body habitus demonstrates the lowest situated diaphragm.

   F. The _____ body habitus has an abdominal cavity that has length and width between the sthenic and asthenic habitus.

   G. The _____ body habitus would require the highest central ray centering to include the diaphragm.

   H. The _____ body habitus would require the lowest central ray centering to include the entire thoracic cavity.

   I. The _____ body habitus would require two crosswise 14- × 17-inch IRs to include the entire peritoneal cavity.

   J. The _____ body habitus would demonstrate a thoracic cavity image with the greatest superoinferior length.

26. Identify which body habitus type is being demonstrated in each of the following projections.

Figure 1-19

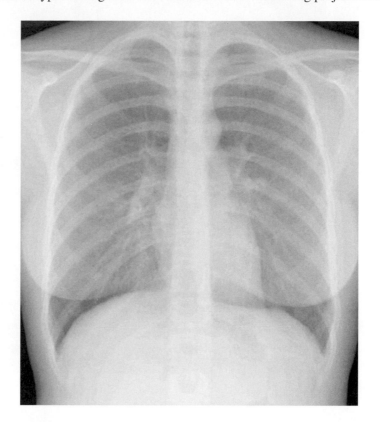

A. Figure 1-19: _____

Figure 1-20

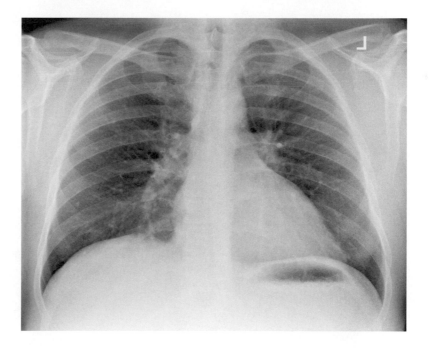

B. Figure 1-20: _____

Figure 1-21

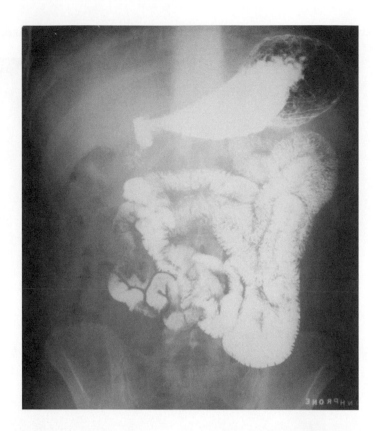

C. Figure 1-21: _____

Figure 1-22

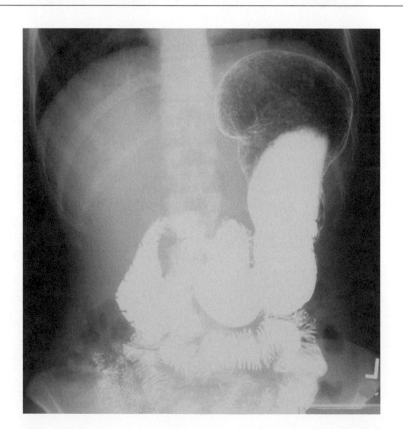

D. Figure 1-22: _____

27. Describe why it is necessary to have the IR extend beyond the joint spaces by 1 to 2 inches (2.5 to 5 cm) when imaging long bones, such as the forearm, humerus, lower leg, and femur.

_____

_____

28. Evaluate the accuracy of the placement of the anatomic structures on the IR in Figure 1-23.

Figure 1-23

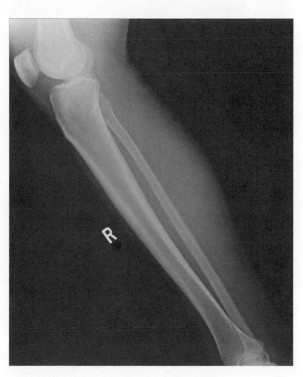

_____

_____

29. Evaluate the accuracy of IR choice and placement of the anatomic structures in Figure 1-24.

Figure 1-24

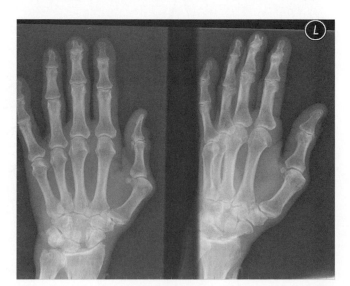

_____

_____

30. Good collimation practices (A) _____ (increase/decrease) patient dosage and (B) _____ (increase/decrease) the visibility of recorded details and image contrast by reducing the amount of (C) _____ that reaches the IR.

31. State where the central ray was centered on the projection in Figure 1-25.

Figure 1-25

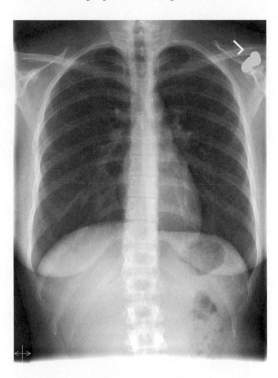

32. The collimator's light field demonstrated on the patient's abdomen in Figure 1-26 measures 8 × 10 inches (18 × 24 cm). Does this mean that the IR placed in the Bucky needs to be only 8 × 10-inches, or should it be larger or smaller?

Figure 1-26

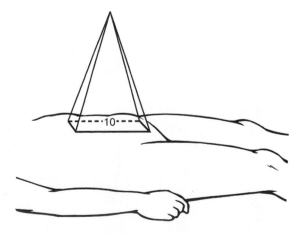

A. _____

B. Defend your answer. _____

_____

33. Evaluate the following projections for good collimation practices and state how poor central ray centering has prevented tighter collimation.

Figure 1-27

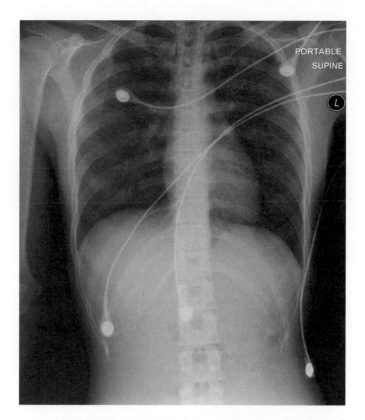

A. Figure 1-27 (AP chest): _____

Figure 1-28

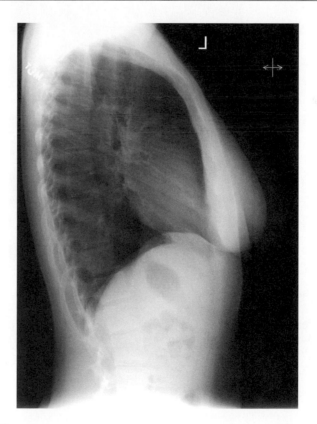

B. Figure 1-28 (lateral chest): _____

Figure 1-29

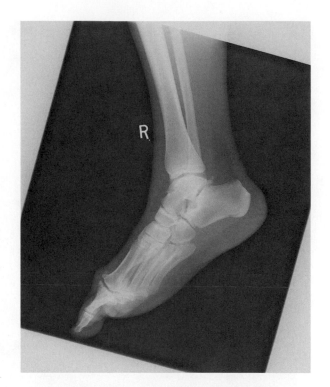

C. Figure 1-29 (lateral foot): _____

Figure 1-30

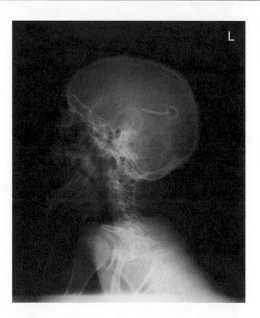

D. Figure 1-30 (lateral skull): _____

34. Where should the marker be positioned on the IR for an AP lumbar vertebral projection that was obtained using a 14- × 17-inch (35- × 43-cm) IR and a 10- × 15-inch (25- × 38-cm) collimation field?

_____

35. Tighter collimation was obtained on one of the AP clavicular projections in Figure 1-31 with the tube column rotated and the other was obtained with the collimator head rotated. Indicate below the clavicular projection that was obtained with the tube column rotated and the projection obtained with the collimator head rotated.

Figure 1-31

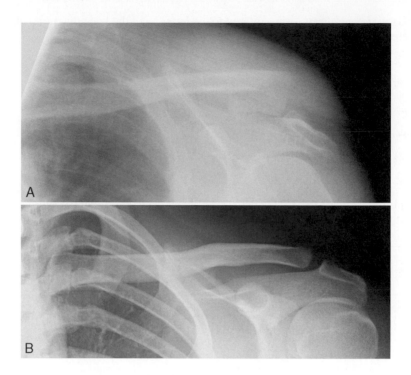

A. Tube column rotation: _____ (A or B)

B. Collimator head rotation: _____ (A or B)

C. Defend your answers to A and B above. _____

_____

36. When imaging a specific body structure within the torso, how can one determine whether the collimating field is close to that structure without clipping it?

_____

_____

37. Use the lateral knee diagram in Figure 1-32 to answer the following questions.

Figure 1-32

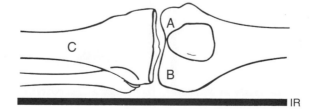

A. If a perpendicular central ray were centered to letter A on the knee diagram, where would letter A be positioned in reference to letter B on the resulting radiographic image?

_____

B. If a perpendicular central ray were centered to the letter C on the knee diagram, where would letter A be positioned in reference to letter B on the resulting image?

(1) _____

Will both letter A and letter B be projected the same distance?

(2) _____ (Yes/No)

Defend your answer.

(3) _____

_____

C. If the central ray were angled 15 degrees caudally and centered to letter A on the knee diagram, where would letter A be positioned in reference to letter B on the image?

(1) _____

How would the image change if the central ray angulation were increased to 45 degrees?

(2) _____

D. If the central ray were angled 15 degrees caudally and centered to letter C on the knee diagram, where would letter A be positioned in reference to letter B on the image?

_____

_____

38. Eight soup cans were arranged on top of a 14- × 17-inch IR as shown in Figures 1-33 and 1-34. A perpendicular central ray (CR) was centered to the center of the IR. The circles shown indicate the bottom of the eight 4-inch (10 cm) tall soup cans'. Draw a second circle for each of the cans to indicate where the top of the soup can will be located. You must consider (1) the direction that the top of the can will be projected because of diverged beams that will be used to record them and (2) the degree of off-centering from the bottom of the can that will be demonstrated when compared with the other cans.

Figure 1-33

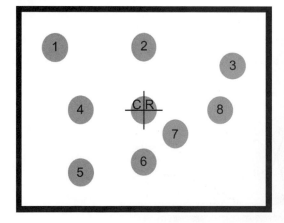

Figure 1-34

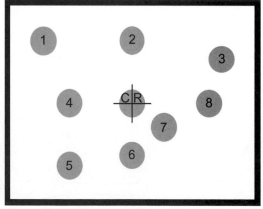

A. On Figure 1-33, draw the circles for an SID of 72 inches (180 cm).

B. On Figure 1-34, draw the circles for an SID of 40 inches (100 cm).

39. The AP chest projection in Figure 1-35 was taken using a 48-inch SID and a perpendicular central ray. With this as your reference point, answer the following:

Figure 1-35

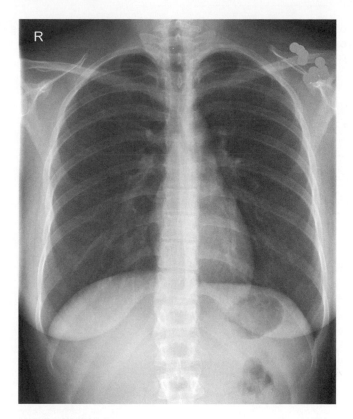

A. If the central ray were inadvertently angled 10 degrees toward the right side of the patient, where would the sternoclavicular joints be located in reference to the vertebral column on the resulting AP chest projection?

_____

B. If the central ray were angled 10 degrees cephalically, where would the sternoclavicular joints be located in reference to the third thoracic vertebral body?

_____

C. How would your answers to A and B be different if a 72-inch SID were used?

_____

D. How would your answers to A and B be different if the heart shadow were used as your reference point instead of the sternoclavicular joints?

_____

40. To minimize shape distortion on an image, keep the part positioned (A) _____ (parallel, perpendicular) to the IR and the central ray (B) _____ (parallel, perpendicular) to both the part and IR.

41. List the two types of shape distortion.

A. _____

B. _____

42. Which type of shape distortion will result in one axis of the part appearing disproportionately longer on the image than the opposite axis? _____

43. For the central ray, part, and IR setups for the AP foot projection in the following figures, state the type of shape distortion that will result.

Figure 1-36

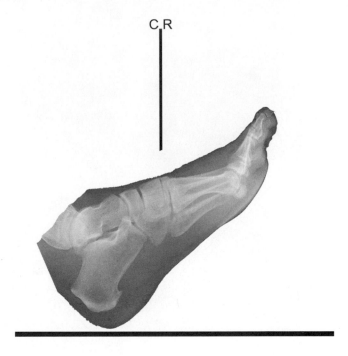

A. Figure 1-36: _____

Figure 1-37

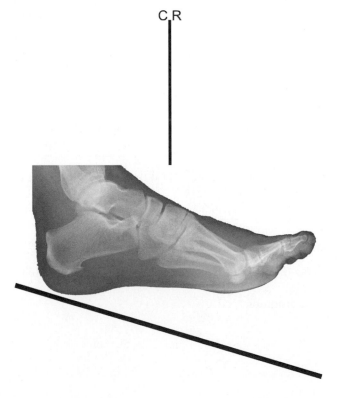

B. Figure 1-37: _____

Figure 1-38

C R

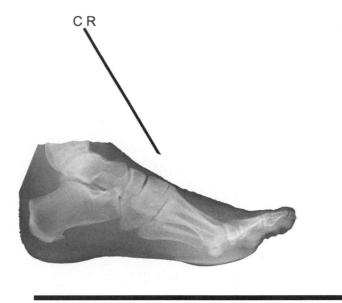

C. Figure 1-38: _____

44. Figure 1-39 demonstrates AP projections of a humeral bone that has been size- and shape-distorted. Identify the type of distortion demonstrated on each projection. If you identify elongation or foreshortening, state the aspect of the bone (proximal or distal humerus) that was positioned farther from the IR.

Figure 1-39

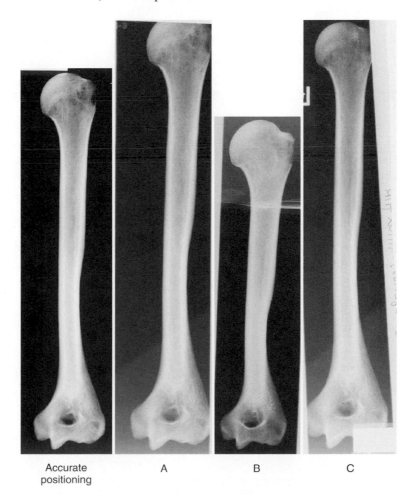

Accurate positioning   A   B   C

A. _____

B. _____

_____

C. _____

_____

45. Which of the following radiographic images will have the greater image magnification? _____

   A. Image 1 was exposed at a 72-inch SID and a 3-inch OID.

   B. Image 2 was exposed at a 72-inch SID and a 4-inch OID.

46. Which of the following radiographic images will have the greater image magnification? _____

   A. Image 1 was exposed at a 72-inch SID and a 2-inch OID.

   B. Image 2 was exposed at a 40-inch SID and a 2-inch OID.

47. To prevent magnification on a radiographic image, the anatomic structure of interest is positioned as _____ (close to/far away from) the IR as possible.

48. List how an anatomic structure can be magnified.

   A. _____

   B. _____

49. List three ways of identifying similarly appearing structures from one another on a radiographic image.

   A. _____

   B. _____

   C. _____

50. If two structures are demonstrated without superimposition on a mispositioned radiographic image, and they should be superimposed on an accurately positioned image of this projection, how does one determine how much to adjust the patient to obtain an optimal image if both structures move in opposite directions when adjusted?

   A. _____

   _____

How does one determine how much to adjust the patient to obtain an optimal image if only one structure moved when the patient was adjusted?

   B. _____

   _____

51. Estimate the degree of patient obliquity demonstrated in the diagrams in Figure 1-40.

Figure 1-40

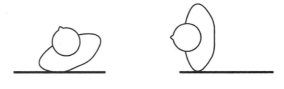

A. _____   B. _____   C. _____

D. _____   E. _____

52. Estimate the degree of flexion demonstrated on the following figures.

Figure 1-41

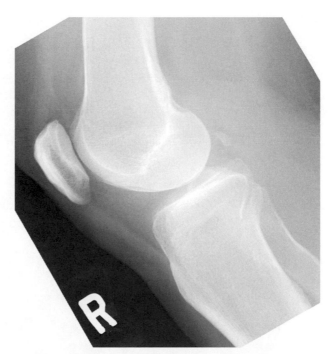

A. _____ degrees (Figure 1-41)

Figure 1-42

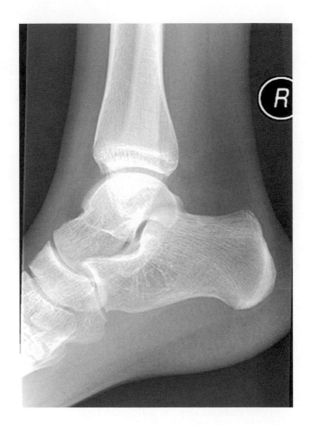

B. _____ degrees (Figure 1-42)

Figure 1-43

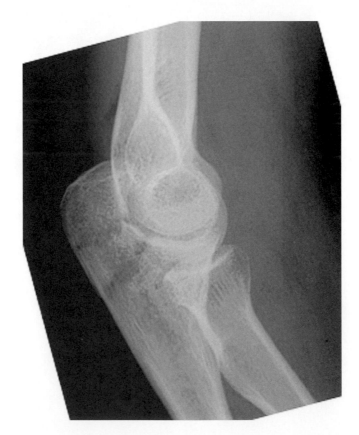

C. _____ degrees (Figure 1-43)

Figure 1-44

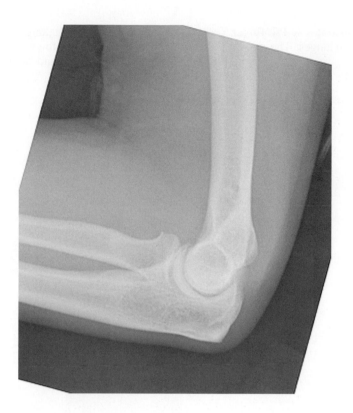

D. _____ degrees (Figure 1-44)

53. Draw a line to indicate the central ray on the AP knee setup in Figure 1-45 so that the resulting AP knee projection will demonstrate an open knee joint space.

Figure 1-45

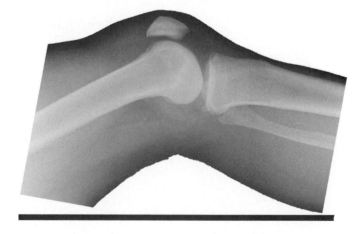

54. Figure 1-46 demonstrates a PA finger projection with closed interphalangeal (IP) joints and foreshortened middle and distal phalanges. The patient was unable to fully extend the finger for the examination. Explain how the central ray and part should be positioned to obtain open IP joints and demonstrate the phalanges without foreshortening.

Figure 1-46

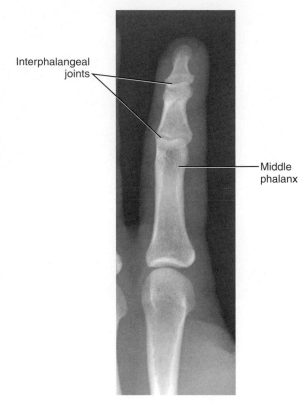

Interphalangeal joints

Middle phalanx

A. _____

Explain how the technologist would have to adjust the central ray to obtain open IP joints and nonforeshortened phalanges if the patient were unable to adjust the hand.

B. _____

_____

55. An angled central ray projects the structure situated (A) _____ (closer to/farther from) the IR farther

than a structure situated (B) _____ (closer/farther) to/from the IR.

56. Figure 1-47 demonstrates an accurately and poorly positioned lateral hand projection. On the poorly positioned image, the fifth metacarpal is situated 1 inch (2.5 cm) anterior to the second through fourth metacarpals. The second through fifth metacarpals should be superimposed on an optimal lateral hand projection. The physical skeleton distance between the second and fifth metacarpals is 2.5 inches (6.25 cm).

Figure 1-47

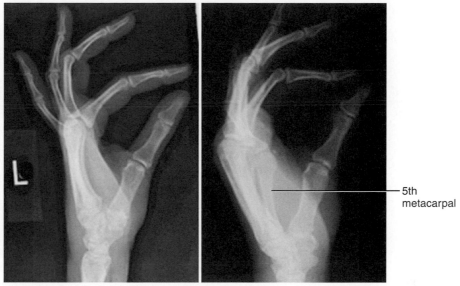

Accurate positioning

5th metacarpal

A. State how and by how much the patient's positioning could be adjusted to obtain an optimal projection. The second and fifth metacarpals will move in opposite directions from each other when the hand is rotated.

_____

_____

B. State how the central ray could be directed toward the hand and the amount of angulation needed to obtain an optimal projection if the patient was unable to adjust positioning.

_____

_____

_____

57. Figure 1-48 demonstrates an accurately and a poorly positioned lateral knee projection. On the poorly positioned projection the lateral femoral condyle is situated 2 inches (5 cm) anterior to the medial femoral condyle. The condyles should be superimposed on an optimal lateral knee projection. The physical skeleton distance between the femoral condyles is 2.5 inches (6.25 cm).

Figure 1-48

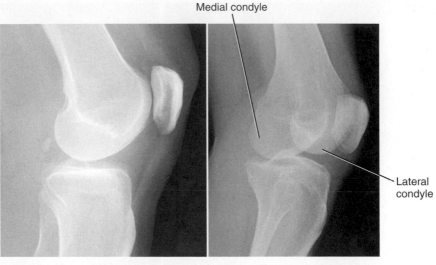

Medial condyle

Lateral condyle

Accurate positioning

A. State how and by how much the patient's positioning could be adjusted to obtain an optimal projection. The lateral and medial condyles will move in opposite directions from each other when the knee is rotated.

_____

B. State how the central ray could be directed toward the knee and the amount of angulation needed to obtain an optimal projection if the patient was unable to adjust positioning.

_____

_____

_____

58. Figure 1-49 demonstrates an accurately and a poorly positioned lateral ankle projection. On the poorly positioned projection, the lateral talar dome is situated 0.25 inch (0.6 cm) posterior to the medial dome. The talar domes should be superimposed on an optimal lateral ankle projection. The physical skeleton distance between the talar domes is 1 inch (2.5 cm).

Figure 1-49

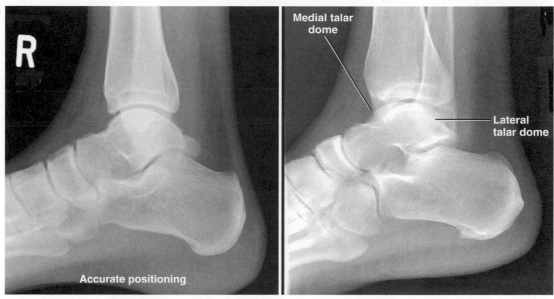

Accurate positioning

Medial talar dome

Lateral talar dome

A. State how and by how much the patient's positioning could be adjusted to obtain an optimal projection. The lateral and medial talar domes will move in opposite directions from each other when the ankle is rotated.

_____

B. State how the central ray could be directed toward the ankle and the amount of angulation needed to obtain an optimal projection if the patient was unable to adjust positioning.

_____

_____

_____

59. A (A) _____ (large/small) focal spot size is used for fine detail demonstration because a detail that is

(B) _____ (larger/smaller) than the focal spot size used to produce the image will not be demonstrated.

60. List four ways in which voluntary motion can be controlled.

A. _____

B. _____

C. _____

D. _____

61. When can normal voluntary motion be considered involuntary motion?

_____

62. How can abdominal motion that is involuntary be controlled?

_____

63. How can voluntary and involuntary motion be distinguished from each other on an AP abdomen projection?

_____

_____

64. State whether the following situations are examples of voluntary or involuntary motions.

   A. The patient was extremely short of breath because of asthma and unable to hold it.

   _____

   B. After being in a car accident, the patient being imaged was unable to stop shaking.

   _____

65. How can a double-exposed film-screen image be distinguished from a film-screen image that has motion?

_____

_____

66. State whether the following projections demonstrate motion or double-exposure.

   Figure 1-50

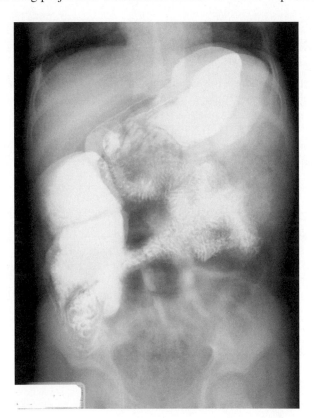

   A. Figure 1-50: _____

Figure 1-51

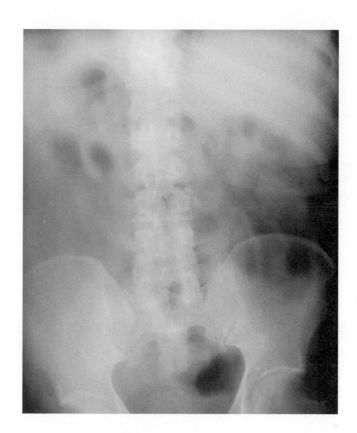

B. Figure 1-51: _____

Figure 1-52

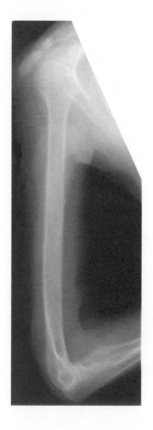

C. Figure 1-52: _____

67. How can one distinguish between poor screen-film contact and patient motion?

_____

_____

68. Which of the following radiographic images will have the sharpest recorded details? _____

    A. Image 1 was exposed at a 40-inch SID and a 3-inch OID.

    B. Image 2 was exposed at a 72-inch SID and a 3-inch OID.

69. Gonadal shielding is recommended under which three conditions?

    A. _____ ____

    B. _____ ____

    C. _____ ____

70. What gonadal organs should be shielded on a female patient? _____

71. Draw a shield on the female pelvic diagram in Figure 1-53 to indicate proper shield placement for the patient.

Figure 1-53

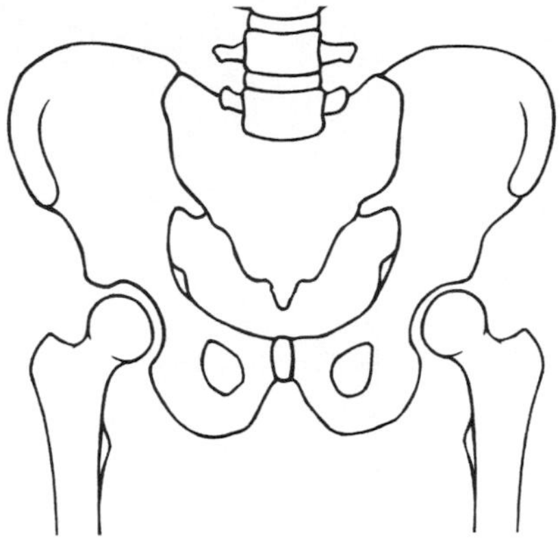

72. Describe how palpable pelvic structures are used to position a flat contact shield on a female patient accurately.

_____

_____

73. Why should the size of the contact shield used for protecting the female patient be seriously considered?

_____

_____

74. Which gonadal organs are shielded on the male patient?

    A. _____

    Where are they located?

    B. _____

75. Approximately where is the top of the shield positioned when shielding the male gonadal organs?

_____

76. Draw a shaded shield on the male pelvic diagram in Figure 1-54 to indicate proper shield placement for the patient.

Figure 1-54

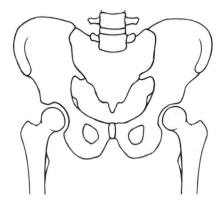

77. Evaluate the female gonadal shielding used on the pelvic projection in Figure 1-55.

Figure 1-55

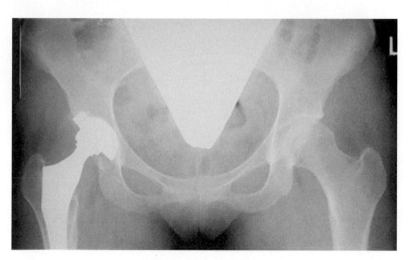

_____

_____

78. Evaluate the pediatric male gonadal shielding used on the femur projection in Figure 1-56.

Figure 1-56

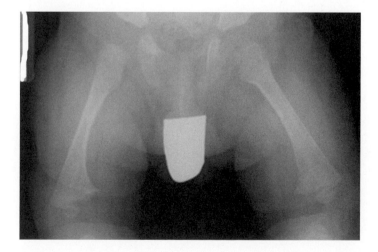

_____

_____

79. Evaluate the pediatric female gonadal shielding used on the pelvic projection in Figure 1-57.

_____

_____

Figure 1-57

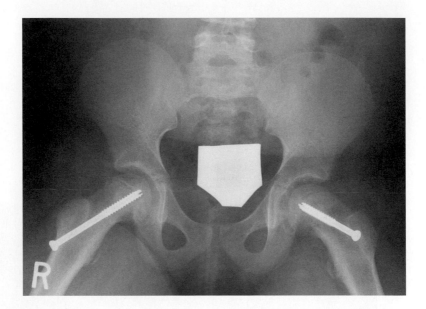

80. State how to shield a patient who is in a lateral projection.

_____

_____

81. Radiosensitive cells such as the _____ (A), _____(B), _____(C), and

_____ (D) should be shielded whenever they lie within _____-inches (E) of the primary
beam.

82. The image in Figure 1-58 demonstrates poor radiation protection practices. Which type of error is demonstrated?

Figure 1-58

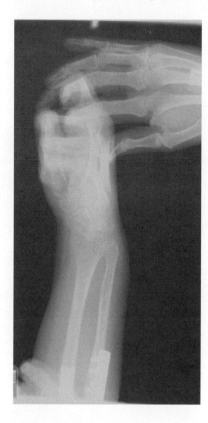

A. _____

How could this examination be taken without this error?

B. _____

_____

83. The technologist sets up for a routine AP abdomen projection on an obese patient using the mobile radiography unit. The resulting source-skin distance (SSD) is 10 inches (25 cm). Using appropriate radiation protection practices, state how the setup should be adjusted prior to exposing the image.

_____

_____

84. Which technical factor is primarily used to regulate image density?

_____

_____

85. How can one distinguish an underexposed radiograhic image from an underpenetrated image?

_____

_____

86. How much mAs adjustment should be made if a conventional screen-film image requires repeating because of poor positioning and the image is slightly darker than optimal but not repeatable because of it?

_____

87. How much mAs adjustment should be made if a conventional screen-film image definitely requires repeating because the image is too light?

_____

88. The PA oblique (scapular Y) shoulder projection in Figure 1-59 was obtained to rule out abnormalities of the scapular body on a 30-year-old woman who complained of shoulder pain. Evaluate the image for proper density, contrast, and penetration and state a new manual technique that should be used to obtain an optimal image. The original manual technique was 73 kVp at 20 mAs.

Figure 1-59

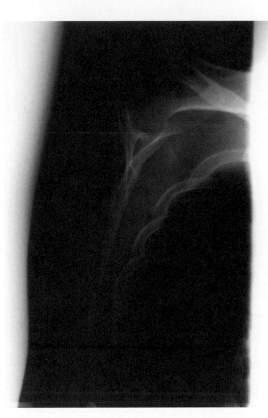

A. Density evaluation: _____

B. Contrast evaluation: _____

C. Penetration evaluation: _____

D. New technique: _____ kVp at _____ mAs

89. The lateral wrist projection in Figure 1-60 was obtained to rule out abnormalities of the carpal bones on a 40-year-old man who has wrist pain following a fall on the ice. Evaluate the projection for proper density, contrast, and penetration and state a new manual technique that should be used to obtain an optimal projection. The original manual technique was 53 kVp at 8 mAs.

Figure 1-60

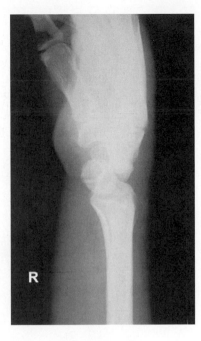

A. Density evaluation: _____

B. Contrast evaluation: _____

C. Penetration evaluation: _____

D. New technique: _____ kVp at _____ mAs

90. The AP abdominal projection in Figure 1-61 was obtained to rule out an obstruction on a 52-year-old man complaining of abdominal pain. Evaluate the projection for proper density, contrast, and penetration and state a new manual technique that should be used to obtain an optimal projection. The original manual technique was 73 kVp at 50 mAs.

Figure 1-61

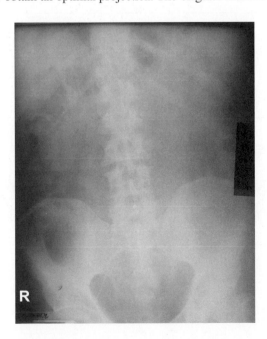

A. Density evaluation: _____

B. Contrast evaluation: _____

C. Penetration evaluation: _____

D. New technique: _____ kVp at _____ mAs

91. The lateral knee projection in Figure 1-62 was obtained to rule out abnormalities of the knee on an 83-year-old woman who complained of knee pain. Evaluate the projection for proper density, contrast, and penetration and state a new manual technique that should be used to obtain an optimal projection. The original manual technique was 60 kVp at 6 mAs.

Figure 1-62

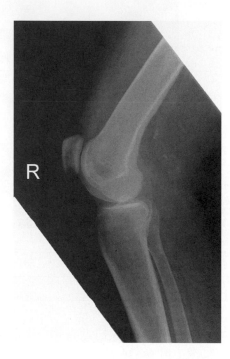

A. Density evaluation: _____

B. Contrast evaluation: _____

C. Penetration evaluation: _____

D. New technique: _____ kVp at _____ mAs

92. Which technical factor is used to regulate penetration and image contrast in screen-film radiography? _____

93. If an image had to be repeated because it was underpenetrated and the density was 2 times (100%) too light, the kVp should be

(A) _____ (increased/decreased) by (B) _____ % to obtain an optimal image.

94. Which disease type causes the tissues to increase mass density or thickness and become more radiopaque? _____

95. State the technical adjustment needed with the patient condition in the first column and state whether it is an additive or destructive disease, to indicate whether the technical adjustment should be increased or decreased by the amount indicated.

	Technical Adjustment	Additive or Destructive
A. Ascites	_____	_____
B. Emphysema	_____	_____
C. Pleural effusion	_____	_____
D. Osteoporosis	_____	_____
E. Osteoarthritis	_____	_____
F. Pneumothorax	_____	_____
G. Pneumonia	_____	_____
H. Bowel obstruction	_____	_____
I. Osteochondroma	_____	_____
J. Rheumatoid arthritis	_____	_____
K. Pulmonary edema	_____	_____
L. Cardomegaly	_____	_____

96. Indicate whether the following statements are true (T) or false (F) as they relate to proper AEC usage by placing a T or F in front of the statement.

_____ A. Set the kVp at optimum for the body part being imaged to obtain appropriate part penetration and contrast scale.

_____ B. If the kVp is so low that the part is inadequately penetrated, the density control button should be increased to +2.

_____ C. Exposures taken with an exposure time that is less than the minimum response time will result in overexposed, dark images.

_____ D. The mA station should be increased when the minimum response time halts the exposure before adequate image density is obtained.

_____ E. The backup time should be set at 150% to 200% of the expected manual exposure time.

_____ F. If the backup time is set at a time that is too low, the exposure will prematurely stop, resulting in an underexposed, light image.

_____ G. An overexposed image results when the ionization chamber chosen is located beneath a structure that has a lower atomic number or is thinner or less dense than the structure of interest.

_____ H. If the activated ionization chamber is not completely covered by the anatomy, resulting in a portion of the chamber being exposed with a part of the x-ray beam that does not go through the patient, the resulting image will be underexposed.

_____ I. Scatter radiation may cause the AEC to shut off prematurely.

_____ J. The AEC should not be used when the structure above the ionization chamber varies greatly in thickness.

_____ K. The AEC can be used when radiopaque hardware or a prosthetic device is present, as long as the hardware or device is positioned in the center of the chamber.

_____ L. An 800-speed screen-film system can be used with an AEC unit that has been calibrated for a 400-speed screen-film system as long as the density control is set at +2.

97. Evaluate the following projections for proper AEC usage.

Figure 1-63

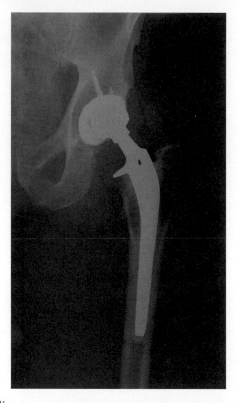

A. AP hip (Figure 1-63): _____

_____

Figure 1-64

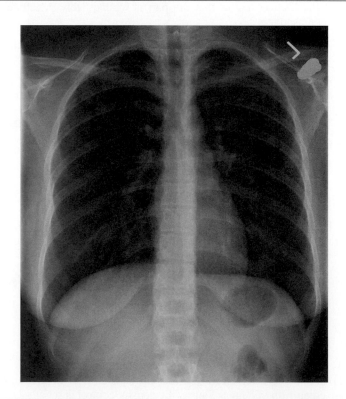

B. PA chest (Figure 1-64): _____

_____

Figure 1-65

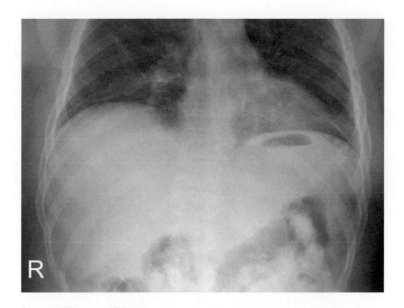

C. AP abdomen, upper image (Figure 1-65): _____

_____

98. An AP pelvis projection obtained in the x-ray department using a 45-inch (113 cm) SID, 80 kVp, and 60 mAs demonstrated adequate density, contrast, and penetration. The next day, the same projection was requested, but because the patient was in traction, the SID needed to be set at 65 inches (163 cm) SID. What should the new mAs be to obtain a quality projection?

_____

99. Increasing the OID may result in a noticeable density loss. The amount of loss is dependent on which two factors?

A. _____

B. _____

100. Use the original technical factors listed below to determine the new mAs that will be needed to produce a quality image if the following changes occurred. Original technical factors: 90 kVp, 80 mAs, 8:1 grid, regular rare earth (400 speed).

A. Nongrid   _____ mAs

B. 6:1 grid   _____ mAs

C. 12:1 grid   _____ mAs

D. 16:1 grid   _____ mAs

E. Medium (300)   _____ mAs

F. High (800)   _____ mAs

101. State if and by how much the mAs should be adjusted because of increased collimation in the following situations.

A. A PA chest projection was requested to demonstrate the pulmonary arterial catheter. The technologist used 80 kVp at 3 mAs and the resulting image demonstrated adequate density and low contrast, making it difficult to visualize the catheter tip in the right atrium. To reduce the effects of scatter radiation and demonstrate the catheter tip, the technologist returned to take a second projection, collimating to the area of interest (8 × 10 inches). Which technique should be used for the second projection?

_____

_____

B. Two PA hand projections were obtained on the same patient's hand. A 10- × 12-inch (25 × 30 cm) IR was needed to include the entire hand on the first projection and the technique used was 60 kVp at 20 mAs. The second projection was collimated to a 2- × 4-inch (5 × 10 cm) field size to include only the first finger. What technique should be used for the second projection?

_____

_____

102. Evaluate the compensating filter placement on the AP foot projection in Figure 1-66.

Figure 1-66

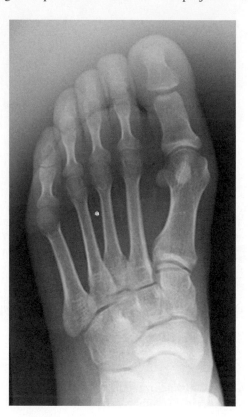

_____

_____

103. Indicate whether the following statements are true (T) or false (F) as they relate to the anode heel effect by placing a T or F in front of the statement.

_____ A. The anode heel effect can be used effectively to produce uniform density between the toes and foot when obtaining an AP foot projection.

_____ B. To incorporate the anode heel effect for a forearm image, the wrist should be placed at the anode end of the tube.

_____ C. To incorporate the anode heel effect for a lower leg image, the ankle should be placed at the cathode end of the tube.

_____ D. To incorporate the anode heel effect for an AP thoracic vertebra projection, the cephalic end of the patient should be at the anode end of the tube.

_____ E. The anode heel effect can be used to produce uniform density across the longitudinal axis of the anatomic part because the photons directed toward the cathode will go through a thick portion of the anode.

104. List the subject contrast differences that cause differential absorption and radiographic contrast.

   A. _____

   B. _____

   C. _____

105. Indicate whether images on patients with the following will display high (H) or low (L) subject contrast.

   _____ A. Strong muscles

   _____ B. Dense bones

   _____ C. Fluid retention because of disease or injury

   _____ D. Porous bones

   _____ E. High fat

   _____ F. Bones of infants

   _____ G. Obesity

106. Evaluate the radiographic contrast on the AP pelvis projection in Figure 1-67 and state how the original technical factors should be adjusted to demonstrate appropriate contrast for a pelvis image.

   Figure 1-67

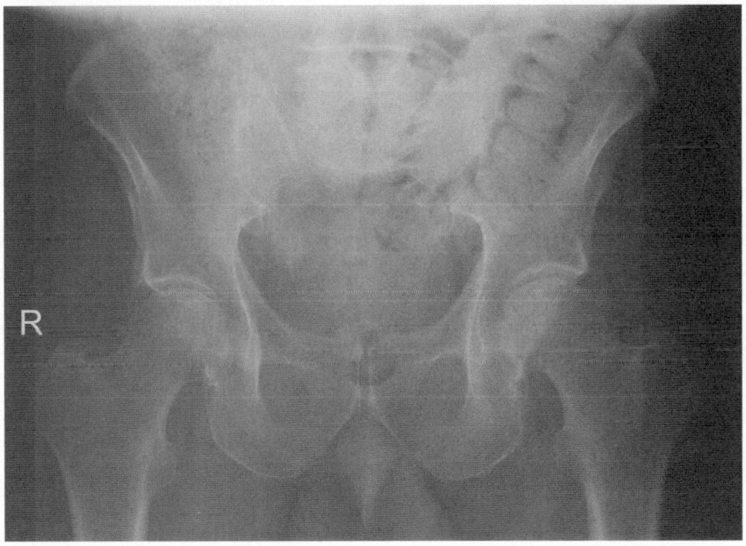

   Original technical factors: 85 kVp at 40 mAs

   New technical factors: (A) _____ kVp at (B) _____ mAs

107. How can the amount of scatter radiation reaching the IR be controlled?

   A. _____

   B. _____

   C. _____

108. Figure 1-68 demonstrates a well-collimated axiolateral (inferosuperior) shoulder projection that demonstrates excessive scatter radiation along the outside of the collimated border. Describe a technique that could be followed to reduce the negative effects of this scatter on the visiblity of the recorded details.

Figure 1-68

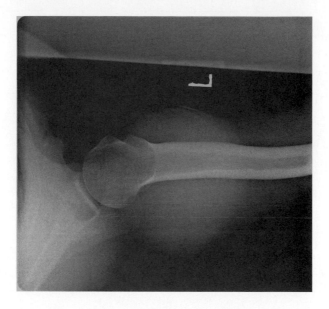

_____

_____

109. Describe the following artifact categories.

A. Anatomic artifact: _____

B. Double-exposure: _____

C. External artifact: _____

D. Internal artifact: _____

E. Equipment-related artifact: _____

F. Improper film handling and processing artifact: _____

110. State the artifact category for each of the artifacts listed below.

A. A fountain pen is visualized on a PA chest projection. _____

B. A hand is demonstrated on an AP hip projection. _____

C. A prosthesis is demonstrated on an AP shoulder projection. _____

D. Grid lines are demonstrated on an axiolateral hip projection. _____

E. Static is demonstrated on a hand projection. _____

111. List the causes of the grid artifacts in Figures 1-69 and 1-70.

Figure 1-69

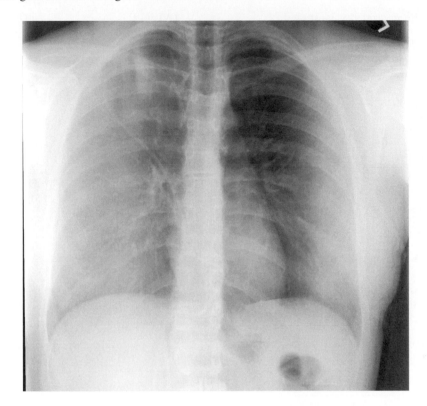

A. Figure 1-69: _____

Figure 1-70

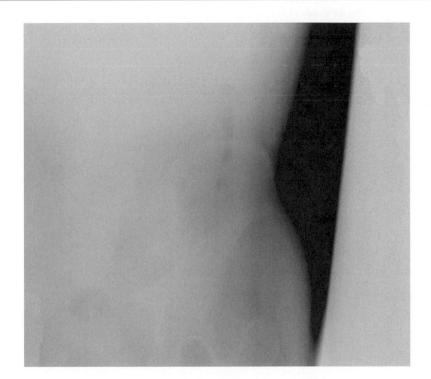

B. Figure 1-70: _____

112. Density loss resulting from poor grid alignment when conventional screen-film radiography is used will be greater on the side the central ray is angled _____ (A) will _____ (B) (increase/decrease) with increased severity of misalignment, and will be more noticeable with _____ (C) (higher/lower) grid ratios.

113. When should an image be repeated because of an artifact? _____

_____

114. What is the difference between an optimal image and an acceptable image?

_____

_____

115. State the goals for performing mobile and trauma imaging.

_____

_____

116. To obtain positioned trauma and mobile projections accurately, the central ray–part–IR must be aligned, as it is routinely for the projection. For each of the projections below, state the "part" that is aligned with the central ray and IR.

    A. Lateral hand: _____

    B. AP elbow: _____

    C. Lateral chest: _____

    D. AP oblique (external rotation) knee: _____

    E. AP axial cranium (Towne method): _____

117. State the technical adjustment needed for trauma patients because of the following.

	kVp adjustment	mAs adjustment
A. Small to medium plaster cast	_____	_____
B. Fiberglass cast	_____	_____
C. Wood backboard	_____	_____
D. Postmortem imaging of head, thorax, and abdomen	_____	_____
E. Upper airway obstruction	_____	_____
F. Wood sliver embedded in soft tissue	_____	_____

118. Using the law of isometry, state the degree of central ray angulation that should be used for the following images.

    A. If the lower leg is at a 40-degree angle with the IR, the central ray should be angled _____ degrees.

    B. If the femur is at a 60-degree angle with the IR, the central ray should be angled _____ degrees.

119. The lateral forearm projection in Figure 1-71 demonstrates a distal ulnar fracture. The patient was unable to position the elbow and wrist in a lateral projection at the same time. Evaluate the accuracy of the arm's alignment.

Figure 1-71

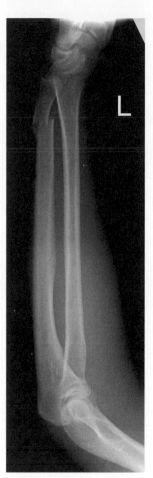

120. Indicate whether the following statements are true (T) or false (F) as they relate to pediatric and obese patient imaging by placing a T or F in front of the statement.

_____ A. When imaging patients younger than 6 years, the kVp value used for adults should be decreased by at least 15% for skull imaging.

_____ B. Decrease the mAs value used for adults by 25% for infants and children aged 0 to 5 years.

_____ C. Clothing should be removed when imaging pediatric patients, if possible, because the lower kVp used increases the chance of clothing artifacts.

_____ D. Using words such as "big" or "lots of help" in hearing distance of an obese patient may make the patient feel unwelcome.

_____ E. Table wheelchair, and cart weight limits should be determined before using them for an obese patient.

_____ F. Obese patients have inherently high subject contrast.

_____ G. Image contrast is affected by the ratio of scatter-to-primary photons that reach the IR when imaging obese patients.

_____ H. For every 2 cm of added tissue thickness, the mAs should be doubled to maintain density.

_____ I. If instead of using mAs to maintain density, the kVp was adjusted by 2 for every centimeter of tissue thickness, the patient would receive less radiation dose.

_____ J. Using a small focal spot when imaging an obese patient may result in patient motion.

1. Use the following clues to complete the crossword puzzle shown in Figure 2-1.

Figure 2-1

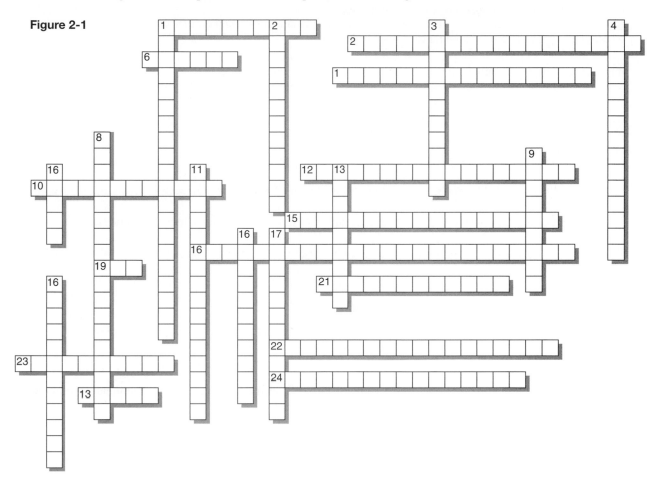

Across

1 Blackening of the areas outside the exposure field after exposure manipulation
5 Receives remnant radiation in DR imaging
6 The layout of pixels in rows and columns
7 Refers to how frequently in a set amount of space the number of details changes
12 Ability of an imaging system to distinguish small adjacent details from each other in the image
14 Process of converting an analog image to binary data
15 Readings that express the amount of light given off by the IP
18 Process distinguishing raw data coming from within the exposure field from that outside the exposure field
19 Data representing the brightness values from the image receptor before rescaling
21 Occurs when IP is not adequately erased before the next image is exposed on it
22 Process of applying algorithms to the raw data to align the histogram with the LUT
23 Degree of lightness or lack of lightness of the pixels in the image
24 Process of collecting x-ray transmission measurements from the patient
25 Grid artifact that causes a wavy line pattern on image

Down

1 Electronic components that store the detected energy in DR imaging
2 Stores trapped electrons prior to being processed
3 Area of the image receptor where the raw data are collected from
4 Used to monitor the radiation output and dose to the patient per volume of tissue irradiated
8 Ability of an imaging system to resolve low-contrast objects on an image
9 Postprocessing manipulation of the image's brightness and contrast
10 A cell within a matrix
11 Anatomic structures of interest
13 Set of rules applied to the raw data to align the image histogram with the LUT
16 The "ideal" reference histogram for the imaged part
17 Assigning each pixel a digital number that represents the amount of light emitted from the surface of IP
20 Range of gray shades that the imaging system can display

2. When using digital imaging, the kilovoltage peak (kVp) should be _____ (increased/decreased) by _____% of that used for screen-film radiography.

3. What is trapped in the imaging plate (IP) and reflects the subject contrast of the body part imaged after a radiographic exposure is obtained using a computed radiography (CR) system?

   _____

4. The light that is converted to an electrical signal in CR imaging is sent to the _____ to be digitized.

5. Pixels that receive less exposure will be assigned values that show _____ (less/more) brightness.

6. Explain why exposure field recognition is important in cassette-based digital systems.

   _____

7. On a histogram graph, what is identified on the following axes?

   A. x-axis: _____

   B. y-axis: _____

8. The volume of interest (VOI) on a histogram graph identifies S1 as the _____ (minimal/maximal) useful signal.

9. Rank the following in the order that each is demonstrated on a histogram, with 1 being farthest to the left on the graph and 5 being farthest to the right.

   A. Air/gas _____

   B. Bone _____

   C. Contrast/metal _____

   D. Fat _____

   E. Soft tissue _____

10. What can cause poor histogram formation and further histogram analysis errors?

   A. _____

   B. _____

   C. _____

   D. _____

   E. _____

   F. _____

   G. _____

11. In regard to automatic rescaling, state the maximum and minimal amounts of rescaling that can occur without degrading image quality.

   A. Overexposures of _____%

   B. Underexposures of _____%

12. Where is the exposure indicator reading taken from on the histogram after the histogram has been developed?

   _____

13. In reference to digital radiography (DR) imaging, during an exposure the thin-film transistor (TFT) receives the remnant radiation and converts it to _____

   _____

14. What determines which small detector elements (DELs) in the TFT have received radiation in DR imaging?

   _____

15. In DR imaging, the examination or body part must be selected _____ (before or after) the image is exposed.

16. In CR imaging, histogram analysis errors can occur because of the image being improperly centered to the image receptor (IR) or because of all collimated borders not being shown or aligned accurately. Why does this error *not*

   occur in DR imaging? _____

   _____

17. Explain where the dose-area product (DAP) indicator is located in relationship to the collimator and the patient.

   _____

18. Shuttering is a great tool to use when the technologist has included more anatomy than necessary on a radiographic

   image. _____ T/F

19. The technologist workstation usually displays a lower quality resolution than the radiologist's monitor. _____ T/F

20. Why is it important to choose the smallest possible IR in CR imaging? _____

   _____

21. When performing DR imaging, to reduce dose to the patient, exposures should not be repeated in the following situations:

A. _____

B. _____

C. _____

22. Evaluate Figure 2-2, which demonstrates a PA axial projection (Caldwell method) of the cranium. It is determined that the exposure index (EI) is 520. The technique used on the projection was 80 kVp at 3 milliampere-seconds (mAs). What new technique would get the EI in the optimal range?

Figure 2-2

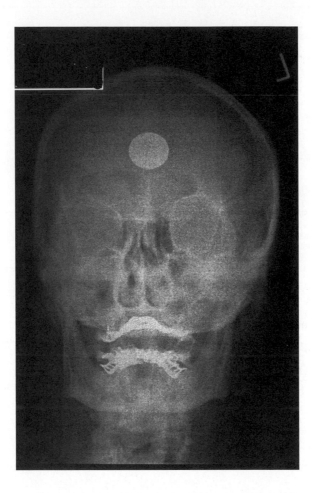

Evaluate the following projections for histogram analysis or artifact errors. State the error demonstrated and describe how you identified the error.

Figure 2-3

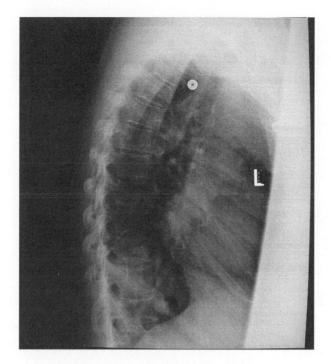

23. Figure 2-3: A lateral T-spine on a 52-year-old woman with an EI of 850.

_____

_____

Figure 2-4

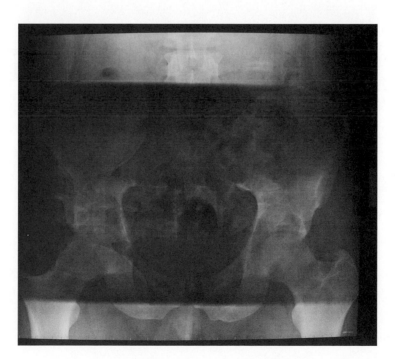

24. Figure 2-4: _____

_____

Figure 2-5

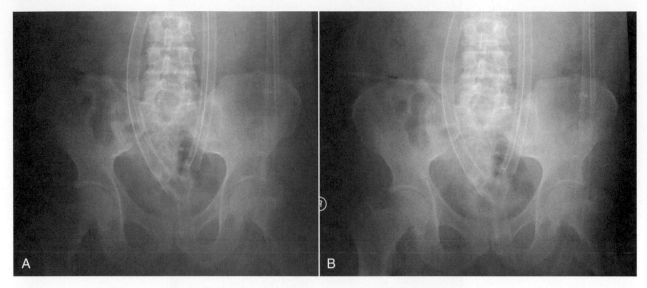

25. Figure 2-5, A and B: Determine which AP abdomen projection was processed under a chest lookup table (LUT) and which was processed under an abdomen LUT. (Hint: look at the contrast of each image.)

_____

_____

Figure 2-6

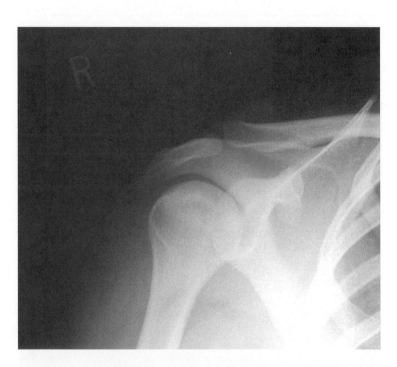

26. Figure 2-6 (AP shoulder projection on a 37-year-old female): Technique used: 75 kVp, center photocell, 40-inch grid.

State the cause of the histogram analysis error. _____

_____

27. The following projections have grid alignment artifacts. For each projection, state the grid alignment artifact that is demonstrated.

Figure 2-7

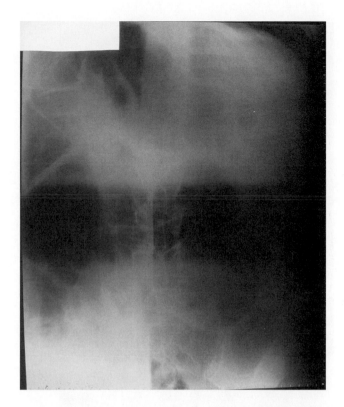

A. Figure 2-7 (mobile AP abdomen): _____

Figure 2-8

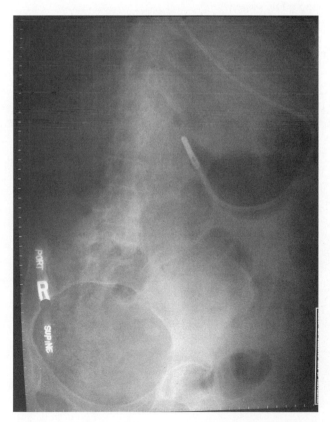

B. Figure 2-8 (mobile AP abdomen on a large patient, using a lengthwise parallel grid):

Figure 2-9

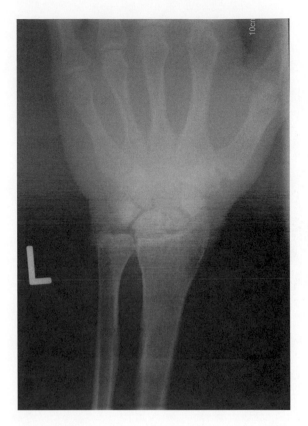

C. Figure 2-9 (PA wrist, using a DR system): _____

28. Identify the artifact that is demonstrated on the AP abdomen projection in Figure 2-10. The projection was obtained using a CR imaging system.

Figure 2-10

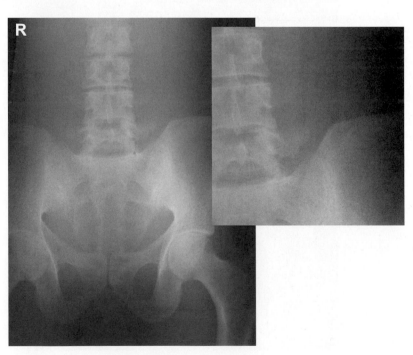

_____

_____

29. Identify the artifact that is demonstrated on the lateral chest projection in Figure 2-11. The projection was obtained using a CR imaging system.

Figure 2-11

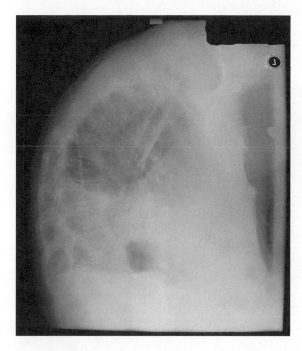

30. Identify the artifact that is demonstrated on the PA chest projection in Figure 2-12. The projection was obtained with a CR imaging system.

Figure 2-12

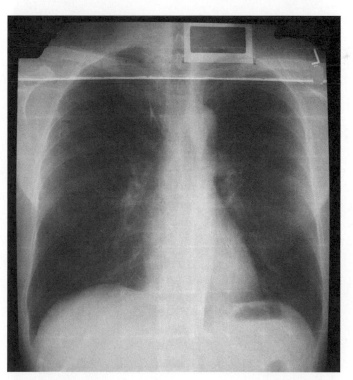

31. Evaluate the following projections for phosphor plate handling artifacts. Choose from the options listed.

1. Dust or dirt
2. Scratches
3. Hair
4. Cassette cleaning solution

Figure 2-13

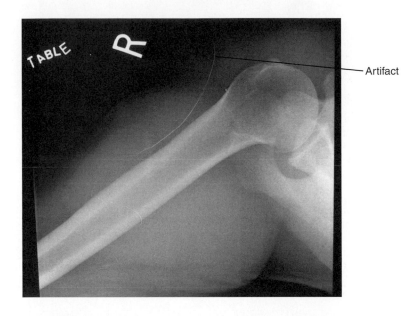

Artifact

A. Figure 2-13: _____

Figure 2-14

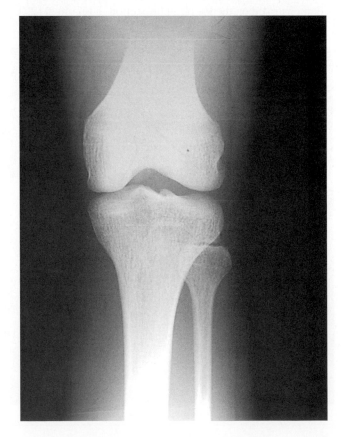

B. Figure 2-14: _____

Figure 2-15

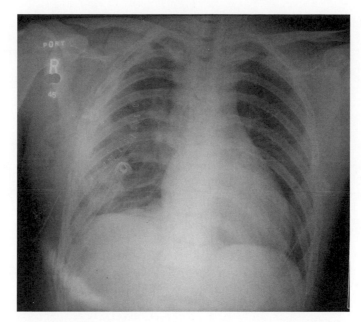

C. Figure 2-15: _____

32. Evaluate the mobile AP hip projection in Figure 2-16 to determine the cause of the artifact shown. The projection was obtained during morning rounds in the intensive care unit of a busy hospital. Between the ordered examinations, the IR was held in a metal basket until all the images taken were brought to the department for developing.

Figure 2-16

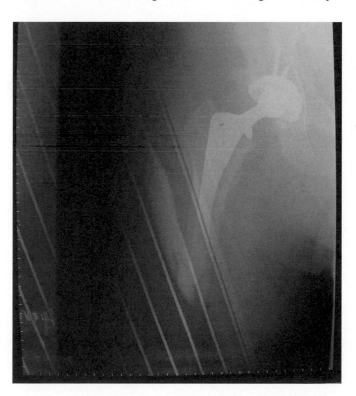

_____

_____

33. During the exposure field recognition process in CR imaging, how does the computer identify the VOI?

_____

34. In CR imaging, how much of the IP should be covered with anatomy to avoid an exposure indicator error?

_____

3 Chest and Abdomen

CHEST STUDY QUESTIONS

1. Describe how the following chest projections should be displayed on a view box or digital monitor.

   A. PA: _____

   B. Lateral (left lateral position): _____

   C. AP axial (lordotic position): _____

   D. PA oblique (RAO): _____

   E. AP (right lateral decubitus): _____

   _____

2. List how to obtain sharply defined recorded details on chest projections.

   A. _____

   B. _____

   C. _____

   D. _____

3. Adequate contrast and density are present on chest projections when which lung structures are clearly demonstrated?

   _____

4. Sufficient penetration has been obtained on chest projections when the _____(A) and

   _____ (B) are seen through the heart and mediastinal structures.

5. Complete Exercise 3-1.

EXERCISE 3-1   Chest Technical Data

ADULT AND PEDIATRIC CHEST TECHNICAL DATA				
Projection	kVp	Grid	AEC Chamber(s)	SID
ADULT CHEST TECHNICAL DATA				
PA				
Lateral				
AP mobile				
AP supine in Bucky				
AP-PA (lateral decubitus)				
AP axial (lordotic)				
AP-PA oblique				
PEDIATRIC CHEST TECHNICAL DATA				
Neonate: AP				
Infant: AP				
Child: PA				
Child: AP				
Neonate: Cross-table lateral				
Infant: Cross-table lateral				
Child: Lateral				
Neonate: AP (lateral decubitus)				
Infant: AP (lateral decubitus)				
Child: AP (lateral decubitus)				

AEC, Automatic exposure control; *SID,* source–image receptor distance.

6. Indicate whether the following statements are true (T) or false (F) as they relate to chest devices, tubes, and catheters by placing a T or F in front of the statement.

_____ A. It is within the technologist's scope of practice to inform the radiologist or attending physician immediately when a mispositioned device, line, or catheter is suspected.

_____ B. The endotracheal tube (ETT) is used to inflate the lung.

_____ C. For adults, the ETT should be positioned 3 to 5 inches (8 to 13 cm) superior to the tracheal bifurcation.

_____ D. The ETT should reside at the level of T4 on the neonate.

_____ E. With head rotation and cervical vertebrae flexion and extension, the ETT tip can move superiorly and inferiorly.

_____ F. The pleural drainage tube is used to remove fluid or air from the lung cavity.

_____ G. For drainage of fluid, the pleural drainage tube is placed laterally at the level of the fifth or sixth intercostal space.

_____ H. The central venous catheter (CVC) is used to allow infusion of substances too toxic for peripheral infusion.

_____ I. Projections taken for CVC placement should visualize the CVC tip extending to the superior vena cava.

_____ J. The pulmonary arterial catheter (PAC) measures atrial pressures, pulmonary artery pressures, and cardiac output.

_____ K. The PAC tip should rest in the superior vena cava.

_____ L. The umbilical artery catheter (UAC) is found in neonates and is used to measure oxygen saturation.

_____ M. The umbilical vein catheter (UVC) is used to deliver fluids and medications.

_____ N. The UVC is radiographically seen on lateral chest projections running adjacent to the vertebral bodies.

_____ O. The pacemaker is used to regulate the heart rate by supplying electrical stimulation to the heart.

_____ P. Lifting the patient's arm whose pacemaker had been inserted within 24 hours of the examination may cause the pacemaker and catheter to dislodge.

_____ Q. The automatic implantable cardioverter defibrillator (ICD) is used to detect arrhythmias and deliver an electrical shock to the heart.

7. Identify the internal tube or line demonstrated in the following projections.

Figure 3-1

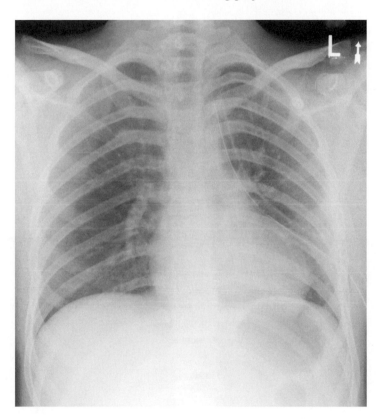

A. Figure 3-1: _____

Figure 3-2

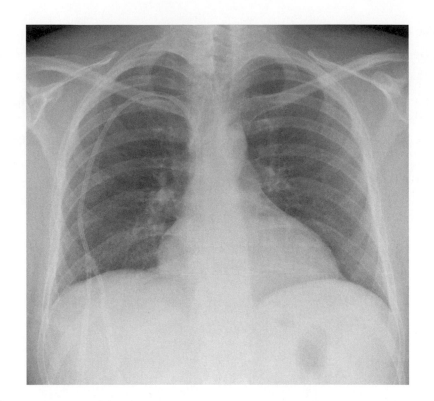

B. Figure 3-2: _____

Figure 3-3

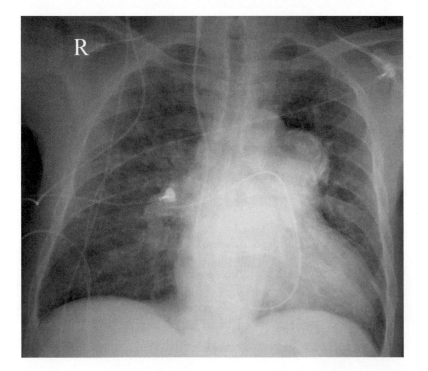

C. Figure 3-3: _____

Figure 3-4

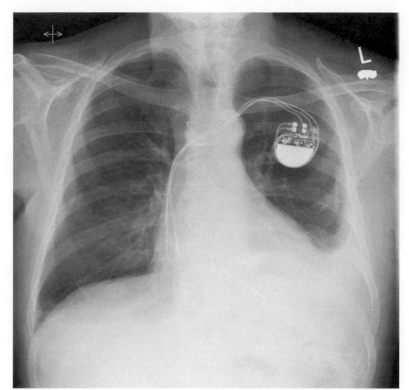

D. Figure 3-4: _____

8. Match the term with its definition.

_____ A. Pleural cavity

_____ B. Pneumothorax

_____ C. Pneumectomy

_____ D. Intraperitoneal

_____ E. Vertebra prominens

_____ F. Apex (apical)

_____ G. Air-fluid line

1. Density line created when fluid and air separate

2. Spinous process of the seventh cervical vertebra

3. Within the abdominal cavity

4. Cavity encasing the lungs

5. Removal of lung

6. Air in pleural cavity

7. Narrow end of a cone-shaped object

9. How must the patient and central ray be positioned for a PA chest projection to obtain the most accurate assessment of air-fluid levels in the thorax?

A. Patient: _____

B. Central ray: _____

10. Identify the pathologic condition demonstrated in the following projections.

Figure 3-5

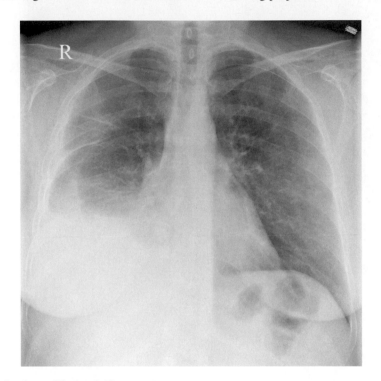

A. Right inferior lung (Figure 3-5): _____

_____

Figure 3-6

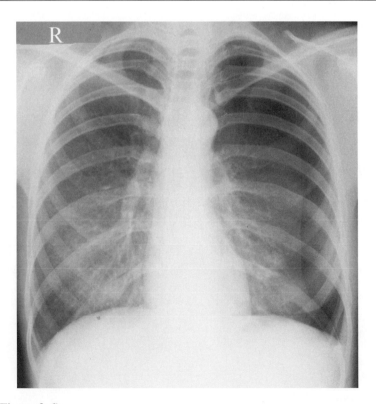

B. Left superior lung (Figure 3-6): _____

_____

Figure 3-7

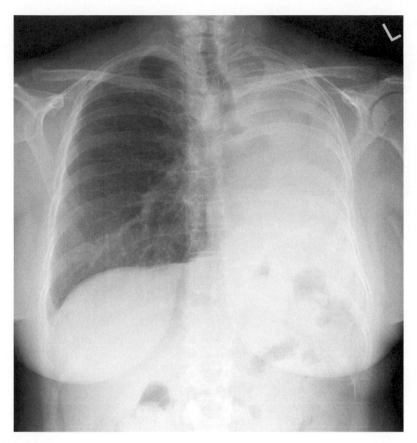

C. Left inferior lung (Figure 3-7): _____

_____

Posteroanterior Projection

11. Complete the statements below, referring to adult PA chest projection analysis criteria

Posteroanterior Chest Projection Analysis Criteria

- The _____ (A) thoracic vertebra is at the center of the exposure field.

- Both lungs, from apices to _____ (B), are included within the collimated field.

- Distances from the vertebral column to the sternal clavicular ends are _____ (C), and lengths of the right and left corresponding posterior ribs are equal.

- Clavicles are positioned on the same _____ (D) plane.

- Scapulae are located _____ (E) the lung field.

- Manubrium is superimposed by the _____ (F) vertebra, with 1 inch (2.5 cm) of apical lung field visible above the clavicles.

- The _____ (G) posterior ribs are visualized above the diaphragm.

12. Identify the labeled anatomy on the PA chest projection in Figure 3-8.

Figure 3-8

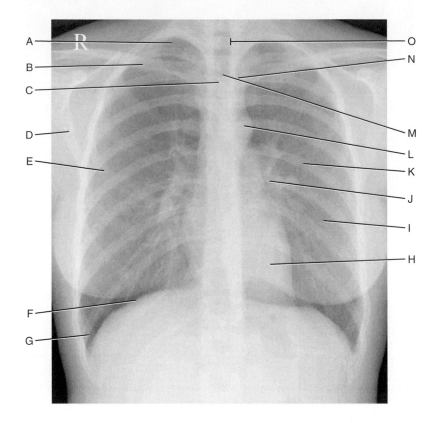

A. _____	F. _____	K. _____
B. _____	G. _____	L. _____
C. _____	H. _____	M. _____
D. _____	I. _____	N. _____
E. _____	J. _____	O. _____

13. List the three dimensions in which the lungs expand and contract during inspiration and expiration.

    A. _____

    B. _____

    C. _____

14. The _____ dimension of the thorax expands the most during inspiration.

15. List two situations that could prevent full lung expansion while taking chest projections.

    A. _____

    B. _____

16. Which body type requires the image receptor (IR) to be placed crosswise when a PA chest projection is taken?

    A. _____

    Describe the lung shape of such a patient.

    B. _____

17. Which body types will require the IR to be placed lengthwise when a PA chest projection is taken?

A. _____, _____

Describe the lung shapes of such patients.

B. _____

18. When it is difficult to decide whether the IR should be placed crosswise or lengthwise for a PA chest projection, what method can be used to determine whether the transverse IR dimension is sufficient?

_____

_____

19. State how the patient is positioned to prevent rotation on a PA chest projection.

_____

_____

20. Refer to Figure 3-9.

Figure 3-9

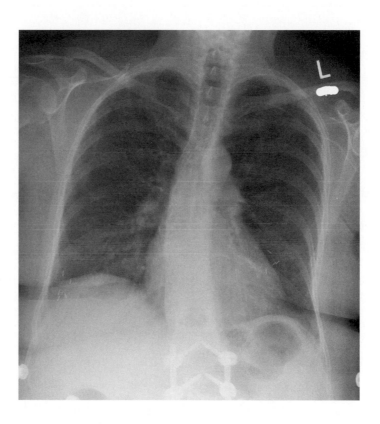

A. What spinal condition is demonstrated in the PA chest projection in Figure 3-9? _____

B. Can patient positioning be adjusted to offset this rotated appearance on such a patient? _____

C. How can this condition be distinguished from rotation on a PA chest projection?

_____

_____

_____

21. How is the patient positioned to place the clavicles on the same horizontal plane on a PA chest projection?

_____

22. How is the patient positioned for a PA chest projection to place the scapulae outside the lung field?

_____

23. The level at which the manubrium is visible on the vertebral column and the amount of apical lung field demonstrated above the clavicles are determined by the tilt of the patient's _____ (A) plane. When this plane is vertical, the manubrium will be at the level of the _____ (B) thoracic vertebra, and approximately _____ (C) inch(es) of the apices will be demonstrated above the clavicles.

24. On an accurately positioned PA chest projection, the clavicles should be horizontal. Which two aspects of the setup procedure could be mispositioned to result in somewhat vertically running clavicles?

   A. _____

   B. _____

25. Why will an increase in lung aeration be obtained when a PA chest projection is taken with the patient in an upright position versus a supine or seated position?

_____

_____

26. Which two positioning procedures will provide a PA chest projection with the greatest amount of vertical lung field?

   A. _____

   B. _____

27. Why are chest projections exposed after the patient has taken the second full inspiration?

_____

28. List two patient conditions that may indicate the need for an expiration chest projection to be taken.

   A. _____

   B. _____

29. On an expiration PA chest projection, the diaphragm will be positioned _____ (A) (higher, lower), _____ (B) posterior ribs will be demonstrated above the diaphragm, the heart shadow will appear _____ (C) and _____ (D), and the projection density will be _____ (E) (lighter, darker).

30. For an accurately positioned PA chest projection, a _____ (A) central ray is centered to the _____ (B) plane at a level approximately 7. 5 inches (18 cm) inferior to the _____ (C).

31. Which anatomic structures are included on an accurately positioned PA chest projection?

_____

For the following descriptions of PA chest projections with poor positioning, state how the patient would have been mispositioned for such a projection to result.

32. The vertebral column is superimposed over the right sternoclavicular (SC) joint, whereas the left SC joint is demonstrated without vertebral superimposition.

_____

33. The clavicles are not positioned on the same horizontal plane. The lateral clavicular ends are elevated. The manubrium is at the same level as the fourth thoracic vertebra.

_____

34. The right scapula is demonstrated within the superolateral lung field.

_____

35. The clavicles are horizontal, the manubrium is situated at the level of the fifth thoracic vertebra, and more than 1 inch (2. 5 cm) of the chest apex is demonstrated superior to the clavicles.

_____

36. The manubrium is situated at the level of the first thoracic vertebra, and less than 1 inch (2. 5 cm) of the chest apex is demonstrated superior to the clavicles.

_____

37. The projection demonstrates the first through eighth posterior ribs above the diaphragm.

_____

For the following PA chest projections with poor positioning, state which anatomic structures are misaligned and how the patient should be repositioned for an optimal projection to be obtained.

Figure 3-10

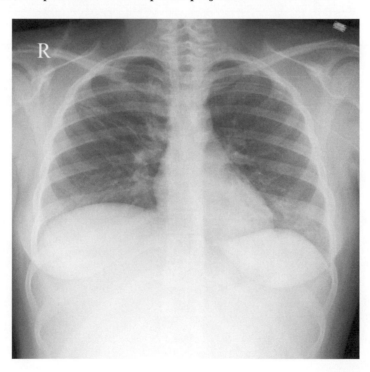

38. Figure 3-10: _____

_____

_____

_____

Figure 3-11

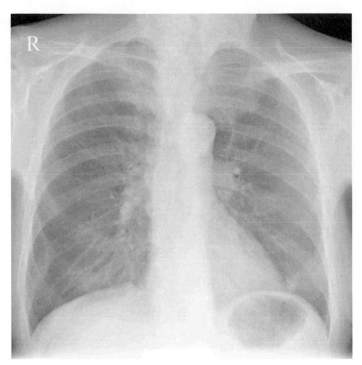

39. Figure 3-11: _____

_____

_____

_____

Figure 3-12

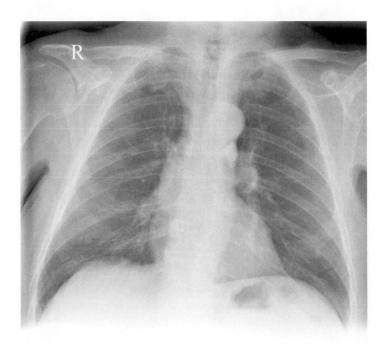

40. Figure 3-12: _____

_____

_____

_____

Figure 3-13

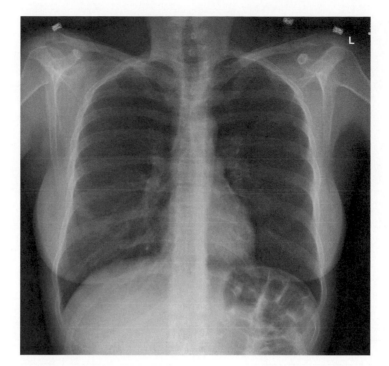

41. Figure 3-13: _____

_____

_____

_____

Figure 3-14

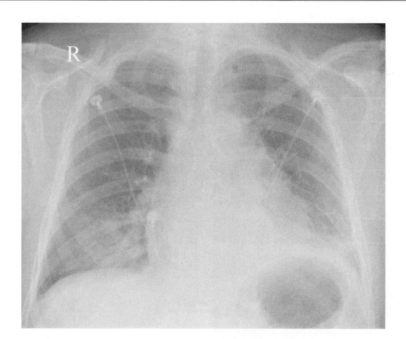

42. Figure 3-14: _____

_____

_____

_____

Figure 3-15

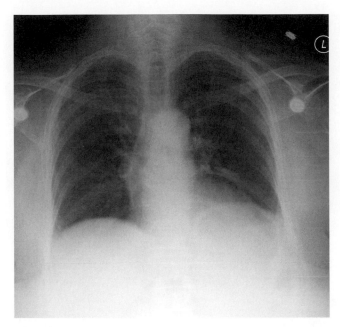

43. Figure 3-15: _____

_____

_____

_____

Lateral Projection (Left Lateral Position).

44. Identify the labeled anatomy in Figure 3-16.

Figure 3-16

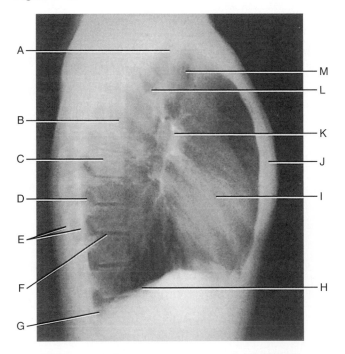

A. _____

B. _____

C. _____

D. _____

E. _____

F. _____

G. _____

H. _____

I. _____

J. _____

K. _____

L. _____

M. _____

45. Complete the statements below, referring to lateral chest projection analysis criteria.

Lateral Chest Projection Analysis Criteria

• The midcoronal plane, at the level of the _____ (A) thoracic vertebra, is at the center of the exposure field.

• Right and left posterior ribs are nearly superimposed, demonstrating not more than a _____ (B) of space between them, and the sternum is in profile.

• Lungs are demonstrated without foreshortening, with nearly superimposed _____ (C).

• No humeral soft tissue is seen superimposing the _____ (D) lung apices.

• Anteroinferior lung and heart shadow are well defined.

• Hemidiaphragms demonstrate a gentle, cephalically bowed contour and are inferior to the _____ (E) vertebra.

---

46. How is the patient positioned to prevent rotation on a lateral chest projection?

_____

47. Which side of the thorax will demonstrate the greatest magnification when a left lateral chest projection is taken?

A. _____

Defend your answer.

B. _____

_____

48. How is rotation identified on a lateral chest projection?

_____

_____

49. List two methods that can be used to identify the right and left hemidiaphragms on a lateral chest projection with poor positioning.

A. _____

B. _____

50. Where is the gastric air bubble located on an upright lateral chest projection?

_____

51. Which side of the chest cavity contains most of the heart? _____

52. A rotated lateral chest projection demonstrates the left lung posteriorly, with 2.5 inches (6.25 cm) of space between the posterior ribs. How should the patient be adjusted, and how much movement from the original position should be made?

_____

_____

53. State a method of distinguishing scoliosis from rotation on a lateral chest projection.

_____

_____

54. How is the patient positioned with respect to the IR for a lateral chest projection to prevent lung foreshortening?

_____

_____

55. Which lung and diaphragm are situated higher on the average patient? _____

56. List two expected differences that would be demonstrated between lateral chest projections obtained in a right and left lateral position.

A. _____

_____

B. _____

_____

57. State whether it is best to take a lateral chest projection in a right or left lateral position for the following.

A. To evaluate right lung details: _____

B. To evaluate the heart: _____

C. To evaluate left lung details: _____

58. How is the patient positioned for a lateral chest projection to prevent the humeral soft tissue from being superimposed over the anterior lung apices?

_____

59. It is best to take a lateral chest projection of an obese patient with the patient in a standing position to better demonstrate

the _____ aspect of the lung and heart.

60. How can one determine if full lung aeration has occurred for a lateral chest projection? _____

_____

61. Which two positioning procedures will provide a lateral chest projection with the greatest amount of vertical lung field?

A. _____

B. _____

62. Which thoracic vertebra has the last rib attached to it? _____

63. To center the chest on a lateral chest projection accurately, the central ray is centered to the _____ (A)

plane at a level 8.5 inches (21.25 cm) _____ (B) to the vertebral prominens.

64. Which anatomic structures are included in a lateral chest projection for which the subject was accurately positioned?

_____

_____

For the following descriptions of lateral chest projections with poor positioning, state how the patient would have been mispositioned for such a projection to result.

65. The humeri soft tissue shadows are superimposed over the anterior lung apices.

_____

_____

66. The posterior ribs are separated by more than 0.5 inch (1. 25 cm), and the superior heart shadow is seen extending

beyond the sternum into the anteriorly situated lung. _____

_____

67. One hemidiaphragm is demonstrated superior to the other, and the gastric bubble is situated beneath the superior hemidiaphragm.

_____

_____

For the following lateral chest projections with poor positioning, state which anatomic structures are misaligned and how the patient should be repositioned for an optimal projection to be obtained.

Figure 3-17

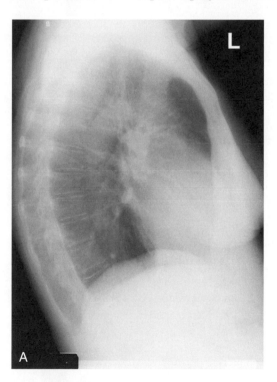

68. Figure 3-17: _____

_____

_____

Figure 3-18

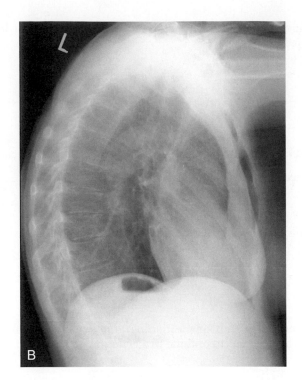

Figure 3-18: _____

_____

_____

Figure 3-19

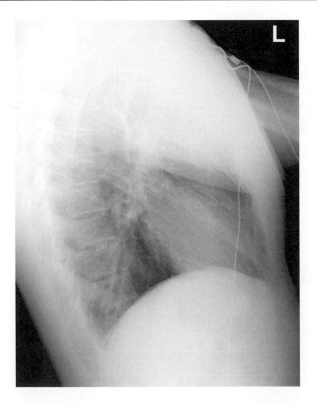

69. Figure 3-19: _____

_____

_____

Figure 3-20

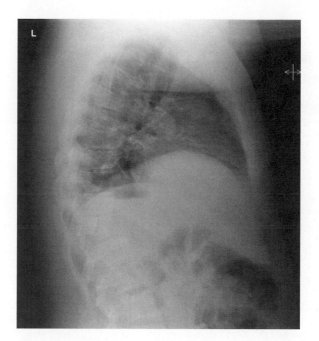

70. Figure 3-20: _____

_____

_____

The following chest case study includes PA and lateral chest projections from the same patient. Evaluate the projections for accurate positioning.

71. Refer to Figure 3-21.

Figure 3-21

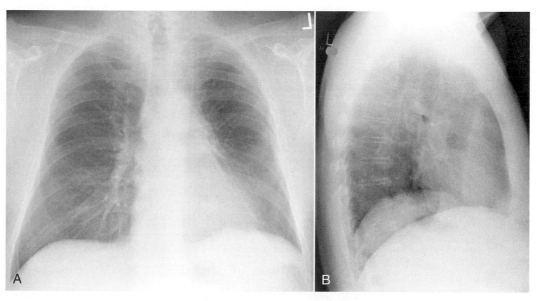

A. _____

_____

_____

B. _____

_____

_____

Anteroposterior Projection (Supine or With Mobile X-Ray Unit)

72. Identify the labeled anatomy in Figure 3-22.

Figure 3-22

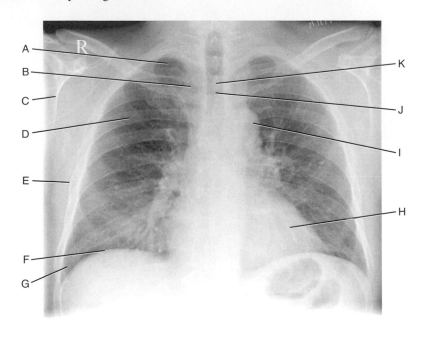

A. _____   F. _____

B. _____   G. _____

C. _____   H. _____

D. _____   I. _____

E. _____   J. _____

K. _____

73. Complete the statements below, referring to adult AP chest projection analysis criteria.

Anteroposterior Chest (Supine or Mobile) Projection Analysis Criteria

• Date and time of examination, SID used, degree of patient elevation, and technical factors used are recorded on projection.

• The _____ (A) thoracic vertebra is at the center of the exposure field.

• The distances from vertebral column to the _____ (B) are equal, and the lengths of the right and left corresponding posterior ribs are equal.

• The _____ (C) is superimposed by the fourth thoracic vertebra, with 1 inch

  (2. 5 cm) of apical lung field visible above the _____ (D).

• Clavicles are positioned on the same _____ (E) plane, when possible.

• The _____ (F) are located outside the lung field, when possible.

• The posterior ribs demonstrate a gentle cephalically bowed contour.

• The _____ (G) posterior ribs are visualized above the diaphragm.

SID, Source–image receptor distance.

74. Why is it important to record the time of day on all mobile chest projections?

_____

_____

75. Why is the degree of patient elevation recorded on all mobile chest projections?

_____

_____

76. Why are air-fluid levels undetectable when the patient is supine?

_____

77. The thoracic vertebral column may not be visible through the heart shadow on an AP mobile chest projection because the _____ used is too low.

78. Complete the statements below, referring to mobile AP chest projections.

    A. Why is it safe to position the IR crosswise for almost all mobile AP chest projections on most body types?

_____

_____

    B. Why is it more likely for the lateral edges of the lung field to be clipped if the IR is placed lengthwise for mobile AP chest projections?

_____

_____

79. State how the patient is positioned to prevent rotation on an AP chest projection.

_____

_____

80. How can rotation be identified on an AP chest projection?

_____

_____

81. When the patient's condition allows, the shoulders should be depressed for an AP chest projection. How can this movement be identified on the projection?

_____

82. When an AP chest projection is obtained that demonstrates somewhat vertically appearing clavicles, how can one determine if this appearance is a result of poor central ray alignment or poor shoulder positioning?

_____

_____

_____

83. When the patient's condition allows, how can the scapulae be drawn from the lung field on an AP supine chest projection?

_____

_____

84. Poor central ray alignment on a mobile chest projection will affect the amount of apical lung field demonstrated superior to the clavicles and the contour of the posterior ribs. For each of the following situations, describe the expected change in apical lung visualization and posterior rib contour.

A. The central ray was angled too caudally.

_____

_____

_____

B. The central ray was angled too cephalically.

_____

_____

_____

85. How can the central ray be adjusted to improve the posterior rib contour and eliminate superimposition of the chin on the apices when imaging a kyphotic patient for an AP chest projection?

_____

86. Complete the statements below, referring to a supine AP chest projection.

A. How is the central ray angled for a supine AP chest projection?

_____

B. Why is this angle needed?

_____

87. Why are fewer posterior ribs demonstrated above the diaphragm on a supine AP chest projection than on an upright PA chest projection?

_____

_____

88. How is the patient instructed to breathe to obtain maximum lung aeration?

_____

89. Why is it unnecessary to watch an unconscious patient on a high-frequency ventilator?

_____

90. Accurate centering on an AP chest projection is accomplished by centering the central ray to the _____ (A) plane at a level _____ (B) inches inferior to the _____ (C).

91. Which anatomic structures are included on an accurately positioned AP chest projection? _____

_____

For the following descriptions of AP chest projections with poor positioning, state how the patient would have been mispositioned or the central ray misaligned for such a projection to result.

92. The left SC joint is visible away from the vertebral column, whereas the right SC joint is superimposed over the vertebral column (list both patient and central ray mispositioning that could cause this projection).

_____

_____

_____

93. The manubrium is shown superimposed over the fifth thoracic vertebra with more than 1 inch (2. 5 cm) of the apical lung field visible above the clavicles, and the posterior ribs demonstrate a vertical contour. _____

_____

94. The manubrium is shown superimposed over the third vertebra with less than 1 inch (2. 5 cm) of apical lung field visible above the clavicles, and the posterior ribs demonstrate a horizontal contour.

_____

95. A projection of a patient with severe kyphosis demonstrates the chin superimposed over the apical region, and the posterior ribs demonstrate a vertical contour. _____

_____

_____

For the following AP chest projections with poor positioning, state which anatomic structures are misaligned and how the patient should be repositioned for an optimal projection to be obtained.

Figure 3-23

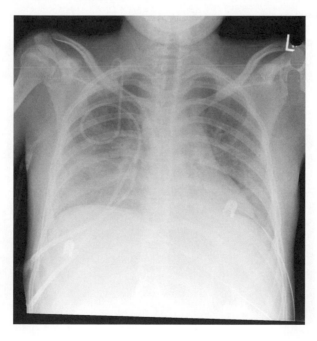

96. Figure 3-23: _____

_____

_____

_____

Figure 3-24

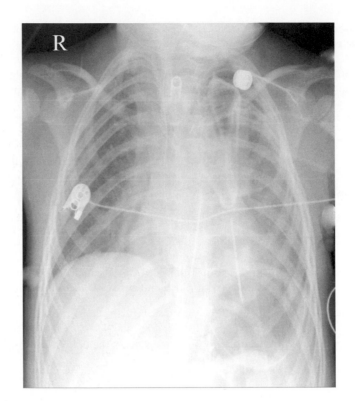

97. Figure 3-24: _____

_____

_____

_____

Figure 3-25

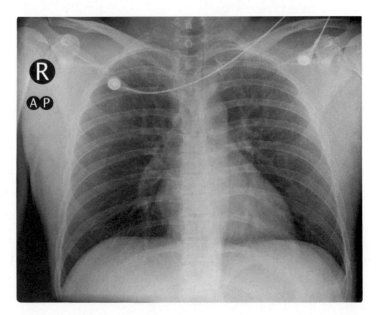

98. Figure 3-25: _____

_____

_____

_____

Anteroposterior or Posteroanterior Projection (Right or Left Lateral Decubitus Position)

99. Identify the labeled anatomy in Figure 3-26.

Figure 3-26

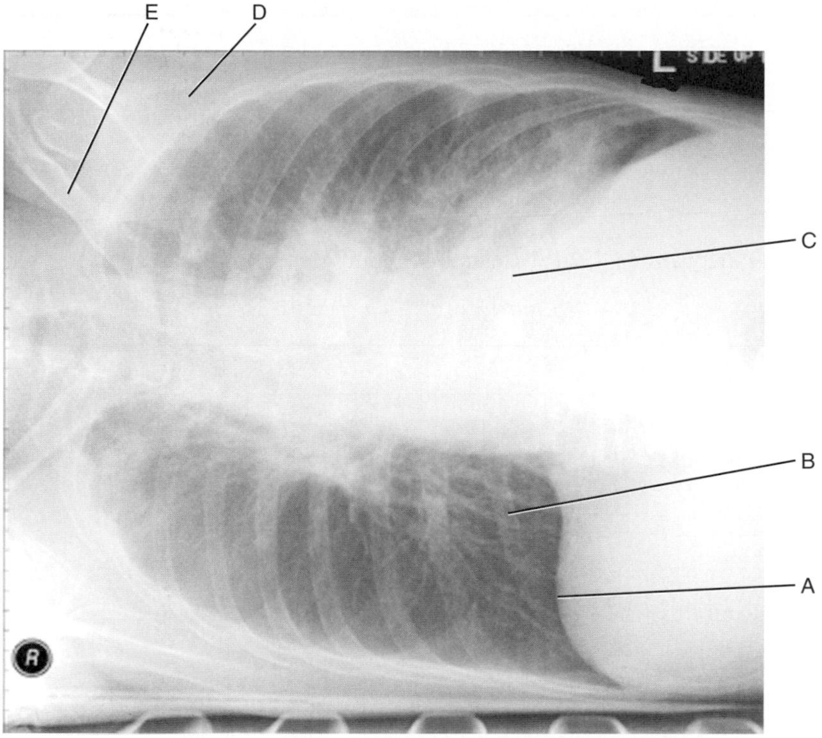

A. _____

B. _____

C. _____

D. _____

E. _____

100. Complete the statements below, referring to adult AP-PA decubitus chest projection analysis criteria.

Anteroposterior-Posteroanterior (Lateral Decubitus) Projection Analysis Criteria
• An arrow or "word" marker identifies the side of the patient positioned _____ (A) from the imaging table or cart.
• The _____ (B) thoracic vertebra is at the center of the exposure field.
• Distances from the _____ (C) to the sternoclavicular ends are equal, and lengths of the right and left corresponding posterior ribs are equal.
• The arms, mandible, and lateral borders of the scapulae are situated _____ (D), and lateral aspects of the clavicles are projected upward.
• Manubrium is superimposed by the _____ (E) vertebra, with 1 inch (2. 5 cm) of apical lung field visible above the (F) _____.
• Nine or 10 posterior ribs are visualized above the _____ (G).
• The lung field adjacent to the cart is demonstrated without superimposition of the cart pad.

101. How is an AP-PA (lateral decubitus) chest projection accurately marked and displayed on the view box or digital monitor?

 A. Marked: _____

 _____

 B. Displayed: _____

 _____

102. The AP-PA (lateral decubitus) projection is primarily performed to confirm the presence of _____ (A) or _____ (B) levels within the pleural cavity.

103. If fluid is present within the pleural cavity on an AP-PA (lateral decubitus) chest projection, where will it be located?

 _____

 _____

104. For each situation below, state whether a right or left AP-PA (lateral decubitus) chest projection should be taken.

 A. Right pneumothorax: _____

 B. Left pleural effusion: _____

105. To avoid rotation on AP-PA (lateral decubitus) chest projections, align the patient's _____

 (A), _____ (B), and _____ (C) perpendicular to the cart.

106. Will an AP or PA (lateral decubitus) chest projection demonstrate the sixth and seventh cervical vertebrae without

 distortion and open intervertebral disk space? _____

107. The lateral scapular borders are situated outside the lung field when the arms are positioned _____ for an AP-PA (lateral decubitus) chest projection.

108. Chest foreshortening can be avoided on an AP-PA (lateral decubitus) chest projection by positioning the _____

 (A) plane) _____ (B) (perpendicular-parallel) to the IR.

109. How can the patient be positioned for an AP-PA (lateral decubitus) chest projection to prevent the cart pad from creating an artifact line along the lung field positioned against it?

 _____

For the following descriptions of AP-PA (lateral decubitus) chest projections with poor positioning, state how the patient would have been positioned for such a projection to be obtained.

110. A PA (lateral decubitus) chest projection demonstrates the vertebral column superimposed over the right SC joint, whereas the left SC joint is demonstrated without vertebral superimposition.

 _____

111. An AP (lateral decubitus) chest projection demonstrates the right SC joint superimposed over the vertebral column, whereas the left SC joint does not demonstrate vertebral superimposition.

 _____

112. An AP (lateral decubitus) chest projection demonstrates the manubrium at the level of the second thoracic vertebra.

 _____

For the following AP-PA (lateral decubitus) chest projections with poor positioning, state which anatomic structures are misaligned and how the patient should be repositioned for an optimal projection to be obtained.

Figure 3-27

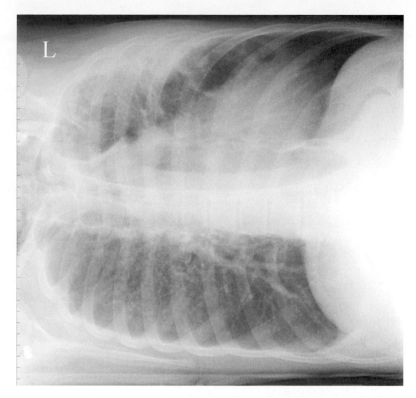

113. Figure 3-27 (AP projection): _____

_____

_____

_____

Figure 3-28

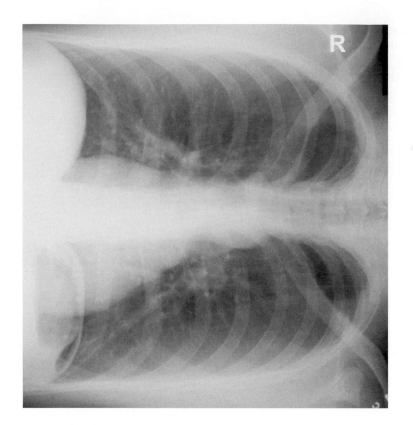

114. Figure 3-28 (AP projection): _____

_____

_____

_____

Anteroposterior Axial Projection (Lordotic Position)

115. Identify the labeled anatomy in Figure 3-29.

Figure 3-29

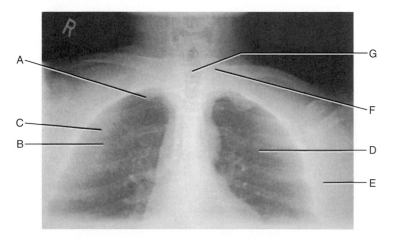

A. _____

B. _____

C. _____

D. _____

E. _____

F. _____

G. _____

116. Complete the statements below, referring to adult AP axial (lordotic) chest projection analysis criteria.

Anteroposterior Axial (Lordotic) Chest Projection Analysis Criteria

• The _____ (A) lung field is at the center of the exposure field.

• Sternoclavicular ends of clavicles are projected _____ (B) to the lung apices, and the first through

fourth ribs lie _____ (C) and are almost superimposed.

• The _____ (D) borders of the scapulae are drawn away from the lung field, and the superior angles of scapulae are demonstrated away from lung apices.

• The distances from the _____ (E) to the sternoclavicular ends are equal.

• The clavicles are positioned on the same (F) _____ plane.

---

117. The AP axial chest projection is taken to visualize the _____.

118. Describe three methods that can be used to position the clavicles superior to the lung apices.

A. _____

_____

B. _____

_____

C. _____

_____

119. An AP axial chest projection with poor positioning demonstrates the medial clavicles superimposed over the lung apices. Which two positional changes can be made to obtain a projection with accurate positioning?

A. _____

B. _____

120. How must the patient be positioned to draw the lateral borders of the scapulae out of the lung field and the superior angles away from the lung apices?

_____

121. How can rotation be identified on an AP axial chest projection?

_____

122. An accurately centered AP axial chest projection is accomplished by centering the central ray to the

_____ (A) plane halfway between the _____ (B) and _____ (C).

123. Which anatomic structures are included on an AP axial chest projection with accurate positioning?

_____

For the following descriptions of AP axial chest projections with poor positioning, state how the patient would have been mispositioned or the central ray misaligned for such a projection to be obtained.

124. The clavicles are superimposed over the lung apices, and the anterior ribs appear inferior to their corresponding posterior ribs.

_____

_____

125. The lateral borders of the scapulae are demonstrated within the lung field, and the superior scapular angles are demonstrated within the apical region.

_____

126. The right SC joint is superimposed over the vertebral column, whereas the left joint is demonstrated without being superimposed over the vertebral column.

_____

For the following AP axial chest projection with poor positioning, state which anatomic structures are misaligned and how the patient should be repositioned for an optimal projection to be obtained.

Figure 3-30

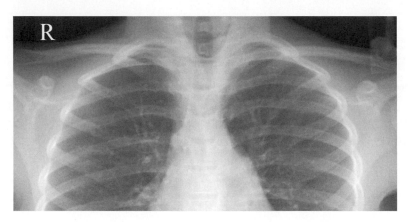

127. Figure 3-30: _____

_____

_____

Posteroanterior Oblique Projection (Right and Left Anterior Oblique Positions)

Figure 3-31

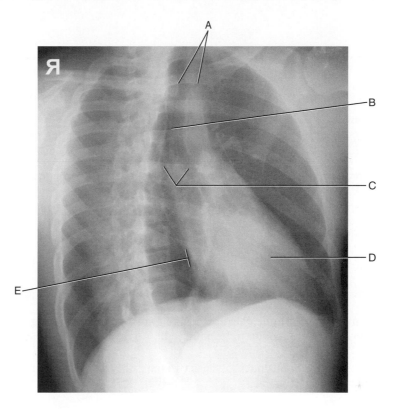

128. Identify the labeled anatomy in Figure 3-31.

A. _____

B. _____

C. _____

D. _____

E. _____

129. Complete the statements below, referring to adult PA oblique chest projection analysis criteria.

Posteroanterior Oblique Chest Projection Analysis Criteria
• The right and left _____ (A) are at the center of the exposure field.
• The _____ (B) are demonstrated without spinal superimposition, with approximately _____ (C) as much lung field demonstrated on one side of the thoracic vertebrae as on the other side.
• The _____ (D) is superimposed by the fourth thoracic vertebra, with 1 inch (2. 5 cm) of apical lung field visible above the clavicles.
• The _____ (E) posterior lungs are visualized above the diaphragm

130. Which body plane is used to determine if the patient has been adequately rotated for an oblique chest projection?

_____

131. For a PA oblique chest projection taken in an LAO position, the patient needs to be rotated _____ degrees to demonstrate the heart shadow without vertebral column superimposition.

132. For the AP-PA oblique chest projections indicated below, state which side of the thorax will be best demonstrated.

    A. AP oblique (RPO position): _____

    B. PA oblique (LAO position): _____

133. The AP oblique chest projection (RPO position) corresponds with which PA oblique projection? _____

134. A PA oblique chest projection with accurate centering is accomplished by centering the central ray at a level 7.5 inches (18 cm) inferior to the _____.

135. Which anatomic structures are included on a PA oblique chest projection with accurate positioning?

_____

For the following descriptions of PA oblique chest projections with poor positioning, state how the patient would have been mispositioned for such a projection to be obtained.

136. A 45-degree oblique projection demonstrates less than two times the lung field on one side of the thoracic vertebrae than on the other side.

_____

137. A 45-degree oblique projection demonstrates more than two times the lung field on one side of the thoracic vertebrae than the other side.

_____

138. A 60-degree PA oblique projection (LAO position) demonstrates superimposition of the vertebral column and heart shadow.

_____

For the following PA oblique chest projections with poor positioning, state which anatomic structures are misaligned and how the patient should be repositioned for an optimal projection to be obtained.

Figure 3-32

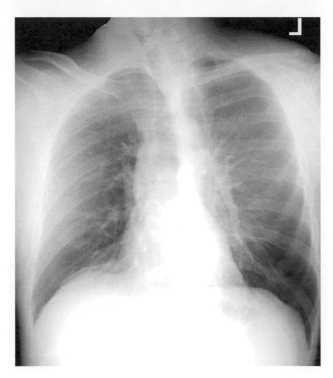

139. Figure 3-32: _____

_____

_____

_____

Figure 3-33

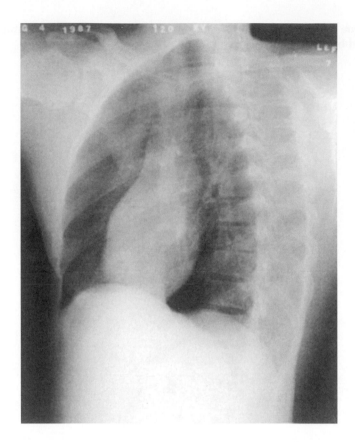

140. Figure 3-33: _____

_____

_____

_____

PEDIATRIC CHEST

141. Why do neonatal and infant chest projections demonstrate less projection contrast than adult chest projections?

_____

142. Discuss the importance of the neonate's or infant's face being positioned forward and the cervical vertebrae being in a neutral position when the patient undergoes imaging for ETT placement. _____

_____

_____

Neonate and Infant: Anteroposterior Projection (Supine or With Mobile X-Ray Unit)

143. Identify the labeled anatomy in Figure 3-34.

Figure 3-34

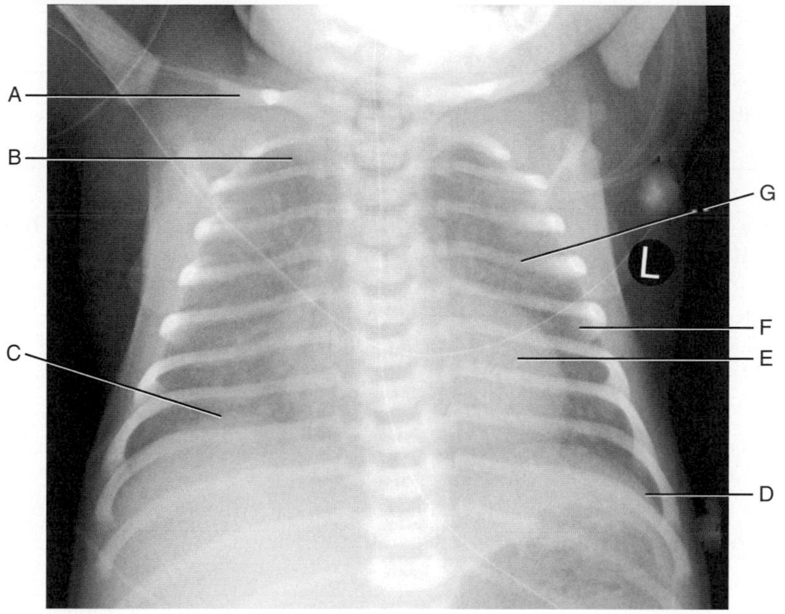

A. _____

B. _____

C. _____

D. _____

E. _____

F. _____

G. _____

144. Complete the statements below, referring to neonate and infant AP chest projection analysis criteria.

Neonate and Infant Anteroposterior Chest Projection Analysis Criteria
• The _____ (A) thoracic vertebra is at the center of the exposure field.
• The distances from the vertebral column to the sternal ends of the clavicles are _____ (B), and the lengths of the right and left corresponding posterior ribs are _____ (C).
• The anterior ribs are projecting _____ (D) and the posterior ribs demonstrate a gentle, _____ (E) bowed contour.
• Neonate: The _____ (F) posterior ribs are demonstrated above the diaphragm, and the lungs demonstrate a fluffy appearance with linear-appearing connecting tissue.
• Infant: The _____ (G) posterior ribs are demonstrated above the diaphragm.
• The _____ (H) does not obscure the airway or apical lung field.

145. Accurate centering is seen on neonatal or infant AP chest projections when a perpendicular central ray is centered to the _____ (A) plane at the level of the _____ (B). The _____ (C) should be included on the projection.

146. Which type of distortion is demonstrated when AP neonatal or infant chest projections demonstrate an excessively lordotic appearance? _____

147. On a neonatal chest projection, what causes the lungs to have a fluffy appearance? _____

148. Explain when the projection should be exposed in the following situations to obtain maximum lung expansion.

    A. Neonate breathing without a ventilator:

    _____

    B. Neonate on a conventional ventilator:

    _____

    C. Neonate on a high-frequency ventilator:

    _____

For the following descriptions of neonatal or infant AP chest projections with poor positioning, state how the patient would have been mispositioned or the central ray misaligned for such a projection to be obtained.

149. The right sternoclavicular end is demonstrated farther from the vertebral column than the left sternoclavicular end, and the right lower posterior ribs are longer than the left. The patient's head is turned toward the right side.

_____

_____

150. The chest demonstrates an excessively lordotic appearance. The anterior ribs are projecting upwardly and the posterior ribs are horizontal. The sixth thoracic vertebra is at the center of the projection.

_____

_____

151. Seven posterior ribs are demonstrated above the diaphragm for a neonatal AP chest projection. The patient was on a conventional ventilator.

_____

_____

152. The patient's chin is superimposed over the airway and apical lung field.

_____

_____

For the following AP neonatal or infant chest projections with poor positioning, state which anatomic structures are misaligned and how the patient should be repositioned for an optimal projection to be obtained.

Figure 3-35

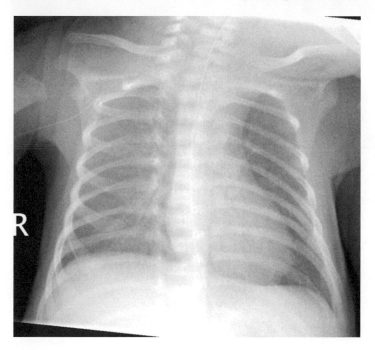

153. Figure 3-35: _____

_____

_____

_____

Figure 3-36

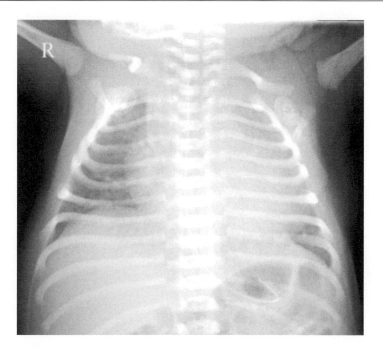

154. Figure 3-36: _____

_____

_____

_____

Figure 3-37

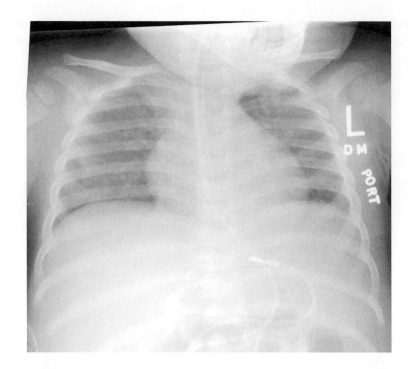

155. Figure 3-37: _____

_____

_____

_____

Figure 3-38

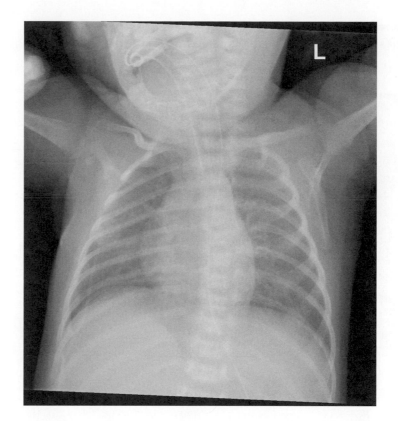

156. Figure 3-38: _____

_____

_____

_____

Child: Posteroanterior and Anteroposterior Projections

157. Identify the labeled anatomy in Figure 3-39.

Figure 3-39

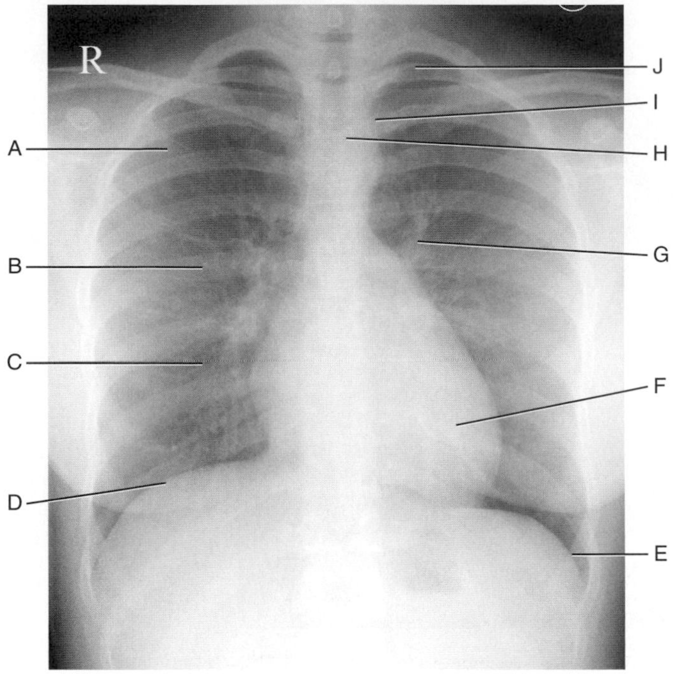

A. _____

B. _____

C. _____

D. _____

E. _____

F. _____

G. _____

H. _____

I. _____

J. _____

For the following descriptions of child PA-AP chest projections with poor positioning, state how the patient would have been mispositioned or the central ray misaligned for such a projection to be obtained.

158. Mobile AP projection: The left sternoclavicular end is visualized without vertebral column superimposition, and the vertebral column is superimposed over the right sternoclavicular end.

_____

_____

159. PA projection: Six posterior ribs are demonstrated above the diaphragm.

_____

_____

160. Mobile AP projection: The manubrium is superimposed over the fifth thoracic vertebra, the posterior ribs demonstrate vertical contour, and more than 1 inch (2. 5cm) of apical lung field is visible above the clavicles.

_____

_____

161. PA projection: The second thoracic vertebra is superimposed over the manubrium.

_____

_____

162. PA projection: The fourth thoracic vertebra is superimposed over the manubrium and the lateral ends of the clavicles are projecting superiorly.

_____

_____

For the following PA-AP child chest projections with poor positioning, state what anatomic structures are misaligned and how the patient should be repositioned for an optimal projection to be obtained.

Figure 3-40

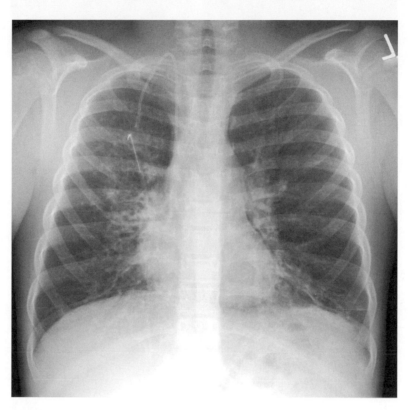

163. Figure 3-40 (PA projection): _____

_____

_____

_____

Figure 3-41

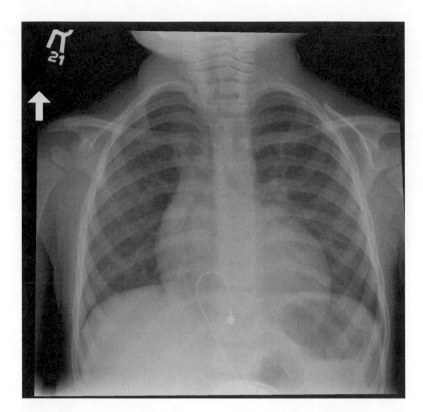

164. Figure 3-41 (PA projection): _____

_____

_____

_____

Figure 3-42

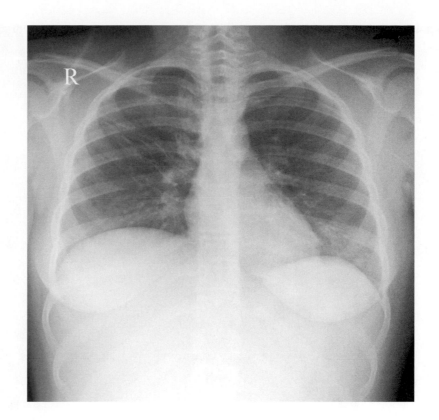

165. Figure 3-42 (PA projection): _____

_____

_____

_____

Figure 3-43

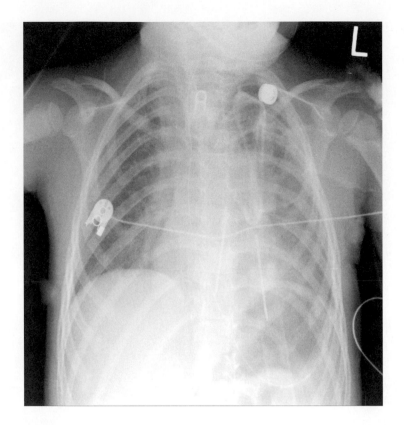

166. Figure 3-43 (AP projection): _____

_____

_____

_____

Figure 3-44

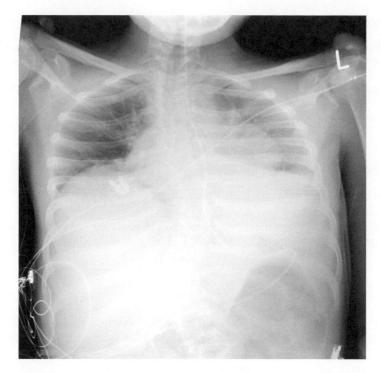

167. Figure 3-44 (AP projection): _____

_____

_____

_____

Neonate and Infant: Cross-Table Lateral Projection (Left Lateral Position)

168. Identify the labeled anatomy in Figure 3-45.

Figure 3-45

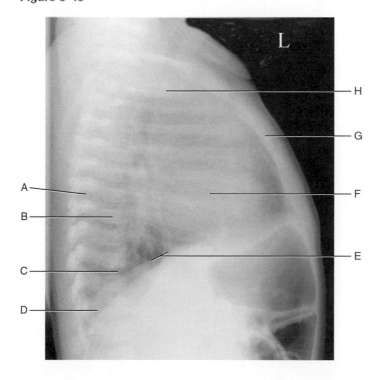

A. _____

B. _____

C. _____

D. _____

E. _____

F. _____

G. _____

H. _____

169. Accurate centering is seen on a neonatal or infant lateral chest projection when the central ray is centered to the

_____ (A) plane at the level just inferior to the _____ (B). The _____ (C) should be included on the projection.

170. List two reasons why cross-table lateral neonatal chest projections are taken instead of overhead projections.

A. _____

B. _____

171. To avoid chest rotation on lateral neonatal and infant chest projections, align an imaginary line connecting the shoulders,

the posterior ribs, and the posterior pelvic wings _____ to the IR.

172. Explain why the 0.5-inch (1. 25-cm) posterior rib separation demonstrated on optimally positioned adult lateral chest projections is not demonstrated on neonatal or infant lateral chest projections.

_____

_____

For the following descriptions of neonatal or infant lateral chest projections with poor positioning, state how the patient would have been mispositioned or the central ray misaligned for such a projection to be obtained.

173. The left posterior ribs are demonstrated posterior to the right posterior ribs.

_____

_____

174. The humeral soft tissue is superimposed over the anterior lung apices.

_____

_____

175. The patient's chin is demonstrated within the collimated field.

_____

_____

176. The hemidiaphragms demonstrate an exaggerated cephalic curvature and are positioned high in the thorax.

_____

_____

For the following neonatal or infant lateral chest projections with poor positioning, state which anatomic structures are misaligned and how the patient should be repositioned for an optimal projection to be obtained.

Figure 3-46

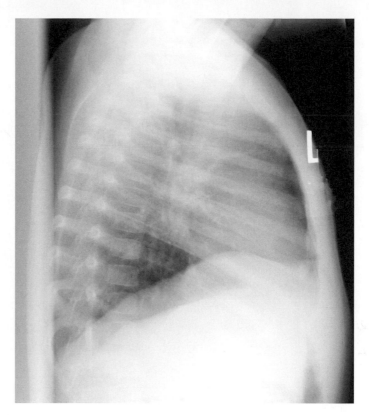

177. Figure 3-46: _____

_____

_____

_____

_____

Figure 3-47

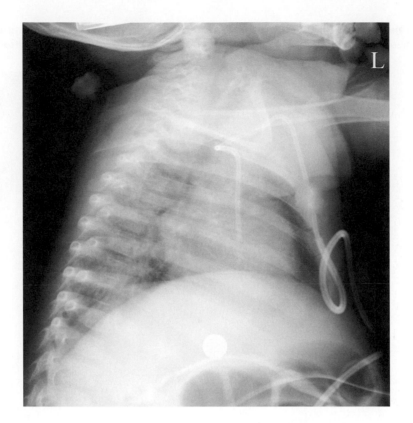

178. Figure 3-47: _____

_____

_____

_____

Child : Lateral Projection (Left Lateral Position)

179. Identify the labeled anatomy in Figure 3-48.

Figure 3-48

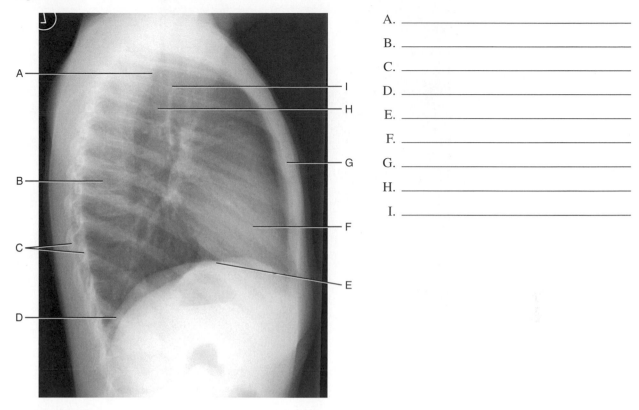

A. _____

B. _____

C. _____

D. _____

E. _____

F. _____

G. _____

H. _____

I. _____

For the following descriptions of child lateral chest projections with poor positioning, state how the patient would have been mispositioned or the central ray misaligned for such a projection to be obtained.

180. More than 0.5 inch (1.25 cm) of separation is demonstrated between the posterior ribs. The gastric air bubble is adjacent to the posteriorly located lung.

_____

_____

181. The hemidiaphragms demonstrate an exaggerated cephalic curve, and they do not cover the entire eleventh thoracic vertebra.

_____

182. The humeral soft tissue is superimposed over the anterior lung apices.

_____

For the following lateral child chest projections with poor positioning, state which anatomic structures are misaligned and how the patient should be repositioned for an optimal projection to be obtained.

Figure 3-49

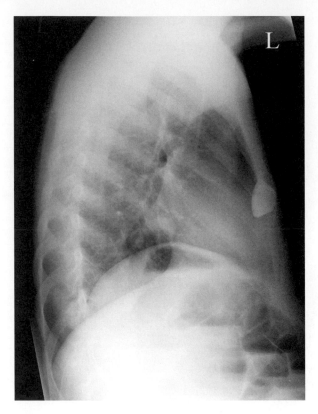

183. Figure 3-49: _____

_____

_____

_____

Figure 3-50

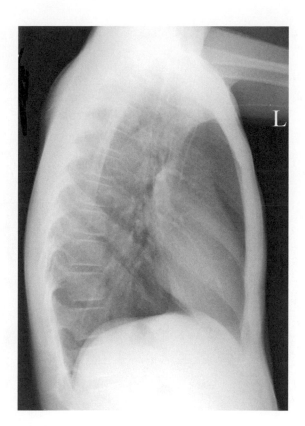

184. Figure 3-50: _____

_____

_____

Figure 3-51

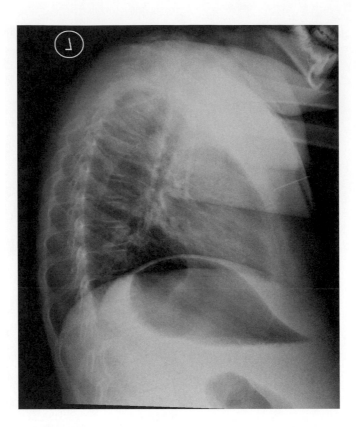

185. Figure 3-51: _____

_____

_____

Neonate and Infant: Anteroposterior Projection (Right or Left Lateral Decubitus Projection)

186. Identify the labeled anatomy in Figure 3-52.

Figure 3-52

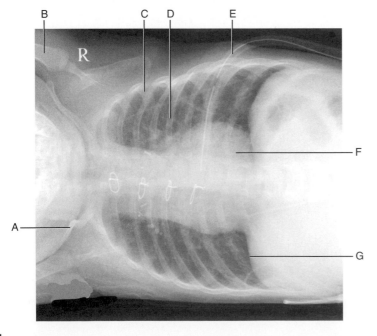

A. _____

B. _____

C. _____

D. _____

E. _____

F. _____

G. _____

187. Complete the statements below, referring to neonate and infant AP (lateral decubitus) chest projection analysis criteria.

Neonate and Infant Anteroposterior (Lateral Decubitus) Chest Projection Analysis Criteria
• The _____ (A) vertebra is at the center of the exposure field.
• Distances from the _____ (B) to the sternal ends of the clavicles are equal, and the lengths of the right and left corresponding posterior ribs are equal.
• The chin and arms are situated outside the lung field, and the lateral aspects of the _____ (C) are projected upward.
• The anterior ribs are projecting _____ (D) and the posterior ribs demonstrate a gentle, _____ (E) bowed contour.
• The _____ (F) posterior ribs are demonstrated above the diaphragm, and the lungs demonstrate a fluffy appearance, with linear-appearing connecting tissue.
• The lung field positioned against the bed or cart is demonstrated without superimposition of the bed or cart pad.
• The _____ (G) plane is seen without lateral tilting.

188. To best demonstrate a pneumothorax on neonatal or infant AP (lateral decubitus) chest projections, the affected side of the patient should be positioned _____.

189. For the upper airway on a neonatal or infant chest projection to be included, the collimation should be open to the

_____.

190. To avoid chest rotation on a neonatal or infant AP (lateral decubitus) chest projection, align an imaginary line connecting the shoulders, the posterior ribs, and the posterior pelvic wings _____ to the IR.

For the following descriptions of neonatal or infant AP (lateral decubitus) chest projections with poor positioning, state how the patient would have been mispositioned or the central ray misaligned for such a projection to be obtained.

191. The right sternoclavicular end is demonstrated farther from the vertebral column than the left sternoclavicular end, and the right posterior ribs are longer than the left.

_____

_____

192. The anterior ribs are projecting cephalically, and the posterior ribs are horizontal.

_____

_____

193. The six posterior ribs are demonstrated superior to the diaphragm.

_____

_____

194. The projection was taken to demonstrate pleural effusion on the right side. Artifact lines are superimposed over the lateral aspect of the right lung.

_____

_____

195. The projection was taken to demonstrate a right-side pneumothorax. The right arm is superimposed over the upper right lateral lung field.

_____

_____

For the following AP (lateral decubitus) neonatal or infant chest projections with poor positioning, state which anatomic structures are misaligned and how the patient should be repositioned for an optimal projection to be obtained.

Figure 3-53

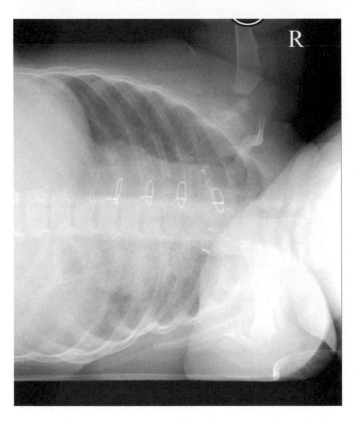

196. Figure 3-53: _____

_____

_____

_____

_____

Figure 3-54

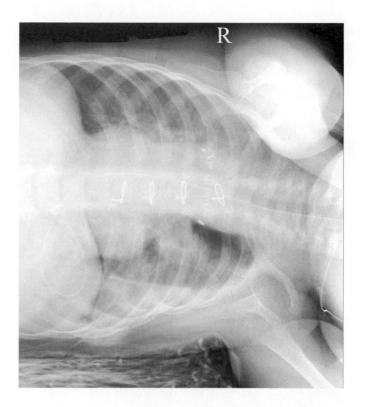

197. Figure 3-54: _____

_____

_____

Figure 3-55

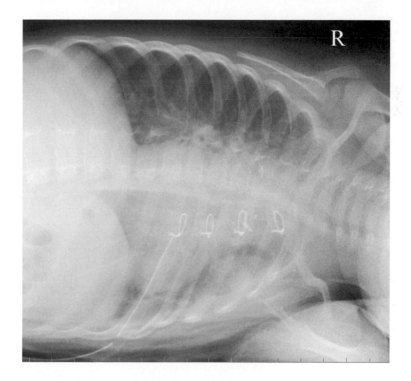

198. Figure 3-55: _____

_____

_____

Child Chest: Anteroposterior or Posteroanterior Projection (Right or Left Lateral Decubitus Position)

199. Identify the labeled anatomy in Figure 3-56.

Figure 3-56

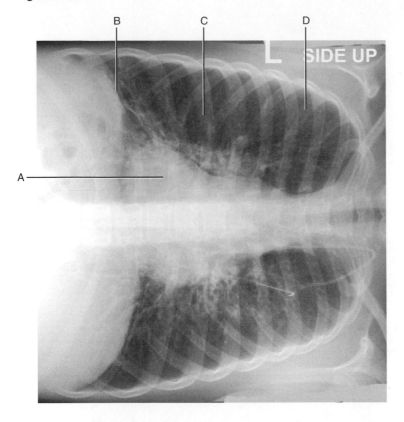

A. _____

B. _____

C. _____

D. _____

For the following descriptions of child AP-PA (lateral decubitus) chest projections with poor positioning, state how the patient would have been mispositioned or the central ray misaligned for such a projection to be obtained.

200. A PA (lateral decubitus) chest projection demonstrates the vertebral column superimposed over the right SC joint.

_____

_____

201. An AP (lateral decubitus) chest projection demonstrates the right SC joint superimposed over the vertebral column, whereas the left SC joint does not demonstrate vertebral superimposition.

_____

_____

202. An AP (lateral decubitus) chest projection demonstrates the manubrium at the level of the second thoracic vertebra.

_____

_____

For the following child AP-PA (lateral decubitus) chest projections with poor positioning, state which anatomic structures are misaligned and how the patient should be repositioned for an optimal projection to be obtained.

Figure 3-57

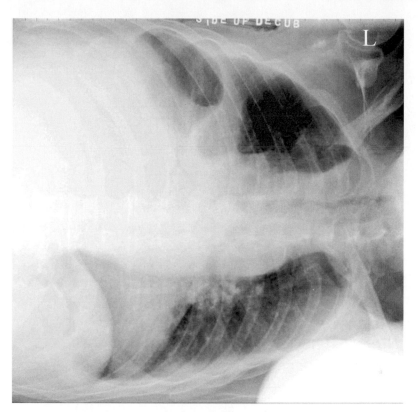

203. Figure 3-57: _____

_____

_____

_____

Figure 3-58

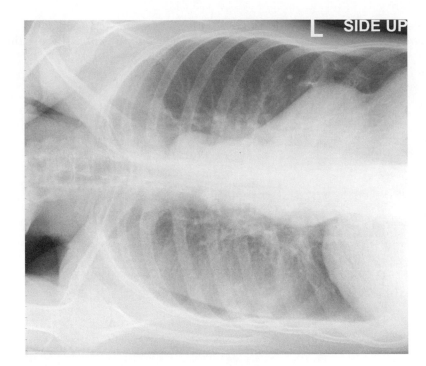

L SIDE UP

204. Figure 3-58: _____

_____

_____

_____

ABDOMEN STUDY QUESTIONS

205. Describe how the following abdomen projections should be displayed on a view box or digital monitor.

    A. AP: _____

    B. AP (left lateral decubitus): _____

206. State two possible causes of voluntary motion on abdomen projections.

    A. _____

    B. _____

207. List three ways in which voluntary motion can be controlled when abdomen projections are taken.

    A. _____

    B. _____

    C. _____

208. State the most common cause of involuntary motion on abdomen projections.

_____

209. How can involuntary motion be controlled on abdomen projections?

_____

210. State whether voluntary or involuntary motion is demonstrated on the following projections.

Figure 3-59

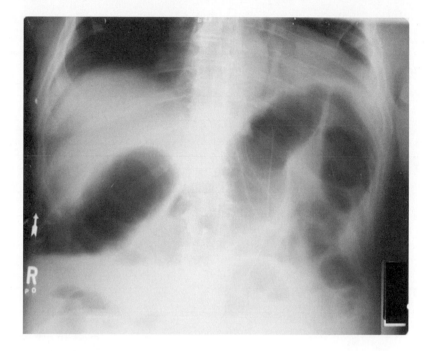

A. Figure 3-59: _____

_____

Figure 3-60

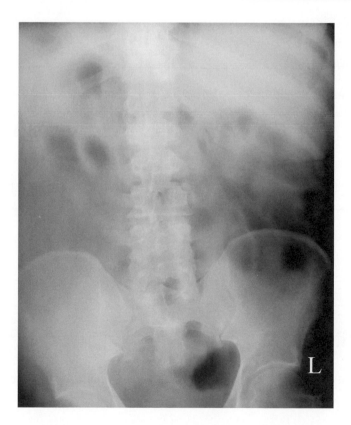

B. Figure 3-60: _____

_____

211. Describe the location of the psoas major muscles.

_____

_____

212. Complete the statements below, referring to the kidneys.

    A. Describe the location of the kidneys. _____

_____

_____

    B. Which kidney is usually demonstrated inferiorly? _____

    C. What causes the inferior location of this kidney? _____

_____

213. List four structures that when optimally demonstrated, ensure that the best possible contrast, density, and penetration have been achieved on an AP abdominal projection.

    A. _____

    B. _____

    C. _____

    D. _____

214. State how the milliampere-seconds (mAs) or kVp level is adjusted for AP abdomen projections of a patient who has a large amount of bowel gas.

    A. mAs: _____

    B. kVp: _____

215. List four possible patient conditions that could require an increase in the routine exposure to obtain adequate projection density.

    A. _____

    B. _____

    C. _____

    D. _____

216. State how the mAs or kVp level is adjusted for AP abdomen projections of a patient with one of the conditions listed in question 215.

    A. mAs: _____

    B. kVp: _____

217. Contrast, density, and penetration should be sufficient to demonstrate the _____ on neonatal and infant AP abdomen projections.

218. Explain why abdominal organs are not well defined on neonatal and infant AP abdomen projections.

_____

_____

219. Complete Exercise 3-2.

EXERCISE 3-2 Abdomen Technical Data				
ADULT AND PEDIATRIC ABDOMEN TECHNICAL DATA				
Projection	kVp	Grid	AEC Chamber(s)	SID
ADULT CHEST TECHNICAL DATA				
AP				
AP (lateral decubitus)				
PEDIATRIC ABDOMINAL TECHNICAL DATA				
Neonate: AP				
Infant: AP				
Child: AP				
Neonate: AP (lateral decubitus)				
Infant: AP (lateral decubitus)				
Child: AP (lateral decubitus)				

AEC, Automatic exposure control; *SID*, source–image receptor distance.

Anteroposterior Projection (Supine and Upright)

220. Identify the labeled anatomy in Figure 3-61.

Figure 3-61

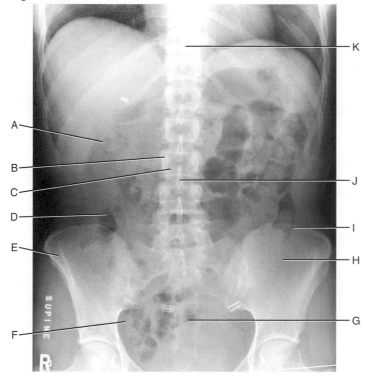

A. _____

B. _____

C. _____

D. _____

E. _____

F. _____

G. _____

H. _____

I. _____

J. _____

K. _____

221. Identify the labeled anatomy in Figure 3-62.

Figure 3-62

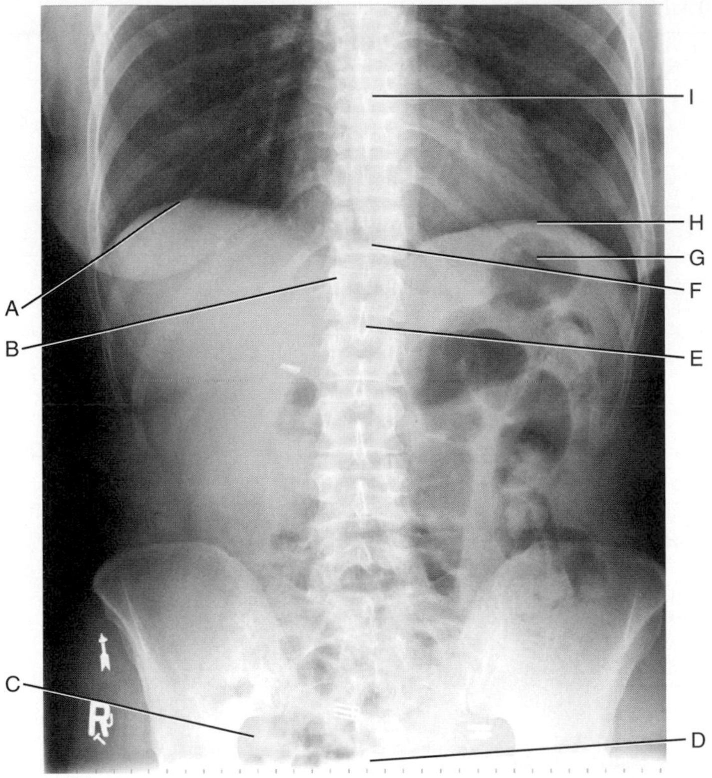

A. _____

B. _____

C. _____

D. _____

E. _____

F. _____

G. _____

H. _____

I. _____

222. Complete the statements below, referring to adult AP abdomen projection analysis criteria.

> **Anteroposterior Abdomen Projection Analysis Criteria**
>
> • Density is uniform across the abdomen.
>
> • Spinous processes are aligned with the midline of the _____ (A), and the distance from the pedicles to the spinous processes is the same on both sides. The sacrum is centered within the inlet of pelvis and is aligned with the _____ (B).
>
> • The long axis of the lumbar vertebral column is aligned with the long axis of the collimated field.
>
> • Diaphragm domes are located superior to the _____ (C) posterior ribs.
>
> • Supine: The _____ (D) lumbar vertebra is at the center of the exposure field.
>
> • Supine: The eleventh thoracic vertebra, the lateral body soft tissues, the iliac wings, and the symphysis pubis are included within the collimated field.
>
> • Upright: The _____ (E) lumbar vertebra is at the center of the exposure field.
>
> • Upright: The ninth thoracic vertebra, lateral body soft tissue, and iliac wings are included within the collimated field.

223. Identify the patient condition that is being demonstrated in Figure 3-63.

Figure 3-63

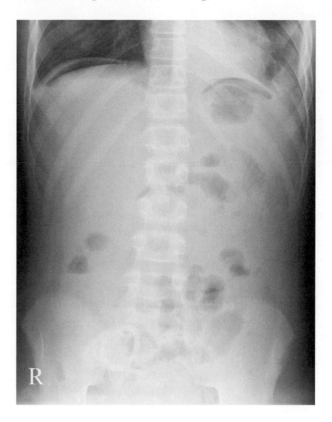

_____

224. How should the patient be positioned to prevent rotation on an AP abdomen projection?

_____

_____

225. Complete the statements below, referring to intraperitoneal air.

    A. To best demonstrate intraperitoneal air, how long should the patient be positioned upright before the projection

       is taken? _____

    B. Why is this time delay necessary? _____

    _____

226. From full inspiration to expiration, the diaphragm position moves from a(n) _____ (A)

(inferior-superior) to _____ (B) (inferior-superior) position. On full expiration the right side of

the diaphragmatic dome will be at the same transverse level as the _____ (C) thoracic vertebra,

whereas on inspiration it is found at the _____ (D) posterior rib.

227. Complete the statements below, referring to respiration for an AP abdomen projection.

    A. What respiration is used for an AP abdominal projection? _____

    B. Why is this respiration used? _____

228. State why it is important that both of the following structures be demonstrated on a supine AP abdomen projection.

    A. Eleventh thoracic vertebra: _____

    _____

    B. Symphysis pubis: _____

    _____

229. Why is it necessary to center 1 inch (2.5 cm) more inferiorly on the male patient than the female patient to include the symphysis pubis?

    _____

    _____

230. For each of the body types listed below, state whether one lengthwise IR or two crosswise IRs should be used for abdomen projections.

    A. Hypersthenic: _____

    B. Sthenic: _____

    C. Asthenic: _____

231. Which anatomic structures are included on the following AP abdomen projections?

    A. Supine: _____

    _____

    B. Upright: _____

For the following descriptions of AP abdomen projections with poor positioning, state how the patient would have been mispositioned or the central ray misaligned for such a projection to be obtained.

232. The distance from the right lumbar vertebral pedicles to the spinous processes is greater than from the left pedicles to the spinous processes.

    _____

    _____

233. The upper abdominal region demonstrates an equal distance from the vertebral pedicles to the spinous processes on each side, and the lower abdominal region demonstrates the sacrum and symphysis pubis without alignment. The sacrum is rotated toward the right pelvic inlet.

    _____

    _____

234. The supine abdomen projection does not include the symphysis pubis or inferior peritoneal cavity.

    _____

    _____

For the following AP abdomen projections with poor positioning, state which anatomic structures are misaligned and how the patient should be repositioned for an optimal projection to be obtained.

Figure 3-64

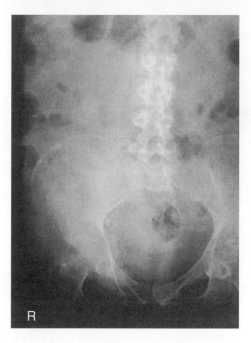

235. A supine abdomen projection was requested (Figure 3-64): _____

_____

_____

_____

Figure 3-65

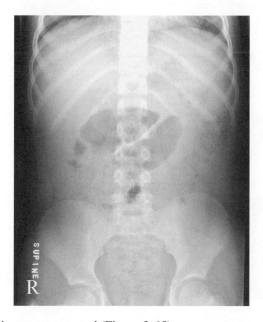

236. A supine abdomen projection was requested (Figure 3-65): _____

_____

_____

_____

Figure 3-66

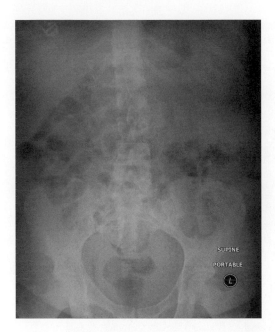

237. A supine abdomen projection was requested (Figure 3-66): _____

_____

_____

_____

Figure 3-67

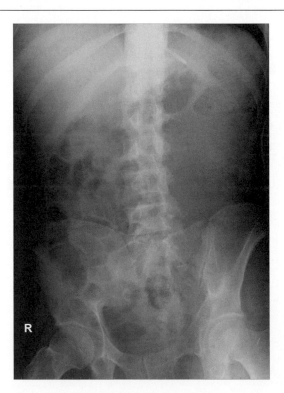

238. A supine abdomen projection was requested (Figure 3-67): _____

_____

_____

_____

Figure 3-68

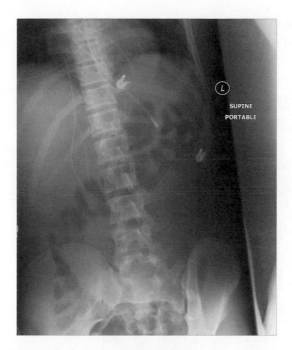

239. A supine abdomen projection was requested (Figure 3-68): _____

_____

_____

_____

Figure 3-69

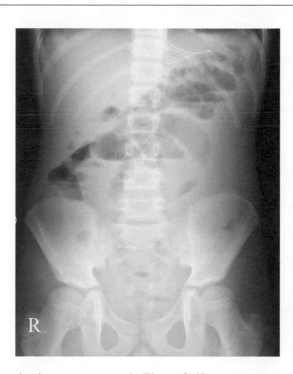

240. An upright abdomen projection was requested. (Figure 3-69): _____

_____

_____

_____

Anteroposterior Projection (Left Lateral Decubitus Position)

241. Identify the labeled anatomy in Figure 3-70.

Figure 3-70

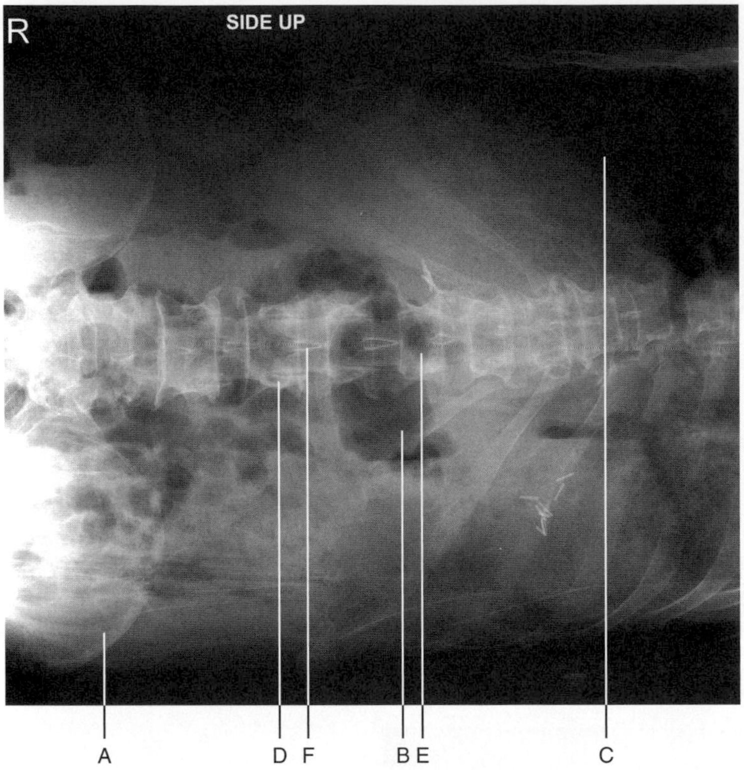

A. _____

B. _____

C. _____

D. _____

E. _____

F. _____

242. Complete the statements below, referring to adult AP (lateral decubitus) abdomen projection analysis criteria.

Anteroposterior (Lateral Decubitus) Abdomen Projection Analysis Criteria

- An arrow or "word" marker, indicating that the right side of the patient is positioned up and away from the imaging table or cart, is present.

- Density is uniform across the abdomen.

- Spinous processes are aligned with the midline of the _____ (A), and the distance from

  the pedicles to the _____ (B) is the same on both sides. The sacrum is centered within the inlet of pelvis and is aligned with the symphysis pubis.

- Diaphragm domes are located superior to the _____ (C) posterior ribs.

- The _____ (D) lumbar vertebra is at the center of the exposure field.

- Right hemidiaphragm, ninth thoracic vertebra, right lateral body soft tissue, and iliac wings are included within the collimated field.

---

243. A patient's requisition states that an AP (lateral decubitus) abdomen projection be taken to rule out ascites. Describe how to determine the technique factors to use for this patient.

_____

_____

244. How is a compensating filter positioned to obtain uniform projection density on a patient with excessive abdominal soft tissue on an AP (lateral decubitus) abdomen projection?

_____

_____

245. For an AP (lateral decubitus) abdomen projection, the _____ (A) side of the patient is positioned against the imaging

table or cart. Why is this side chosen? (B) _____

_____

246. How is the patient positioned for an AP (lateral decubitus) abdomen projection to prevent rotation?

_____

_____

247. Placing a pillow between the patient's knees for an AP (lateral decubitus) abdomen projection will prevent

_____

_____

248. To obtain optimal intraperitoneal air demonstration, the patient should remain in the decubitus position for

_____ (A) minutes before the AP (lateral decubitus) projection is taken. Why is this time delay necessary? (B)

_____

_____

249. Intraperitoneal air is most often found beneath the _____ on an AP (lateral decubitus) abdomen projection with proper positioning.

250. Describe the shape of a patient's body that will result in the intraperitoneal air being demonstrated over the right iliac wing on a properly positioned AP (lateral decubitus) abdomen projection.

_____

_____

251. What respiration is used for an AP (lateral decubitus) abdomen projection? _____

252. Which anatomic structures are included on an AP (lateral decubitus) abdomen projection with accurate positioning?

_____

_____

253. State when gonadal shielding is used on female and male patients for imaging the abdomen in an AP (lateral decubitus) projection.

A. Female: _____

B. Male: _____

For the following descriptions of AP (lateral decubitus) abdomen projections with poor positioning, state how the patient would have been mispositioned or the central ray misaligned for such a projection to be obtained.

254. The projection demonstrates a greater distance from the left lumbar vertebral pedicles to the spinous processes than from the right pedicles to the spinous processes.

_____

255. The projection demonstrates the upper abdominal region with equal distances from the vertebral pedicles to the spinous processes on each side, and the lower abdominal region demonstrates the sacrum and symphysis pubis without alignment. The sacrum is rotated toward the left pelvic inlet.

_____

_____

256. The projection demonstrates a clipped right diaphragmatic dome.

_____

For the following AP (lateral decubitus) abdomen projection with poor positioning, state which anatomic structures are misaligned and how the patient should be repositioned for an optimal projection to be obtained.

Figure 3-71

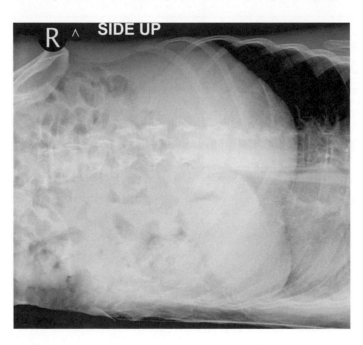

257. Figure 3-71: _____

_____

_____

_____

Neonate and Infant: Anteroposterior Projection

258. Identify the labeled anatomy in Figure 3-72.

Figure 3-72

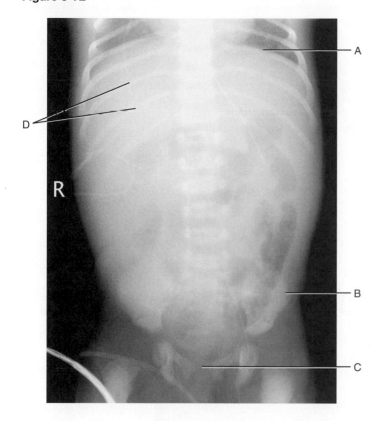

A. _____

B. _____

C. _____

D. _____

259. Complete the statements below, referring to neonate and infant AP abdomen projection analysis criteria.

Anteroposterior Abdomen Projection Analysis Criteria
• The right and left inferior posterior ribs and the iliac wings are symmetrical.
• The diaphragm domes are superior to the _____ (A) posterior rib.
• The long axis of the lumbar vertebral column is aligned with the long axis of the collimated field.
• The _____ (B) vertebra is at the center of the exposure field.
• The diaphragm, abdominal structures, and symphysis pubis are included in the collimation field.

260. To center a neonatal and infant AP abdomen projection accurately, the central ray is centered to the _____ (A) plane at a level _____ (B) inches _____ (C) to the _____ (D).

For the following descriptions of neonatal or infant AP abdomen projections with poor positioning, state how the patient would have been mispositioned or the central ray misaligned for such a projection to be obtained.

261. The diaphragm is not included on the projection.

_____

_____

262. The patient's upper vertebral column is tilted toward the left side.

_____

263. The left inferior posterior ribs are longer than the posterior ribs on the right side.

_____

264. The right iliac wing is wider than the left wing.

_____

265. The diaphragm is at the level of the ninth posterior rib.

_____

For the following AP neonatal or infant abdomen projections with poor positioning, state which anatomic structures are misaligned and how the patient should be repositioned for an optimal projection to be obtained.

Figure 3-73

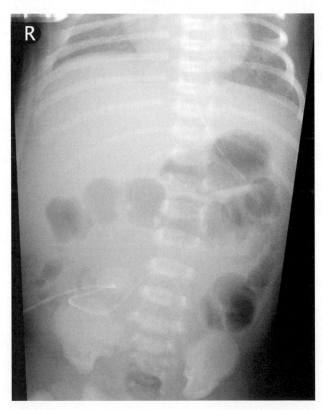

266. Figure 3-73: _____

_____

_____

_____

Figure 3-74

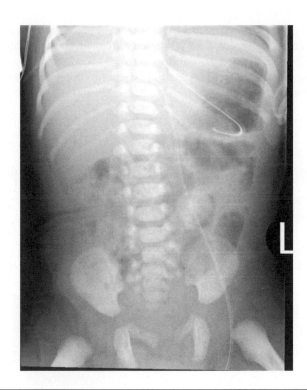

267. Figure 3-74: _____

_____

_____

_____

Child: Anteroposterior Projection

268. Identify the labeled anatomy in Figure 3-75.

Figure 3-75

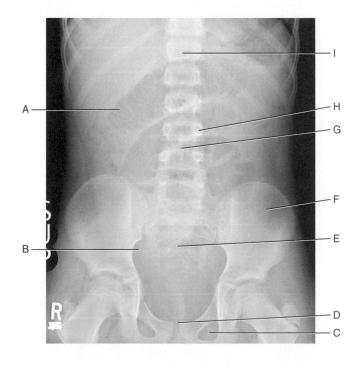

A. _____

B. _____

C. _____

D. _____

E. _____

F. _____

G. _____

H. _____

I. _____

For the following descriptions of child AP abdomen projections with poor positioning, state how the patient would have been mispositioned or the central ray misaligned for such a projection to be obtained.

269. The distance from the right lumbar vertebral pedicles to the spinous processes is greater than the distance from the left pedicles to the spinous processes.

_____

_____

270. The left inferior posterior ribs are longer than the right, and the left iliac wing is wider than the right.

_____

_____

For the following AP child abdomen projections with poor positioning, state which anatomic structures are misaligned and how the patient should be repositioned for an optimal projection to be obtained.

Figure 3-76

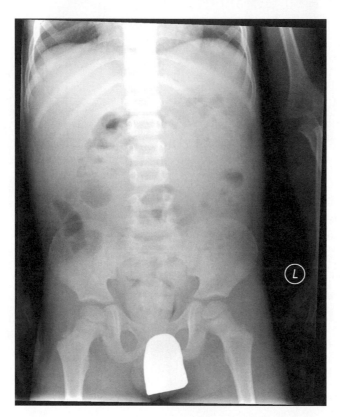

271. Figure 3-76 (supine abdomen): _____

_____

_____

_____

Figure 3-77

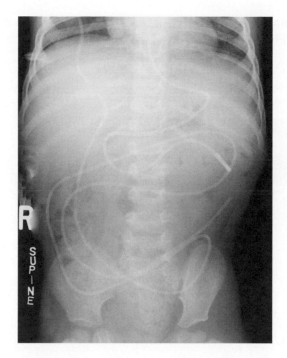

272. Figure 3-77 (supine abdomen): _____

_____

_____

_____

Figure 3-78

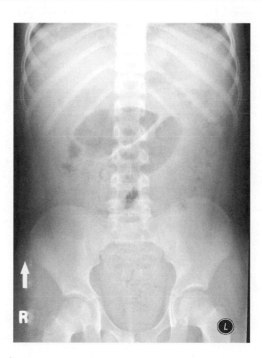

273. Figure 3-78 (upright abdomen): _____

_____

_____

_____

Neonate and Infant: Anteroposterior Projection (Left Lateral Decubitus Position)

274. Identify the labeled anatomy in Figure 3-79.

Figure 3-79

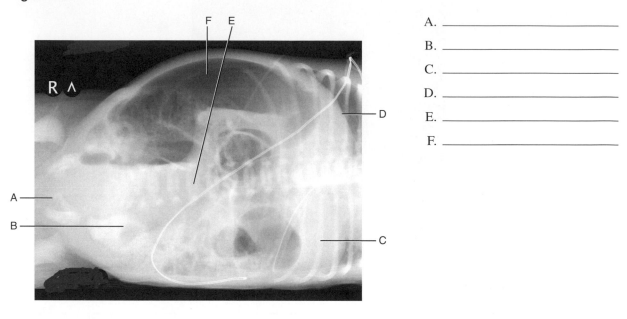

A. _____

B. _____

C. _____

D. _____

E. _____

F. _____

275. Explain why the left side of the patient is placed adjacent to the bed or cart when the patient is positioned for neonatal or infant AP (lateral decubitus) abdomen projections.

_____

_____

276. For a neonatal and infant AP (lateral decubitus) abdomen projection a horizontal central ray is centered to the

_____ (A) plane at a level _____ (B) inches _____

(C) to the _____ (D).

For the following descriptions of neonatal or infant AP (lateral decubitus) abdominal projections with poor positioning, state how the patient would have been mispositioned or the central ray misaligned for such a projection to be obtained.

277. The left iliac wing is narrower than the right iliac wing.

_____

_____

278. The diaphragm is not included on the projection.

_____

_____

279. The right posterior ribs are longer than the posterior ribs on the left side.

_____

_____

For the following neonatal or infant AP (lateral decubitus) abdominal projections with poor positioning, state which anatomic structures are misaligned and how the patient should be repositioned for an optimal projection to be obtained.

Figure 3-80

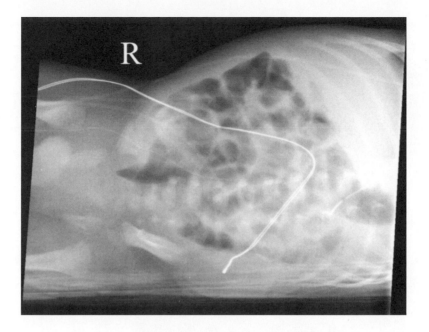

280. Figure 3-80: _____

_____

_____

Figure 3-81

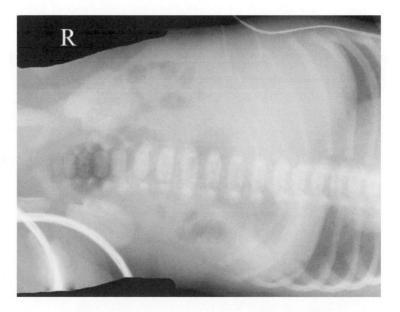

281. Figure 3-81: _____

_____

_____

Child: Anteroposterior Projection (Left Lateral Decubitus Position)

282. Identify the labeled anatomy in Figure 3-82.

Figure 3-82

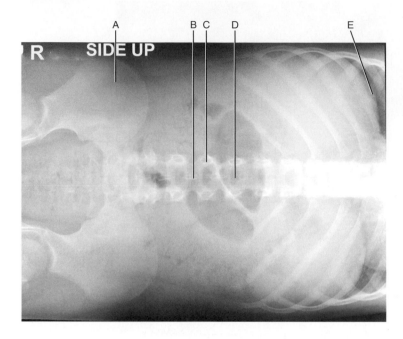

A. _____

B. _____

C. _____

D. _____

E. _____

283. Identify the patient condition demonstrated on the projection in Figure 3-83.

Figure 3-83

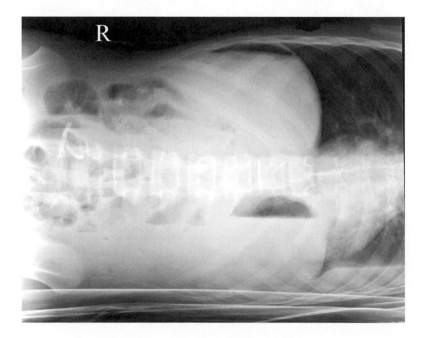

For the following descriptions of child AP (lateral decubitus) abdomen projections with poor positioning, state how the patient would have been mispositioned or the central ray misaligned for such a projection to be obtained.

284. The diaphragm is at the level of the ninth posterior rib. The child was on a conventional ventilator.

_____

_____

285. The distance from the left lumbar vertebral pedicles to the spinous processes is greater than that from the right pedicles to the spinous processes.

_____

_____

For the following child AP (lateral decubitus) projections with poor positioning, state which anatomic structures are misaligned and how the patient should be repositioned for an optimal projection to be obtained.

286. Figure 3-83: _____

_____

_____

Figure 3-84

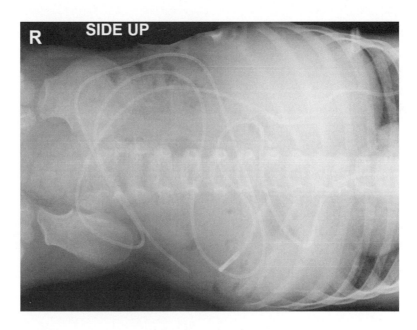

287. Figure 3-84: _____

_____

_____

4 Upper Extremity

STUDY QUESTIONS

Finger

1. Describe how the following upper extremity projections would be displayed on a view box or digital monitor.

   A. AP oblique hand: _____

   B. PA hand: _____

   C. PA oblique wrist: _____

   D. AP forearm: _____

   E. Lateral humerus: _____

2. What is the most frequent cause of recorded detail that lacks sharpness on a projection?

   A. _____

   List four methods of controlling this problem.

   B. _____

   C. _____

   D. _____

   E. _____

3. A _____ (high/low) contrast _____, (high/low) kilovoltage technique will best enhance the bony and soft-tissue structures of the finger.

4. Adequate contrast, density, and penetration have been obtained on an upper extremity projection when

   the _____ (A) patterns and _____ (B) outlines of the phalanges, metacarpals, and carpal bones are demonstrated.

5. Upper extremity projections are obtained using _____ (A) kilovoltage peak (kVp) and _____ (B) source–image receptor distance (SID).

6. Use the following clues to complete the crossword puzzle in Figure 4-1.

Figure 4-1

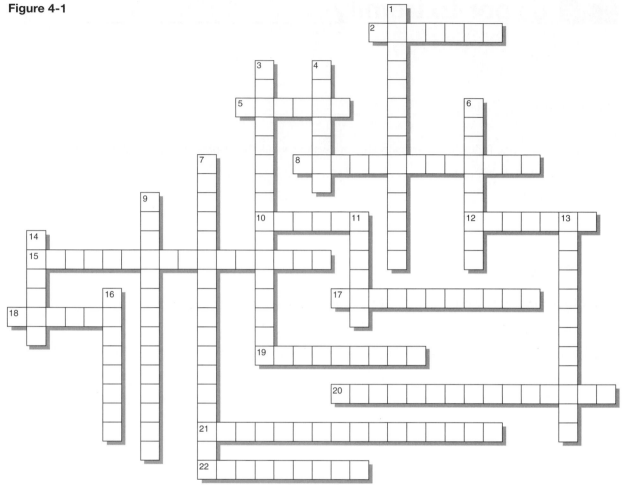

Across

2 Curved or rounded inward
5 Curved or rounded outward
8 Escape of fluid into the joint
10 Accumulation of fatty tissues
12 The patient's side
15 Turn extremity outward
17 Wrist passageway
18 Anterior hand surface
19 Turn hand so palm is facing downward
20 Move the lateral hand toward radial side
21 Turn extremity inward
22 Straightening of a joint

Down

1 Supporting material with calcaneous bone
3 Accumulation of fat that is anterior to radius
4 Movement that bends a joint
6 Backward bending
7 Accumulation of fat located lateral to the radius
9 Move hand toward the ulnar surface
11 Situated away from the source
13 A joint
14 Inner side of an extremity
16 Close to the source

Finger: Posteroanterior Projection

7. Identify the labeled anatomy in Figure 4-2.

Figure 4-2

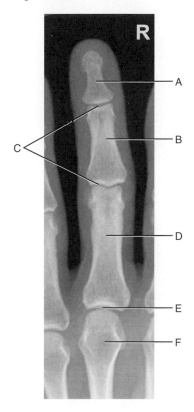

A. _____

B. _____

C. _____

D. _____

E. _____

F. _____

8. Complete the statements below, referring to PA finger projection analysis criteria.

Posteroanterior Finger Projection Analysis Criteria

• The long axis of the finger is aligned with the long axis of the collimated field.

• The soft tissue width and midpoint concavity are _____(A) on both sides of the phalanges.

• There is no soft tissue overlap from adjacent digits.

• The IP and _____ (B) joints are demonstrated as open spaces, and the phalanges are not foreshortened.

• The _____ (C) joint is at the center of the exposure field.

• The entire digit and half of the _____ (D) are included within the collimated field.

IP, Interphalangeal.

9. A finger projection has been requested for a patient with severe rheumatoid arthritis. The patient has a ring on the affected finger that cannot be removed. What procedure should be followed?

_____

_____

10. To prevent finger rotation on a PA finger projection, the patient's hand should be positioned _____ against the IR.

11. In which direction is the finger most frequently rotated when rotation occurs on a PA finger projection?

A. _____

Why?

B. _____

12. On a rotated PA projection, the side of the finger that is rolled _____ (farther from/closer to) (A) the IR will demonstrate the greatest phalangeal midshaft concavity and the _____ (B) soft tissue thickness.

13. Which of the finger metacarpals is the longest? _____

14. Which of the finger metacarpals is the shortest? _____

15. The long axis of the affected digit is aligned with the long axis of _____ (A) for a PA finger projection to prevent clipping of the distal _____ (B) or distal _____ (C).

16. How is the patient positioned for a PA finger projection to prevent soft tissue overlap of adjacent fingers onto the affected finger? _____.

17. To accomplish open joint spaces on a PA finger projection, the central ray must be aligned _____ (perpendicular/parallel) (A) to the joint space and the IR must be aligned _____ (B) to the joint space.

18. If the finger is flexed for the PA projection, the joint spaces will be _____ (A) and the phalanges will be _____ (B).

19. On a patient whose finger is flexed, open IP joint spaces can be obtained by _____ (A) the hand and elevating the proximal metacarpals until the joint of interest is aligned _____ (B) to the IR.

20. Accurate central ray centering is seen on a PA finger projection by centering a _____ (A) central ray to the _____ (B) joint.

21. Included within the collimated field on a PA finger projection with accurate positioning are the _____ (A) and half of the _____ (B).

22. Accurate transverse collimation has been obtained when the collimated borders are _____ _____.

For the following descriptions of PA finger projections with poor positioning, state how the patient would have been mispositioned for such a projection to be obtained.

23. The projection demonstrates unequal soft tissue width and midshaft concavity on each side of the phalanges. The side of the phalanges with the least amount of concavity is facing the longest finger metacarpal.

_____

24. The projection demonstrates closed IP and metacarpophalangeal (MP) joints, and the distal and middle phalanges are foreshortened.

_____

For the following PA finger projections with poor positioning, state which anatomic structures are misaligned and how the patient should be repositioned for an optimal projection to be obtained.

Figure 4-3

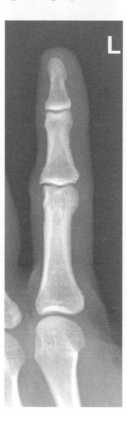

25. Figure 4-3: _____

_____

_____

_____

_____

Figure 4-4

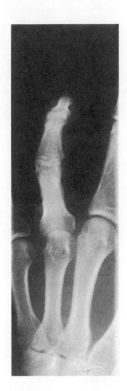

26. Figure 4-4: _____

_____

_____

_____

_____

Finger: Posteroanterior Oblique Projection

27. Identify the labeled anatomy in Figure 4-5.

Figure 4-5

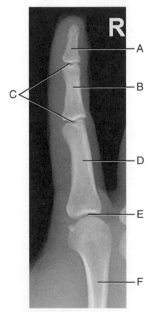

A. _____

B. _____

C. _____

D. _____

E. _____

F. _____

28. Complete the statements below, referring to PA oblique finger projection analysis criteria.

> **Posteroanterior Oblique Finger Projection Analysis Criteria**
>
> - The long axis of the finger is aligned with the long axis of the collimated field.
>
> - _____ (A) as much soft tissue width is demonstrated on one side of the digit as on the other side, and more _____ (B) is seen on one aspect of the phalangeal midshafts than the others.
>
> - There is no soft tissue overlap from adjacent digits.
>
> - The IP and MP joints are demonstrated as _____ (C), and the phalanges are not foreshortened.
>
> - The _____ (D) joint is at the center of the exposure field.
>
> - Entire digit and half of the metacarpal are included within the collimated field.

IP, Interphalangeal; *MP*, metacarpophalangeal.

29. What do the following initials stand for?

A. OID: _____

B. PIP: _____

C. IP: _____

D. MP: _____

30. The affected finger is rotated _____ degrees from the PA projection for a PA oblique finger projection.

31. In which direction are the patient's hand and finger rotated for a PA oblique projection when imaging the third through fifth fingers?

A. _____

For the second finger?

B. _____

Why might the second finger be rotated differently?

C. _____

32. Why is it important to align the long axis of the affected digit with the long axis of the collimator's light field for a PA oblique finger projection?

_____

_____

33. Why should the fingers be slightly spread before a PA oblique finger projection is taken?

_____

34. To obtain open IP and MP joint spaces, the finger needs to be fully _____ (A) and positioned _____ (B) to the image receptor (IR).

35. When imaging the third and fourth fingers, why is it often necessary to position a sponge beneath the distal phalanx?

_____

36. Accurate central ray centering on a PA oblique finger projection is accomplished by centering a _____

   (A) central ray to the _____ (B) joint.

37. Which anatomic structures are included on a PA oblique finger projection with accurate positioning?

   _____

For the following descriptions of PA oblique finger projections with poor positioning, state how the patient would have been mispositioned for such a projection to be obtained.

38. The soft tissue width and midshaft concavity are almost equal on each side of the digit.

   _____

39. More than twice as much soft tissue width is present on one side of the phalanges as on the other. One aspect of the midshafts of the phalanges is concave, and the other aspect is slightly convex.

   _____

40. The soft tissue from the adjacent digit is superimposed over the affected digit's soft tissue.

   _____

41. The projection demonstrates closed IP joint spaces, and the distal and middle phalanges are foreshortened.

   _____

For the following PA oblique finger projections with poor positioning, state which anatomic structures are misaligned and how the patient should be repositioned for an optimal projection to be obtained.

Figure 4-6

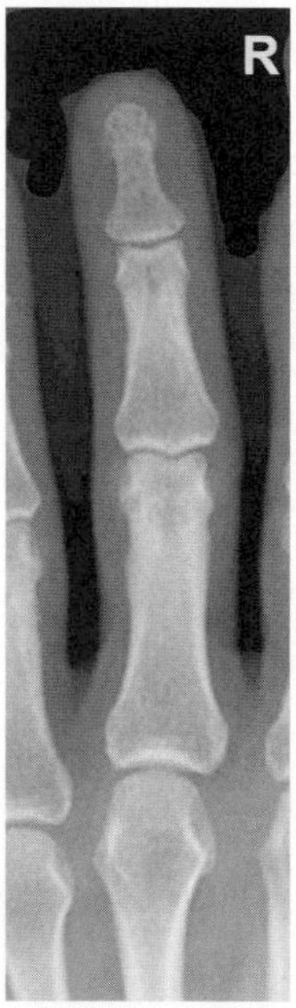

42. Figure 4-6 (third digit): _____

   _____

   _____

   _____

   _____

Figure 4-7

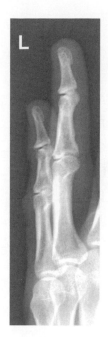

43. Figure 4-7 (fourth digit): _____

_____

_____

_____

_____

Figure 4-8

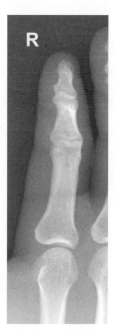

44. Figure 4-8 (second digit): _____

_____

_____

_____

_____

Finger: Lateral Projection

45. Identify the labeled anatomy in Figure 4-9.

Figure 4-9

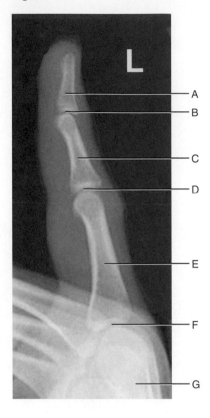

A. _____

B. _____

C. _____

D. _____

E. _____

F. _____

G. _____

46. Complete the statements below, referring to lateral finger projection analysis criteria.

Lateral Finger Projection Analysis Criteria
• The long axis of the finger is aligned with the long axis of the collimated field.
• The _____ (A) aspect of the middle and proximal phalanges demonstrates midshaft concavity, and the _____ (B) aspects of the phalanges show slight convexity.
• There is no soft tissue overlap from adjacent digits.
• The IP joints are demonstrated as open spaces, and the phalanges are not foreshortened.
• The _____ (C) is at the center of the exposure field.

IP, Interphalangeal.

47. How many degrees from the PA projection should the finger be rotated for a lateral finger projection with accurate positioning? _____

48. For each of the following fingers, state how the hand is rotated (internally/externally) from the PA projection to properly position the finger for a lateral projection.

   A. Second finger: _____

   B. Third finger: _____

   C. Fourthfinger:_____

   D. Fifth finger: _____

49. What determines how the hand is rotated for question 48?

   _____

50. How is the patient's hand positioned for a lateral finger projection to prevent soft tissue overlap of the adjacent fingers onto the affected finger and to demonstrate the affected finger's proximal phalanx best?

   _____

51. Which anatomic structures are included on a lateral finger projection with accurate positioning?

   _____

52. Describe the positioning error that is demonstrated on the projection in Figure 4-10.

   Figure 4-10

   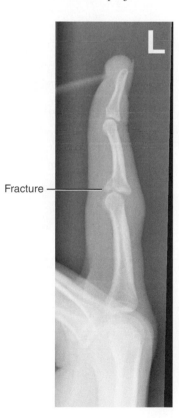

   Fracture

   _____

   _____

For the following descriptions of lateral finger projections with poor positioning, state how the patient would have been mispositioned for such a projection to be obtained.

53. The proximal phalanges of the unaffected fingers overlap the proximal phalanx of the affected finger.

_____

54. Concavity is demonstrated on both sides of the middle and proximal phalangeal midshafts.

_____

55. The IP joint spaces are closed, and the phalanges are foreshortened.

_____

For the following lateral finger projections with poor positioning, state which anatomic structures are misaligned and how the patient should be repositioned for an optimal projection to be obtained.

Figure 4-11

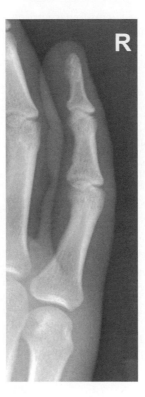

56. Figure 4-11: _____

_____

_____

_____

Figure 4-12

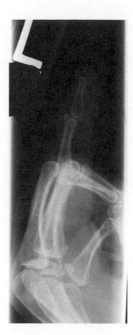

57. Figure 4-12: _____

_____

_____

_____

Thumb: Anteroposterior Projection

58. Identify the labeled anatomy in Figure 4-13.

Figure 4-13

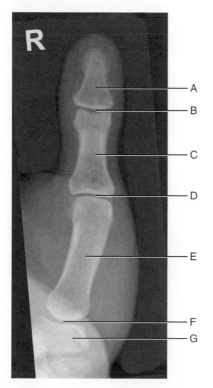

A. _____

B. _____

C. _____

D. _____

E. _____

F. _____

G. _____

59. Complete the statements below, referring to AP thumb projection analysis criteria.

Anteroposterior Thumb Projection Analysis Criteria

- The _____ (A) on both sides of phalanges and metacarpal midshafts is equal. There is equal _____ (B) width on each side of phalanges.

- The long axis of _____ (C) is aligned with the long axis of the collimated field.

- There is no soft tissue overlap from adjacent digits.

- The IP, MP, and CM joints are demonstrated as _____ (D), and the phalanges are not foreshortened.

- Superimposition of the _____ (E) soft tissue over the proximal first metacarpal and the CM joint is minimal.

- The _____ (F) is at the center of the exposure field.

- The entire digit and CM joint are included within the collimated field.

CM, Carpometacarpal; IP, interphalangeal; MP, metacarpophalangeal.

60. For the thumb to be positioned in an AP projection, the hand is _____ (internally/externally) (A) rotated and the thumbnail is positioned _____ (B) against the IR.

61. When the thumb is rotated away from an AP projection, the amount of phalangeal midshaft concavity increases on the side positioned _____ (farther/closer) from/to the IR.

62. Why is it important to align the long axis of the first digit with the collimator's longitudinal light line for an AP thumb projection?

_____

63. To obtain open joint spaces on an AP thumb projection, the patient's thumb is fully _____ and the central ray is accurately aligned and centered to the thumb.

64. How is the hand positioned to prevent the medial palm soft tissue and possibly the fourth and fifth metacarpals from being superimposed over the proximal metacarpal? _____

_____

65. Accurate central ray centering on an AP thumb projection is accomplished by centering a _____ (A) central ray to the _____ (B) joint.

66. The MP joint is located at the level where the palm interconnecting skin attaches to the _____.

67. List the anatomic structures that are included within the collimated field on an AP thumb projection with accurate positioning. _____

_____

For the following descriptions of AP thumb projections with poor positioning, state how the patient would have been mispositioned for such a projection to be obtained.

68. The soft tissue width and the concavity of the phalangeal and metacarpal midshafts on each side are not equal. The side demonstrating the more concavity is facing toward the second through fifth digits, and the thumbnail is facing away from the second through fifth digits.

   _____

69. The projection demonstrates a foreshortened distal phalanx and a closed distal interphalangeal (DIP) joint space.

   _____

70. The fifth metacarpal and the medial palm soft tissue are superimposed over the proximal first metacarpal and carpometacarpal (CM) joints.

   _____

For the following AP thumb projections with poor positioning, state which anatomic structures are misaligned and how the patient should be repositioned for an optimal projection to be obtained.

Figure 4-14

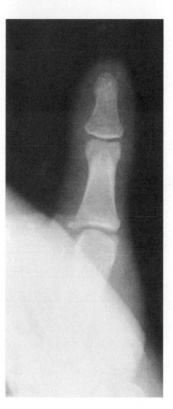

71. Figure 4-14: _____

   _____

   _____

   _____

Figure 4-15

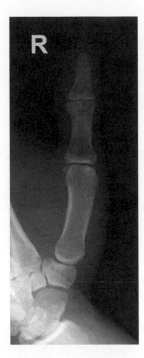

72. Figure 4-15: _____

_____

_____

_____

Thumb: Lateral Projections

73. Identify the labeled anatomy in Figure 4-16.

Figure 4-16

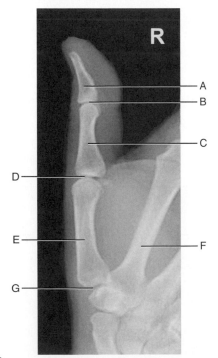

A. _____

B. _____

C. _____

D. _____

E. _____

F. _____

G. _____

74. Complete the statements below, referring to lateral thumb projection analysis criteria.

Lateral Thumb Projection Analysis Criteria

• The _____ (A) aspect of the proximal phalanx and metacarpal demonstrates midshaft concavity, and the _____ (B) aspect of the proximal phalanx and metacarpal demonstrates slight convexity.

• The long axis of the thumb is aligned with the long axis of the collimated field.

• There is no soft tissue overlap from adjacent digits.

• The IP, MP, and CM joints are demonstrated as open spaces, and the phalanges are not foreshortened.

• The proximal first metacarpal is only slightly superimposed by the proximal _____ (C) metacarpal.

• The first _____ (D) is at the center of the exposure field.

• The entire digit and CM joint are included within the collimated field.

CM, Carpometacarpal; *IP*, interphalangeal; *MP*, metacarpophalangeal.

75. To obtain a lateral projection of the thumb, rest the patient's hand flat against the IR and then _____ it until the thumb rolls into a lateral position.

76. How should the thumb be aligned for a lateral thumb projection to enable you to collimate tightly without clipping required anatomy? _____

_____

77. How should the thumb be positioned to obtain open joint spaces and demonstrate the phalanges without foreshortening? _____

_____

78. Abducting the thumb will decrease the amount of _____ superimposition of the CM joint.

79. Accurate central ray centering on a lateral thumb projection is accomplished by centering a _____ (A) central ray to the _____ (B) joint, which is located at the level at which the palm interconnecting skin attaches _____ (C).

80. List the anatomic structures that are included within the collimated field on a lateral thumb projection with accurate positioning. _____

_____

For the following descriptions of lateral thumb projections with poor positioning, state how the patient would have been mispositioned for such a projection to be obtained.

81. The second and third proximal metacarpals are superimposed over the first proximal metacarpal.

_____

82. The anterior and posterior aspects of the proximal phalanx and metacarpal midshafts demonstrate concavity. The first proximal metacarpal is demonstrated without superimposition of the second and third proximal metacarpals.

For the following lateral thumb projections with poor positioning, state which anatomic structures are misaligned and how the patient should be repositioned for an optimal projection to be obtained.

Figure 4-17

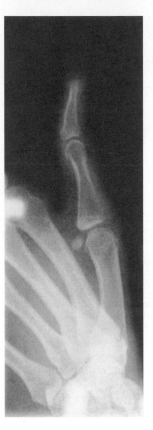

83. Figure 4-17: _____

_____

_____

_____

Figure 4-18

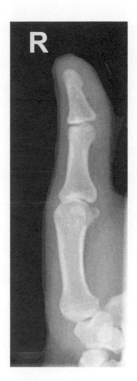

84. Figure 4-18: _____

_____

_____

_____

Thumb: Posteroanterior Oblique Projection

85. Identify the labeled anatomy in Figure 4-19.

Figure 4-19

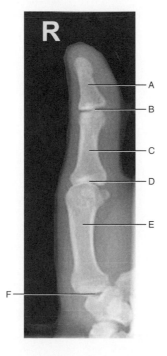

A. _____

B. _____

C. _____

D. _____

E. _____

F. _____

86. Complete the statements below, referring to PA oblique thumb projection analysis criteria.

Posteroanterior Oblique Thumb Projection Analysis Criteria
• _____ (A) as much soft tissue and more phalangeal and metacarpal midshaft concavity are present on the side of the thumb next to the fingers than on the other side.
• The long axis of the _____ (B) is aligned with the long axis of the collimated field.
• The IP, MP, and CM joints are demonstrated as open spaces, and the phalanges are not foreshortened.
• The _____ (C) is at the center of the exposure field.

CM, Carpometacarpal; *IP,* interphalangeal; *MP,* metacarpophalangeal.

87. The affected thumb is rotated _____ degrees for accurate positioning for a PA oblique thumb projection.

88. The thumb is placed in a PA oblique projection when the patient's hand is _____ (A) and the palm surface is placed _____ (B) against the IR.

89. Which anatomic structures are included on a PA oblique thumb projection with accurate positioning?

_____

90. Accurate transverse collimation has been obtained on a thumb projection when the collimated borders are within

_____.

For the following description of a PA oblique thumb projection with poor positioning, state how the patient would have been mispositioned for such a projection to be obtained.

91. The midshafts of the proximal phalanx and metacarpal demonstrate slight convexity on the posterior surfaces and concavity on the anterior surfaces.

_____

For the following PA oblique thumb projections with poor positioning, state which anatomic structures are misaligned and how the patient should be repositioned for an optimal projection to be obtained.

Figure 4-20

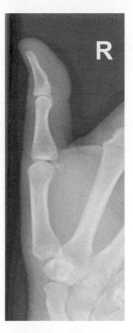

92. Figure 4-20: _____

_____

_____

_____

Figure 4-21

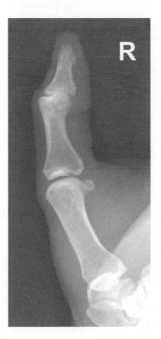

93. Figure 4-21: _____

_____

_____

_____

Hand: Posteroanterior Projection

94. Identify the labeled anatomy in Figure 4-22.

Figure 4-22

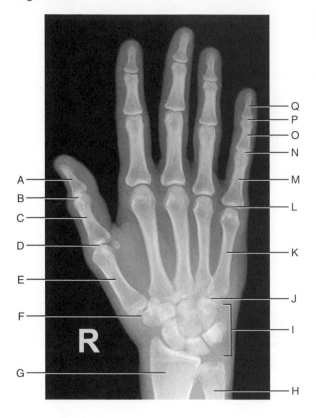

A. _____

B. _____

C. _____

D. _____

E. _____

F. _____

G. _____

H. _____

I. _____

J. _____

K. _____

L. _____

M. _____

N. _____

O. _____

P. _____

Q. _____

95. Complete the statements below, referring to PA hand projection analysis criteria.

Posteroanterior Hand Projection Analysis Criteria

- The soft tissue outlines of the second through fifth phalanges are uniform, the distance between the

  _____ (A) is equal, and the same midshaft concavity is seen on both sides of the

  _____ (B) and metacarpals of the second through fifth digits.

- There is no soft tissue overlap from adjacent digits.

- The _____, _____, and _____ (C) joints are
  demonstrated as open spaces, and the phalanges are not foreshortened. The thumb demonstrates a 45-degree
  oblique projection.

- The _____ (D) is at the center of the exposure field.

---

96. A PA hand projection has been ordered for a patient who is unable to remove a wedding ring. Which procedure

    should be followed? _____

    _____

97. To obtain a PA hand projection, _____ (A) the patient's hand and place it _____ (B) against the IR.

98. Why is internal rotation seldom the cause of a mispositioned PA hand projection?

_____

99. How is the hand aligned with the collimated field for a PA hand projection to obtain maximum collimation? _____

_____

100. What changes in the joint spaces, phalanges, and metacarpals would be expected on a PA hand projection if the hand is in a flexed position when the image was obtained? _____

101. How will the position of the first digit change if the hand is flexed for a PA hand projection?

_____

102. Which anatomic structures are included on an accurately collimated PA hand projection?

_____

_____

For the following descriptions of PA hand projections with poor positioning, state how the patient would have been mispositioned for such a projection to be obtained.

103. The projection demonstrates superimposed third through fifth metacarpal heads and unequal midshaft concavity of the phalanges and metacarpals.

_____

104. The projection demonstrates soft tissue overlap of the third, fourth, and fifth digits.

_____

105. The projection demonstrates closed IP and CM joints and foreshortened phalanges and metacarpals.

_____

For the following PA hand projections with poor positioning, state which anatomic structures are misaligned and how the patient should be repositioned for an optimal projection to be obtained.

Figure 4-23

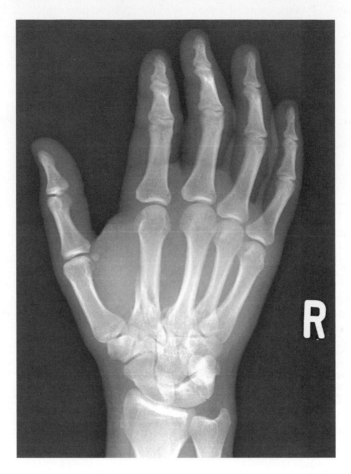

106. Figure 4-23: _____

_____

_____

_____

Figure 4-24

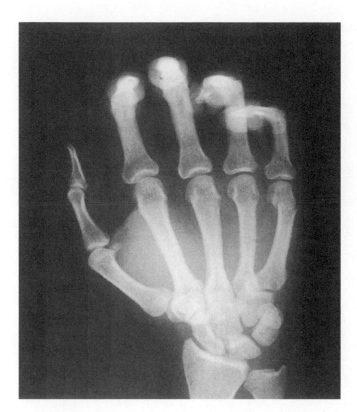

107. Figure 4-24: _____

_____

_____

_____

108. The PA hand projection in Figure 4-24 demonstrates a proximal fifth metacarpal fracture. If the patient could not move the hand from its current position, how should the central ray and IR be adjusted to obtain an optimal PA projection of this fractured metacarpal?

_____

_____

_____

_____

Hand: Posteroanterior Oblique Projection

109. Identify the labeled anatomy in Figure 4-25.

Figure 4-25

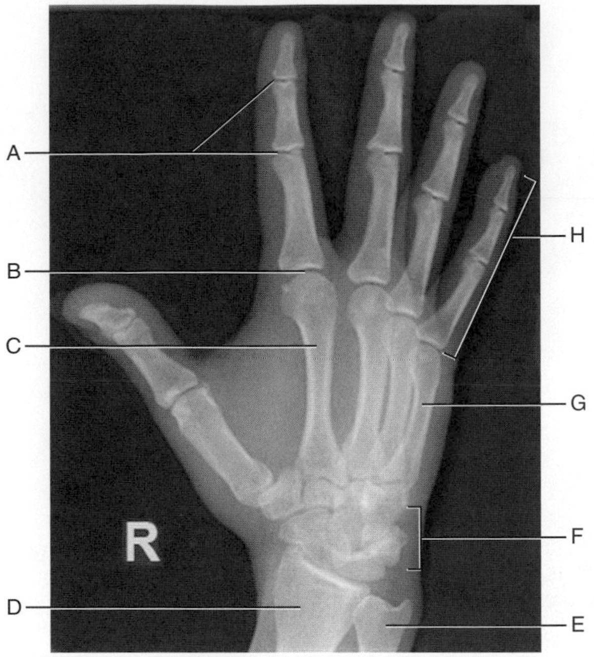

A. _____

B. _____

C. _____

D. _____

E. _____

F. _____

G. _____

H. _____

110. Complete the statements below, referring to PA oblique hand projection analysis criteria.

Posteroanterior Oblique Hand Projection Analysis Criteria
• Each of the second through fifth metacarpal midshafts demonstrate more concavity on one side than on the other and have varying amounts of space between them. The _____ (A) metacarpal heads are not superimposed and the _____ (B) metacarpal heads are slightly superimposed, and a slight space is present between the _____ (C) metacarpal midshafts.
• There is no soft tissue overlap from adjacent digits.
• The IP and MP joints are demonstrated as open spaces, and the phalanges are not foreshortened. The thumb position may vary from a lateral to an oblique projection.
• _____ (D) is at the center of the exposure field.

IP, Interphalangeal; *MP,* metacarpophalangeal.

111. The hand is rotated _____ (A) degrees (B) _____ (internally/externally) (B) from the PA projection for a PA oblique hand projection.

112. Why is it important to view the hand and not the wrist when determining the degree of hand obliquity to use for a PA oblique hand projection?

_____

113. How must the fingers be positioned to demonstrate open IP and MP joints on a PA oblique hand projection?

_____

114. A PA oblique hand projection is ordered to evaluate the healing of a patient's third metacarpal fracture. Is it acceptable to flex the patient's fingers, using them to prop the hand for the projection?

A. _____ (Yes/No)

Why or why not?

B. _____

115. Which anatomic structures are included on an accurately collimated PA oblique hand projection? _____

_____

For the following descriptions of PA oblique hand projections with poor positioning, state how the patient would have been mispositioned for such a projection to be obtained.

116. The metacarpal heads are demonstrated without superimposition, and the spaces between the metacarpal midshafts are almost equal.

_____

117. The third through fifth metacarpal midshafts are superimposed.

_____

118. The projection demonstrates foreshortened phalanges and closed IP joint spaces.

_____

For the following PA oblique hand projections with poor positioning, state which anatomic structures are misaligned and how the patient should be repositioned for an optimal projection to be obtained.

Figure 4-26

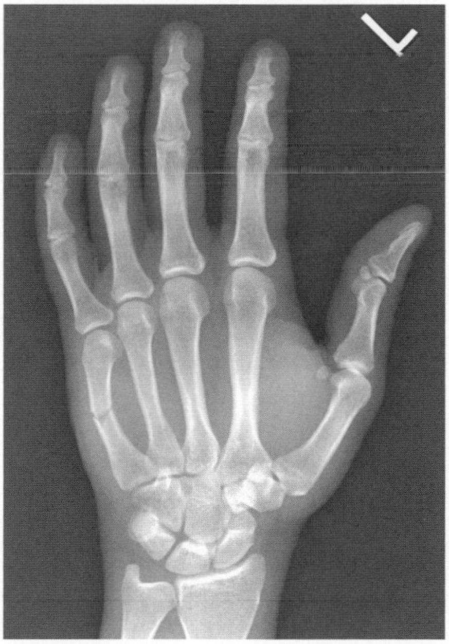

119. Figure 4-26: _____

_____

_____

_____

Figure 4-27

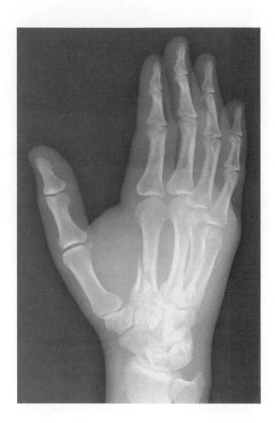

120. Figure 4-27: _____

_____

_____

_____

121. The PA oblique hand projection in Figure 4-26 demonstrates a midshaft fifth metacarpal fracture. If the patient could not move the hand to position it in a PA oblique projection adequately, how should the central ray and IR be adjusted for an optimal PA oblique projection to be obtained?

_____

_____

_____

_____

122. The PA oblique hand projection in Figure 4-27 demonstrates a proximal second metacarpal fracture. If the patient could not move the hand to adequately position it in a PA oblique projection, how should the central ray and IR be adjusted for an optimal PA oblique projection to be obtained?

_____

_____

_____

_____

Hand: Lateral "Fan" Projection (Lateromedial)

123. Identify the labeled anatomy in Figure 4-28.

Figure 4-28

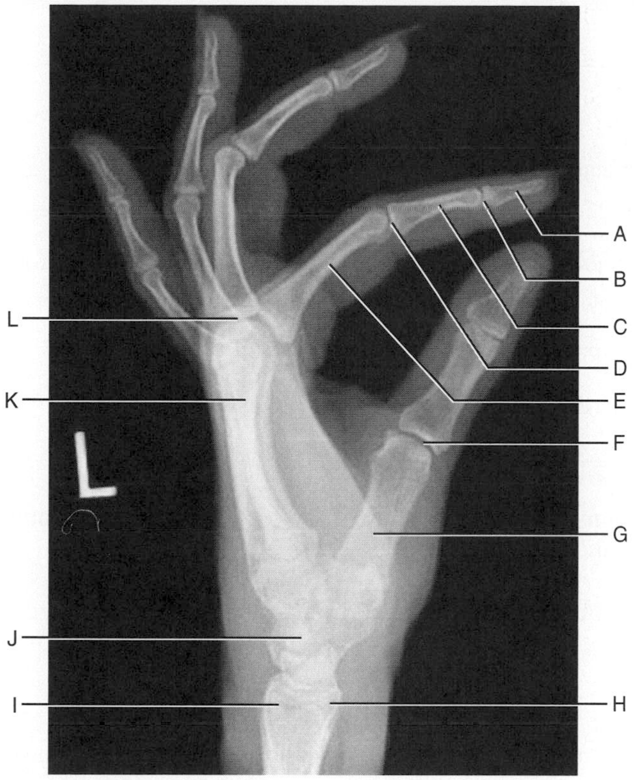

A. _____

B. _____

C. _____

D. _____

E. _____

F. _____

G. _____

H. _____

I. _____

J. _____

K. _____

L. _____

124. Complete the statements below, referring to lateral hand projection analysis criteria.

Lateral Hand Projection Analysis Criteria

- The second through _____ (A) digits are separated, demonstrating little superimposition of the proximal bony or soft tissue structures. The thumb is demonstrated without superimposition of the other digits.

- The second through _____ (B) metacarpals are superimposed.

- The IP joints are open, and the phalanges are not foreshortened.

- The _____ (C) are at the center of the exposure field.

IP, Interphalangeal.

125. Why is it difficult to demonstrate the phalanges and metacarpals simultaneously on a fan lateral hand projection?

_____

_____

126. For a fan lateral hand projection, the digits are most effectively fanned by drawing the second and third fingers

_____ (anteriorly/posteriorly) (A) and the fourth and fifth fingers _____ (anteriorly/posteriorly) (B).

127. In what projection will the first digit be placed for accurate positioning for a lateral hand projection?

_____

128. The fifth metacarpal can be distinguished from the second through fourth metacarpals by its length. It is the

_____ (longest/shortest) (A) of these metacarpals, and the second metacarpal is the _____ (longest/shortest) (B).

129. How should the thumb be positioned to obtain open joint spaces and demonstrate the phalanges without foreshortening on a lateral hand projection?

_____

130. Which anatomic structures are included on an accurately collimated lateral hand projection?

_____

For the following descriptions of lateral hand projections with poor positioning, state how the patient would have been mispositioned for such a projection to be obtained.

131. The second through fifth metacarpal midshafts are demonstrated without superimposition. The shortest metacarpal is demonstrated anterior to the other metacarpals.

_____

132. The second through fifth metacarpal midshafts are demonstrated without superimposition. The longest metacarpal is demonstrated anterior to the other metacarpals.

_____

133. The projection demonstrates superimposed metacarpals and superimposed digits.

_____

For the following lateral hand projections with poor positioning, state which anatomic structures are misaligned and how the patient should be repositioned for an optimal projection to be obtained.

Figure 4-29

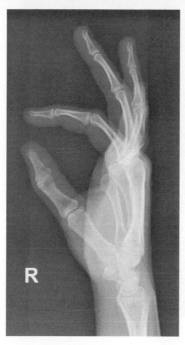

134. Figure 4-29: _____

_____

_____

_____

Figure 4-30

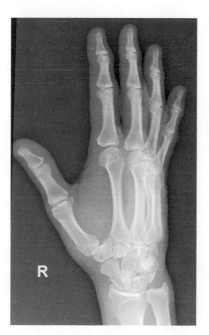

135. Figure 4-30: _____

_____

_____

_____

Figure 4-31

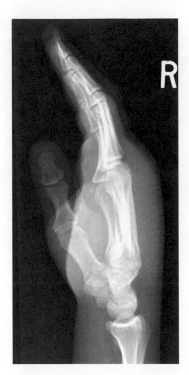

136. Figure 4-31: _____

_____

_____

_____

Wrist: Posteroanterior Projection

137. Identify the labeled anatomy in Figure 4-32.

Figure 4-32

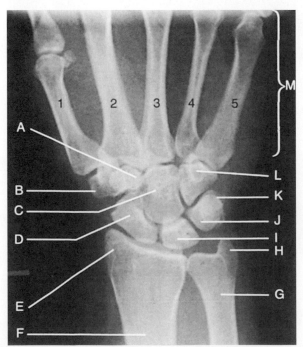

A. _____

B. _____

C. _____

D. _____

E. _____

F. _____

G. _____

H. _____

I. _____

J. _____

K. _____

L. _____

M. _____

138. Complete the statements below, referring to PA wrist projection analysis criteria.

Posteroanterior Wrist Projection Analysis Criteria
• The _____ (A) fat stripe is demonstrated.
• The radial and ulnar styloids are at the extreme lateral and medial edges, respectively, of each bone. The _____ (B) articulation is open, and superimposition of the metacarpal bases is limited.
• The anterior and posterior articulating margins of the radius are almost superimposed, within _____ (C) inch.
• The _____ (D) MC joint spaces are open. The scaphoid is only slightly foreshortened, and the lunate is trapezoidal.
• The long axes of the third metacarpal and midforearm are aligned with the long axis of the collimated field.
• The scaphoid and half of the lunate are positioned distal to the radius.
• _____ (E) are at the center of the exposure field.

MC, Metacarpal.

139. Describe the shape and location of the scaphoid fat stripe. _____
_____

140. Why is the visualization of the scaphoid fat stripe important on a PA wrist projection?
_____

141. To demonstrate the ulnar styloid in profile, the elbow is placed in a _____ (A) projection and the humerus is positioned _____ (B).

142. The _____ (anterior/posterior) (A) margin of the distal radius is demonstrated distal to the _____ (anterior/posterior) (B) margin on a PA wrist projection with accurate positioning.

143. How is the forearm positioned for a PA wrist projection to obtain open radioscaphoid and radiolunate joint spaces?
_____

144. How is a patient with large muscular or thick proximal forearms positioned for a PA wrist projection to prevent demonstrating an excessive amount of the radial articular surface? _____

145. How is the patient positioned for a PA wrist projection to obtain open second through fifth CM joint spaces?
_____

146. When the hand is placed on a flat surface, the wrist will be _____ (flexed/extended) (A), causing the distal scaphoid to shift _____ (anteriorly/posteriorly) (B).

147. Why is the long axis of the third metacarpal and midforearm aligned with the long axis of the collimated field for a PA wrist projection?

A. _____

Where does this alignment position the lunate with respect to the distal radius?

B. _____

148. When the fifth metacarpal and ulna are aligned with the long axis of the collimation field for a PA wrist projection, the distal scaphoid shifts _____ (anteriorly/posteriorly) (A) and is _____ (foreshortened/elongated) (B), and the lunate moves _____ (medially/laterally) (C).

149. The distal scaphoid shifts _____ (anteriorly/posteriorly) when the wrist is ulnar-deviated.

150. Accurate central ray centering on a PA wrist projection is accomplished by centering a _____ central ray to the wrist.

151. Which anatomic structures are included on an accurately collimated PA wrist projection?

_____

152. How should one center the central ray and collimate differently when a PA wrist projection is ordered with the request that more than one fourth of the distal forearm be included? _____

_____

For the following descriptions of PA wrist projections with poor positioning, state how the patient would have been mispositioned for such a projection to be obtained.

153. The ulnar styloid is not demonstrated in profile.

_____

154. The laterally located carpal and metacarpal joints are demonstrated as open spaces, and the medially located carpals and metacarpals are superimposed, closing the medially located carpal joints. The radioulnar joint is closed, and the radial styloid is not in profile.

_____

155. The laterally located carpals and metacarpals are superimposed, the pisiform and hamate hook are well demonstrated, and the radioulnar joint is closed.

_____

156. The posterior margin of the distal radius has been projected too far distal to the anterior margin.

_____

157. The scaphoid is foreshortened and demonstrates a signet ring configuration, the CM joints are obscured, and the lunate is triangular and properly positioned distal to the radius.

_____

158. The scaphoid is elongated, the second through fourth metacarpals are superimposed over the CM joints, and the lunate is triangular and properly positioned distal to the radius.

_____

159. The scaphoid is foreshortened, the lunate is positioned mostly distal to the ulna, the third metacarpal is not aligned with the long axis of the midforearm, and the CM joints are open.

_____

160. The scaphoid is elongated, the lunate is entirely positioned distal to the radius, and the third metacarpal is not aligned with the long axis of the midforearm.

_____

For the following PA wrist projections with poor positioning, state which anatomic structures are misaligned and how the patient should be repositioned for an optimal projection to be obtained.

Figure 4-33

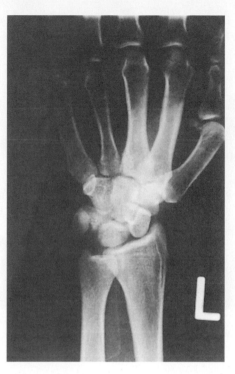

161. Figure 4-33: _____

_____

_____

_____

Figure 4-34

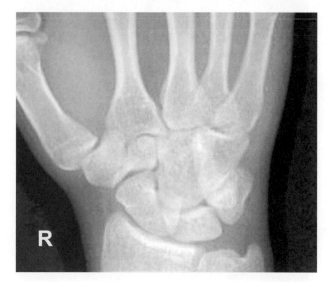

162. Figure 4-34: _____

_____

_____

_____

Figure 4-35

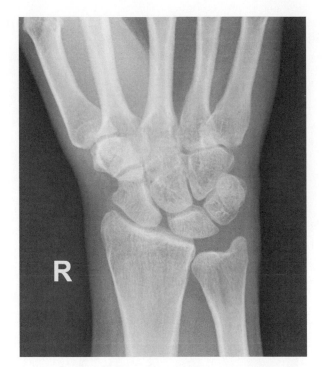

163. Figure 4-35 _____

_____

_____

_____

Figure 4-36

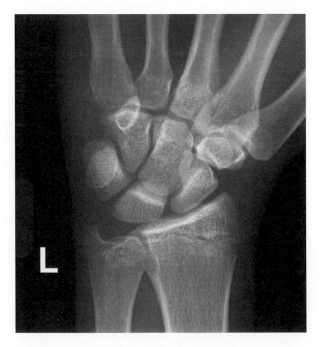

164. Figure 4-36: _____

_____

_____

_____

Wrist: Posteroanterior Oblique Projection

165. Identify the labeled anatomy in Figure 4-37.

Figure 4-37

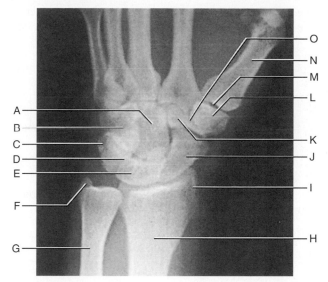

A. _____   I. _____

B. _____   J. _____

C. _____   K. _____

D. _____   L. _____

E. _____   M. _____

F. _____   N. _____

G. _____   O. _____

H. _____

166. Complete the statements below, referring to PA oblique wrist projection analysis criteria.

Posteroanterior Oblique Wrist Projection Analysis Criteria
• The _____ (A) stripe is demonstrated.
• The _____ (B) and _____ (C) are demonstrated without superimposition, and the trapeziotrapezoidal joint space is open.
• The scaphoid tuberosity and waist are demonstrated in profile. Only a small degree of trapezoid and capitate superimposition is present.
• The _____ (D) CM is demonstrated as an open space.
• The long axes of the third metacarpal and midforearm are aligned with the long axis of the collimated field.
• The interior and posterior articulating margins of the radius are almost superimposed (within 0.25 inch [0.6 cm]).
• The _____ (E) is in profile at the far medial edge.
• The _____ (F) are at the center of the exposure field.

CM, Carpometacarpal.

167. Define the term *styloid.* _____

168. What routine degree of patient wrist rotation is required for a PA oblique wrist projection?

A. _____

As a routine, should the wrist be internally or externally rotated from a PA projection?

B. _____

169. What carpal joint space is open on an externally rotated PA oblique wrist projection to indicate that the wrist was adequately rotated? _____

170. For a PA projection of the wrist, the trapezoid and trapezium are superimposed. Which of these carpal bones is located anteriorly?

_____

171. The long axes of which two anatomic structures should be aligned when positioning the patient for a PA oblique wrist projection to ensure that no radial or ulnar deviation will result?

A. _____

B. _____

172. If the forearm is positioned parallel with the IR for a PA oblique wrist projection, how is the distal radius demonstrated on the resulting projection?

_____

173. On a PA oblique wrist projection with accurate positioning, the radioulnar joint space is closed. Which surface of the radius is superimposed over the ulna? _____ (anterior/posterior)

174. Where is the ulnar styloid demonstrated on a PA oblique wrist projection with accurate positioning?

A. _____

How must the patient be positioned for this styloid placement to be obtained?

B. _____

175. Accurate central ray centering on a PA oblique wrist projection is accomplished by centering a _____ central ray to the wrist.

176. Which anatomic structures are included on an accurately collimated PA oblique wrist projection?

_____

For the following descriptions of PA oblique wrist projections with poor positioning, state how the patient would have been mispositioned for such a projection to be obtained.

177. The trapezoid and trapezium demonstrate slight superimposition, obscuring the trapeziotrapezoidal joint space, and trapezoid-capitate superimposition is minimal.

_____

178. The scaphoid is foreshortened, and the scaphoid is situated next to the radius.

_____

179. The posterior margin of the distal radius is more than 0.25 inch (0.6 cm) proximal to the anterior margin.

_____

For the following PA oblique wrist projections with poor positioning, state which anatomic structures are misaligned and how the patient should be repositioned for an optimal projection to be obtained.

Figure 4-38

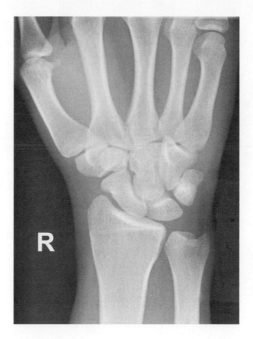

180. Figure 4-38: _____

_____

_____

_____

Figure 4-39

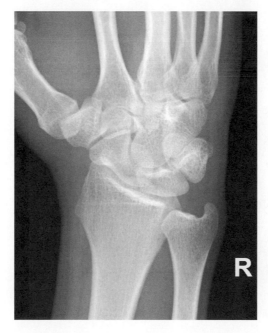

181. Figure 4-39: _____

_____

_____

_____

Figure 4-40

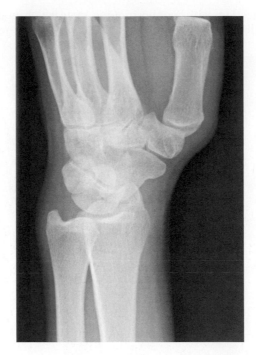

182. Figure 4-40: _____

_____

_____

_____

Figure 4-41

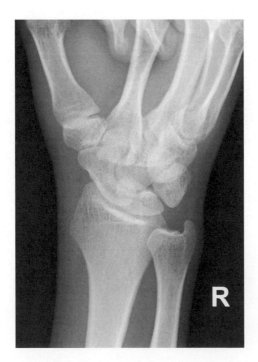

183. Figure 4-41: _____

_____

_____

_____

Wrist: Lateral Projection (Lateromedial)

184. Identify the labeled anatomy in Figure 4-42.

Figure 4-42

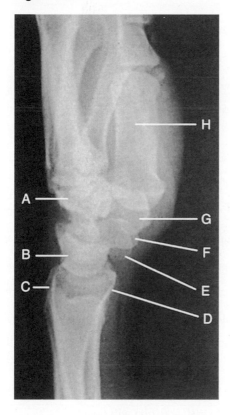

A. _____

B. _____

C. _____

D. _____

E. _____

F. _____

G. _____

H. _____

185. Complete the statements below, referring to lateral wrist projection analysis criteria.

Lateral Wrist Projection Analysis Criteria
• The _____ (A) fat stripe is demonstrated.
• The _____ (B) aspects of the distal scaphoid and pisiform are aligned, and the distal radius and ulna are superimposed.
• The distal aspects of the distal scaphoid and pisiform are aligned.
• The long axis of the _____ (C) is aligned parallel with the forearm.
• The ulnar styloid is demonstrated in profile _____ (D).
• The _____ (E) is demonstrated without superimposition of the first proximal metacarpal.
• The carpal bones are at the center of the exposure field.

186. Describe the shape and location of the pronator fat stripe that is demonstrated on a lateral wrist projection with accurate positioning.

_____

_____

187. Why is the visualization of the pronator fat stripe on a lateral wrist projection of importance? _____
_____

188. Which two sets of anatomic structures should be superimposed on a lateral wrist projection to indicate that a true lateral has been obtained?

A. _____ and _____

B. _____ and _____

189. Which side of the wrist is placed against the IR for a routine lateral wrist projection?

A. _____ (radial/ulnar)

What projection is this?

B. _____ _____

In this projection, is the pisiform or distal scaphoid positioned closer to the IR?

C. _____

190. How are the patient's hand and forearm aligned to prevent radial and ulnar deviation of the wrist for a lateral wrist

projection? _____

_____

191. Ulnar deviation of the wrist causes the distal scaphoid to be demonstrated _____ (proximal/distal) (A) to

the pisiform, and radial deviation causes the distal scaphoid to be demonstrated _____ (proximal/distal)
(B) to the pisiform on a lateral wrist projection.

192. If a lateral wrist projection is obtained on a patient with large muscular or thick proximal forearm without

hanging the proximal forearm off the IR or imaging table, what type of wrist deviation will result? _____

_____

193. For a lateral wrist projection, how is the patient positioned so that the wrist is in a neutral position without wrist extension or flexion?

_____

194. For a lateral wrist projection, how are the humerus and elbow positioned to demonstrate the ulnar styloid in profile?

_____

195. For a lateral wrist projection, how are the humerus and elbow positioned to demonstrate the ulnar styloid projecting

distal to the midline of the ulnar head? _____

_____

196. Will the elbow and humeral positioning described in question 194 or 195 demonstrate the ulna closer to the lunate on

the resulting lateral wrist projection? _____

_____

197. How is the patient positioned to prevent the first proximal metacarpal from being superimposed over the trapezium?

_____

198. Accurate central ray centering on a lateral wrist projection is accomplished by centering a _____ central ray to the wrist.

199. Which anatomic structures are included on an accurately collimated lateral wrist projection? _____

_____

200. Accurate transverse collimation has been obtained when the collimated borders are _____

_____ .

201. State whether the elbow was positioned in an AP or lateral projection for the lateral wrist projections in Figure 4-43.

Figure 4-43

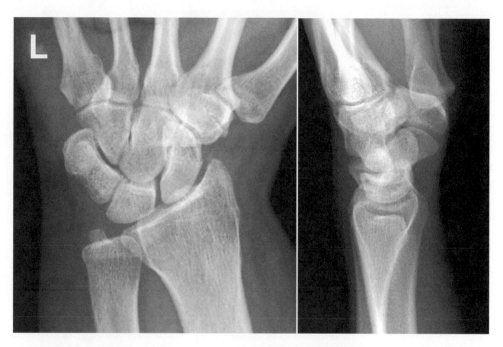

A. _____

B. _____

For the following descriptions of lateral wrist projections with poor positioning, state how the patient would have been mispositioned for such a projection to be obtained.

202. The pisiform is demonstrated anterior to the scaphoid, and the ulna is demonstrated anterior to the radius.

_____

203. The pisiform is demonstrated posterior to the distal scaphoid, and the radius is anterior to the ulna.

_____

204. The pisiform is demonstrated distal to the scaphoid, and the midcarpal bones are centered within the collimated field.

_____

205. The distal scaphoid is demonstrated distal to the pisiform.

_____

206. The ulnar styloid is projecting distal to the midline of the ulnar head. (In some facilities, this may not be considered poor positioning.)

_____

207. The first proximal metacarpal is superimposed over the trapezium.

_____

For the following lateral wrist projections with poor positioning, identify the anatomic structures that are misaligned, state how the patient should be repositioned for an optimal projection to be obtained, and describe the position of the ulnar styloid.

Figure 4-44

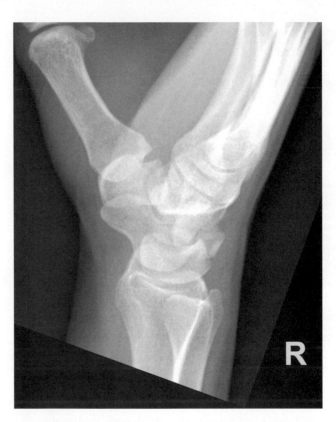

208. Figure 4-44: _____

_____

Ulnar styloid: _____ (profile/midline of ulnar head)

Figure 4-45

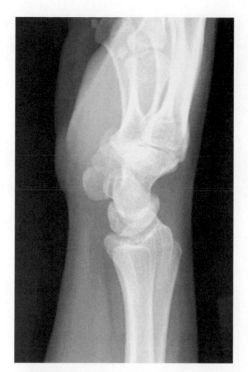

209. Figure 4-45: _____

Ulnar styloid: _____ (profile/midline of ulnar head)

Figure 4-46

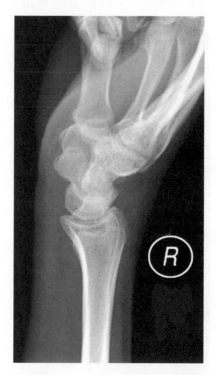

210. Figure 4-46: _____

Ulnar styloid: _____ (profile/midline of ulnar head)

Figure 4-47

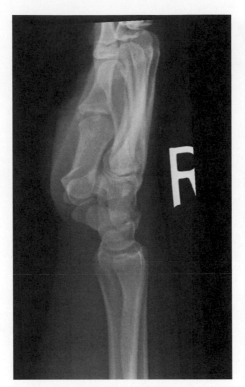

211. Figure 4-47: _____

Ulnar styloid: _____ (profile/midline of ulnar head)

Figure 4-48

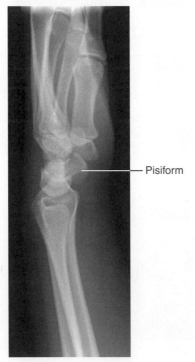

——— Pisiform

212. Figure 4-48: _____

Ulnar styloid: _____ (profile/midline of ulnar head)

213. Figure 4-49: Because of the forearm fracture, the patient was unable to externally rotate the arm enough to obtain an accurately positioned lateral wrist projection. How should the central ray have been adjusted from perpendicular to obtain accurate positioning?

Figure 4-49

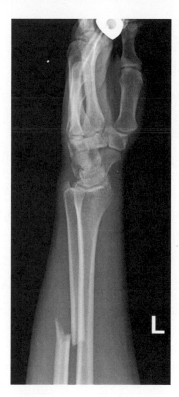

Wrist: Ulnar Deviation, Posteroanterior Axial Projection (Scaphoid)

214. Identify the labeled anatomy in Figure 4-50.

Figure 4-50

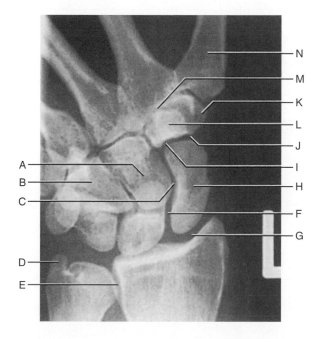

A. _____

B. _____

C. _____

D. _____

E. _____

F. _____

G. _____

H. _____

I. _____

J. _____

K. _____

L. _____

M. _____

N. _____

215. Complete the statements below, referring to PA axial (scaphoid) wrist projection analysis criteria.

> **Posteroanterior Axial (Scaphoid) Wrist Projection Analysis Criteria**
>
> - The _____ (A) fat stripe is demonstrated.
> - The _____ (B) and scaphotrapezoidal joint spaces are open.
> - The long axes of the first metacarpal and radius are aligned.
> - The scaphocapitate and scapholunate joints are open. The ulnar styloid is in profile _____ (C).
> - The radioscaphoid joint space is open.
> - The _____ (D) is at the center of the exposure field.

216. What is the name of the soft tissue structure demonstrated on a PA projection of the wrist that can be used to diagnose joint effusion?

_____

217. Sufficient ulnar deviation of the wrist has been accomplished in the PA axial projection when the long axis of the

_____ (A) and _____ (B) are aligned and the lunate is positioned distal to

the _____ (C).

218. Why does ulnar deviation of the wrist increase the demonstration of the scaphoid on a PA axial projection?

_____

219. For a PA axial projection, how is the patient positioned to obtain open scaphocapitate and scapholunate joint spaces?

_____

220. If the wrist is adequately ulnar-deviated for the PA axial projection, how much and in which direction is the central

ray angled if a fracture of the scaphoid waist is suspected? _____

221. What central ray angulation is used if the patient is unable to ulnar-deviate adequately for a PA axial wrist projection?

A. _____

Why is this adjustment needed?

B. _____

222. Where do most fractures occur on the scaphoid? _____

223. How is the central ray angle adjusted for a PA axial wrist projection if a fracture of the distal scaphoid is suspected?

A. _____

If a proximal scaphoid fracture is suspected?

B. _____

224. If the central ray is not aligned parallel with the fracture site for a PA axial wrist projection, will the fracture line be

clearly visible? _____ (Yes/No)

225. How is the patient positioned for a PA axial wrist projection to obtain an open radioscaphoid joint space?

_____

226. Which anatomic structures are included on a PA axial wrist projection with accurate positioning?

_____

_____

227. For the PA axial wrist projections in Figure 4-51, state whether a distal, waist, or proximal scaphoid fracture is demonstrated and the degree of central ray angulation that should be used to demonstrate each best.

Figure 4-51

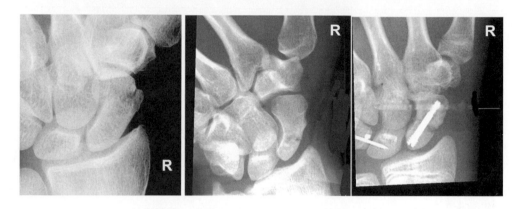

A. _____

B. _____

C. _____

For the following descriptions of PA axial wrist projections with poor positioning, state how the patient would have been mispositioned for such a projection to be obtained.

228. The scaphocapitate and scapholunate joints are closed, and the lunate is superimposed over a portion of the scaphoid.

_____

229. The scaphotrapezium, scaphotrapezoidal, and CM joint spaces are closed.

_____

For the following PA axial wrist projections with poor positioning, state which anatomic structures are misaligned and how the patient should be repositioned for an optimal projection to be obtained.

Figure 4-52

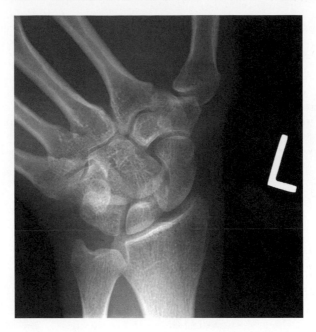

230. Figure 4-52: _____

_____

_____

_____

Figure 4-53

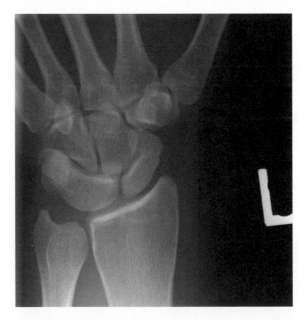

231. Figure 4-53: _____

_____

_____

_____

Figure 4-54

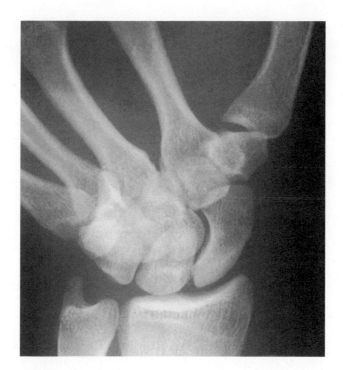

232. Figure 4-54: _____

_____

_____

_____

Wrist Carpal Canal: Tangential, Inferosuperior Projection

233. Identify the labeled anatomy in Figure 4-55.

Figure 4-55

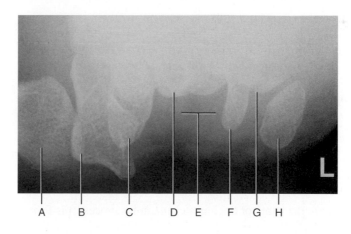

A. _____   E. _____

B. _____   F. _____

C. _____   G. _____

D. _____   H. _____

234. Complete the statements below, referring to tangential, inferosuperior carpal canal projection analysis criteria.

> **Tangential, Inferosuperior Carpal Canal Projection Analysis Criteria**
>
> - The _____ (A) is demonstrated without superimposition of the hamulus of the hamate, and the carpal canal is clearly demonstrated.
> - The carpal canal is visualized in its entirety, and the carpal bones are demonstrated with only slight elongation.
> - The _____ (B) is at the center of the exposure field.

235. The tangential, inferosuperior carpal canal projection is used to evaluate the carpal tunnel for _____

(A) and demonstrate _____ (B) of the pisiform and hamulus of the hamate.

236. The pisiform is demonstrated without superimposition of the hamulus of the hamate on the tangential, inferosuperior

carpal canal projection when _____

237. To show the carpal canal and demonstrate the carpals with only slight elongation on a tangential, inferosuperior

carpal canal projection, the patient's hand is positioned _____ (A)

and the central ray angled _____ (B).

238. When imaging a patient who is unable to extend the wrist enough to place the metacarpals to within 15 degrees of

vertical, the central ray needs to be _____ (increased/decreased) (A). If a 20-degree angle were required to bring the central ray parallel with the patient's palmar surface in this situation, the angle needed for the carpal

canal projection would be _____ (B) and the resulting projection would show the carpals and carpal

canal, although they will be elongated because of the _____ (C).

For the following descriptions of tangential, inferosuperior carpal canal projections with poor positioning, state how the patient would have been mispositioned for such a projection to be obtained.

239. The pisiform is superimposed over the hamulus of the hamate.

_____

240. The carpal canal is not demonstrated in its entirety, and the carpal bones are foreshortened.

_____

241. The metacarpal bases obscure the bases of the hamate's hamulus process, pisiform, and scaphoid.

_____

For the following tangential, inferosuperior carpal canal projections with poor positioning, state which anatomic structures are misaligned and how the patient should be repositioned for an optimal projection to be obtained.

Figure 4-56

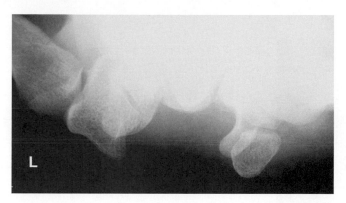

242. Figure 4-56: _____

_____

_____

_____

Figure 4-57

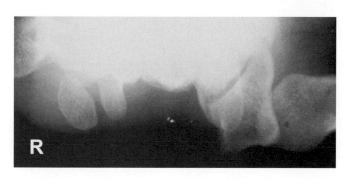

243. Figure 4-57: _____

_____

_____

_____

Figure 4-58

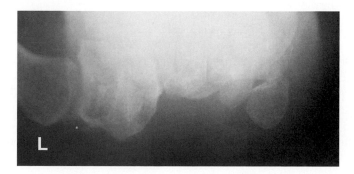

244. Figure 4-58: _____

_____

_____

_____

Forearm: Anteroposterior Projection

245. Identify the labeled anatomy in Figure 4-59.

Figure 4-59

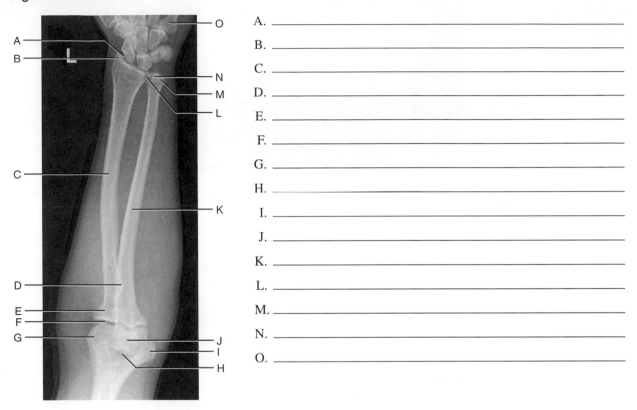

A. _____

B. _____

C. _____

D. _____

E. _____

F. _____

G. _____

H. _____

I. _____

J. _____

K. _____

L. _____

M. _____

N. _____

O. _____

246. How is the forearm positioned with respect to the x-ray tube to take advantage of the anode heel effect? _____

_____

247. Why does the IR need to extend at least 1 inch (2.5 cm) beyond the elbow and wrist joints when the forearm is projectioned in an AP projection?

_____

248. How can the location of the elbow joint be determined?

_____

249. On an AP forearm projection with accurate positioning, the _____ (A) is centered to

the collimated field. This is accomplished by centering a _____ (B) central ray to the

_____ (C).

250. Which anatomic structures are included on an AP forearm projection with accurate positioning?

_____

251. An AP projection of the distal forearm has been obtained when the radial styloid is demonstrated in profile

_____ (medially/laterally) (A) and superimposition of the radius and

_____ (B) is minimal.

252. A patient from the emergency room is unable to position the wrist and elbow in an AP projection simultaneously for an AP forearm projection. How is this patient positioned for the projection?

_____

253. Which specific anatomic structures must be accurately positioned to place the ulnar styloid distal to the midline of the ulnar head for an AP forearm projection?

_____

254. On an AP proximal forearm projection with accurate positioning, the radial head and tuberosity are superimposed

over the ulna by approximately _____ (A) inch and the _____ (B) are demonstrated in profile.

255. Why is the capitulum-radial joint partially or completely obscured on an AP forearm projection?

_____

256. On an AP forearm projection with accurate positioning, the radial tuberosity is demonstrated in profile and the

radius and ulna are visualized _____ with each other.

257. How is the patient positioned to place the radial tuberosity in profile on an AP forearm projection? _____

_____

For the following descriptions of AP forearm projections with poor positioning, state how the patient would have been mispositioned for such a projection to be obtained.

258. The distal forearm demonstrates superimposition of the first and second metacarpal bases and laterally located carpal bones.

_____

259. The AP proximal forearm demonstrates the ulna without radial head and tuberosity superimposition.

_____

260. The radius is crossing over the ulna, and the radial tuberosity is not demonstrated in profile.

_____

261. Describe how the patient was positioned for the AP forearm projection in Figure 4-60.

Figure 4-60

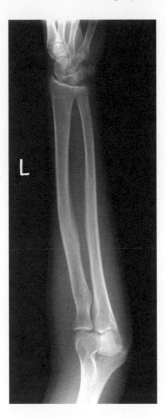

_____

_____

_____

_____

_____

262. The forearm projections in Figure 4-61 demonstrate a distal forearm fracture. Evaluate the accuracy of positioning in these two projections.

Figure 4-61

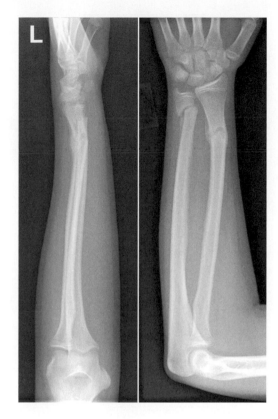

_____

_____

_____

_____

_____

For the following AP forearm projection with poor positioning, state which anatomic structures are misaligned and how the patient should be repositioned for an optimal projection to be obtained.

Figure 4-62

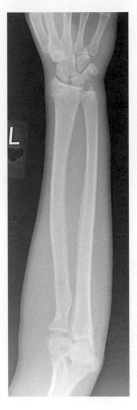

263. Figure 4-62: _____

_____

_____

_____

264. The AP forearm projection in Figure 4-63 demonstrates a midshaft radial fracture. If the patient could not move the forearm to position it in an AP projection adequately, how should the central ray and IR be adjusted for an optimal AP forearm projection to be obtained?

Figure 4-63

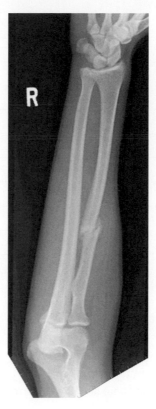

_____

_____

_____

_____

Forearm: Lateral Projection (Lateromedial)

265. Identify the labeled anatomy in Figure 4-64.

Figure 4-64

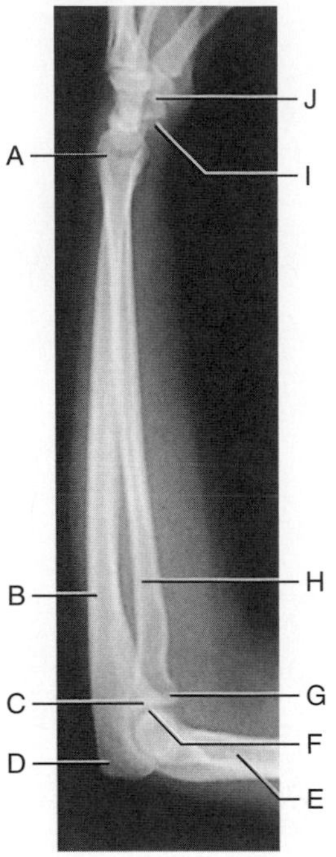

A. _____

B. _____

C. _____

D. _____

E. _____

F. _____

G. _____

H. _____

I. _____

J. _____

266. To take advantage of the anode heel effect, state how the forearm is positioned with respect to the x-ray tube for a lateral forearm projection. _____

_____

267. On a lateral forearm projection with accurate positioning, the _____ is centered within the collimated field.

268. Which anatomic structures are included on an accurately collimated lateral forearm projection?

_____

269. On a lateral forearm projection with accurate positioning, the distal scaphoid is demonstrated _____ (A) to the pisiform, and the distal radius and ulna are _____ (B).

270. What side of the arm is placed against the IR for a lateral forearm projection?

_____

271. On a proximal lateral forearm projection with poor positioning, the ulna is demonstrated posterior to the radius. What will the distal scaphoid and pisiform relationship be?

_____

272. Describe the placement of the ulnar styloid on a lateral forearm projection with accurate positioning.

A. _____

How must the patient be positioned to obtain this ulnar styloid positioning?

B. _____

273. Should the radial tuberosity be demonstrated in profile on a lateral forearm projection with accurate positioning?

A. _____ (Yes/No)

How is the patient positioned to obtain this positioning?

B. _____

274. In patients with average-size forearms, the elbow joint space is open on a lateral forearm projection. What two patient forearm shapes result in a closed elbow joint space?

A. _____

B. _____

275. A lateral forearm projection with poor positioning demonstrates the capitulum distal to the distal surface of the medial trochlea. What is the radial head and coronoid relationship on this projection?

_____

276. A patient from the emergency room is unable to position the wrist and elbow in a lateral position simultaneously for a lateral forearm projection. The requisition states that the examination is being performed to rule out a proximal forearm fracture. How should the patient be positioned for this projection?

_____

_____

277. Evaluate the accuracy of the trauma lateral forearm projection in Figure 4-65. The patient could not position the distal and proximal forearm in a lateral projection at the same time.

Figure 4-65

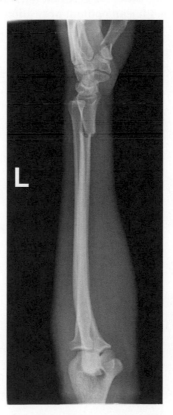

For the following descriptions of lateral forearm projections with poor positioning, state how the patient would have been mispositioned for such a projection to be obtained.

278. The pisiform is demonstrated anterior to the distal scaphoid, and the ulna is anterior to the radius. The proximal forearm demonstrates accurate positioning.

_____

279. The pisiform is visible posterior to the distal scaphoid, and the distal surface of the capitulum is demonstrated proximal to the distal surfaces of the medial trochlea.

_____

_____

280. The ulnar styloid is projecting distal to the midline of the ulnar head.

_____

281. The projection demonstrates the radial tuberosity in profile anteriorly.

_____

282. The radial head is demonstrated too far posterior on the coronoid process. The distal forearm demonstrates accurate positioning.

_____

For the following lateral forearm projection with poor positioning, state which anatomic structures are misaligned and how the patient should be repositioned for an optimal projection to be obtained.

Figure 4-66

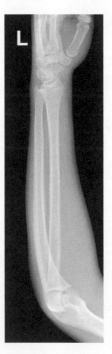

283. Figure 4-66: _____

_____

_____

_____

284. The lateral forearm projection in Figure 4-67 demonstrates a distal radial fracture. The patient's arm was externally rotated as far as possible. How should the central ray and IR be adjusted for an optimal lateral forearm projection to be obtained?

Figure 4-67

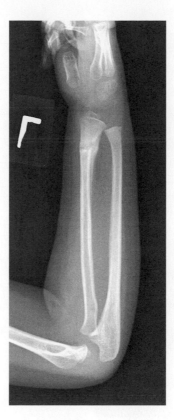

_____

_____

_____

_____

Elbow: Anteroposterior Projection

285. Identify the labeled anatomy in Figure 4-68.

Figure 4-68

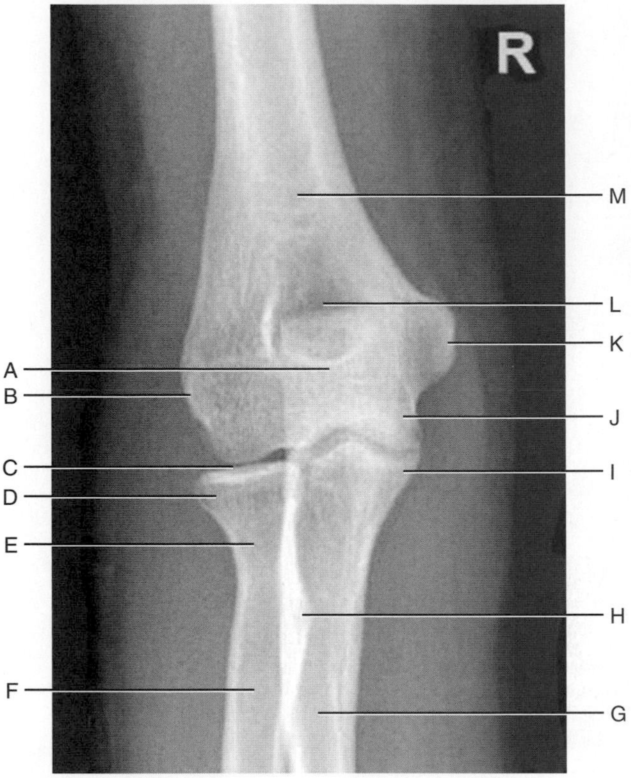

A. _____

B. _____

C. _____

D. _____

E. _____

F. _____

G. _____

H. _____

I. _____

J. _____

K. _____

L. _____

M. _____

286. Complete the statements below, referring to AP elbow projection analysis criteria.

Anteroposterior Elbow Projection Analysis Criteria
• The medial and lateral humeral epicondyles are demonstrated in _____ (A) at the extreme medial and lateral edges of the distal humerus, and the radial head superimposes the lateral aspect of the proximal ulna by _____ (B). The coronoid process is demonstrated on end.
• The radial tuberosity is in profile _____ (C), and the radius and ulna are parallel.
• The elbow joint is open, the radial head articulating surface is not demonstrated, and the olecranon process is situated within the olecranon fossa.
• The _____ (D) is at the center of the exposure field.

287. Which anatomic structures are palpated and positioned at equal distances from the IR to place the elbow in an AP projection?

_____

288. Which humeral epicondyle rotates out of profile with only a slight degree of elbow rotation? _____

289. If the humeral epicondyles are accurately positioned for an AP elbow projection, what other structures can be manipulated to change the degree of radial tuberosity visualization?

_____

290. What two aspects of the positioning procedure need to be accurately set up to demonstrate the capitulum-radial joint space as an open space on an AP elbow projection?

A. _____

B. _____

291. A poorly positioned AP elbow projection demonstrates a closed capitulum-radial joint space. How can one determine

if this closure was a result of poor central ray placement or elbow flexion? _____

_____

_____

292. How is the patient positioned for an AP elbow projection if the elbow is unable to extend at least 30 degrees?

_____

_____

293. Accurate central ray centering on an AP elbow projection is accomplished by centering a _____

(A) central ray _____ (B) _____ (C) to the medial epicondyle. Why is it

easier to palpate the medial epicondyle than the lateral epicondyle (D)? _____

294. Which anatomic structures are included on an accurately collimated AP elbow projection?

_____

295. What patient condition is demonstrated on the projection in Figure 4-69?

Figure 4-69

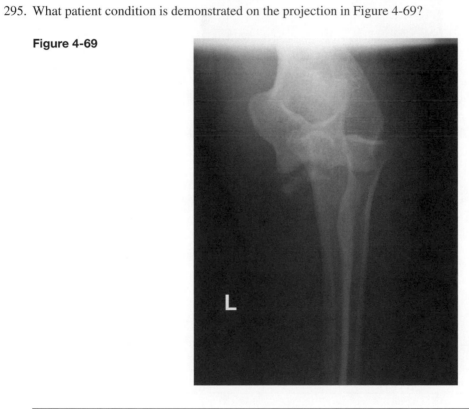

_____

_____

_____

For the following descriptions of AP elbow projections with poor positioning, state how the patient would have been mispositioned for such a projection to be obtained.

296. The radial head is superimposing approximately 0.5 inch (1 cm) of the ulna.

_____

297. The ulna is demonstrated without radial head superimposition.

_____

298. The projection demonstrates the radius crossing over the ulna, and the radial tuberosity is not shown in profile.

_____

299. The projection demonstrates a foreshortened proximal forearm and a closed capitulum-radial joint space.

_____

For the following AP elbow projections with poor positioning, state which anatomic structures are misaligned and how the patient should be repositioned for an optimal projection to be obtained.

Figure 4-70

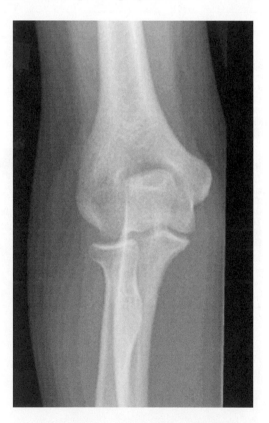

300. Figure 4-70: _____

_____

_____

_____

Figure 4-71

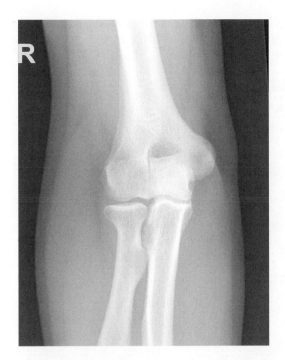

301. Figure 4-71: _____

_____

_____

_____

Figure 4-72

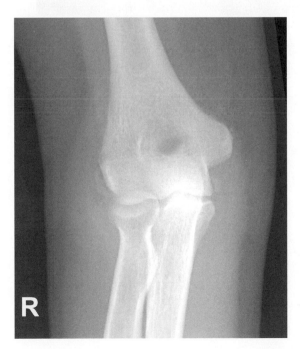

302. Figure 4-72: _____

_____

_____

_____

303. The AP projection in Figure 4-73 demonstrates a proximal radial fracture. If the patient could not move the arm to position it adequately for an AP projection, how should the central ray and IR be adjusted for an optimal AP elbow projection to be obtained?

Figure 4-73

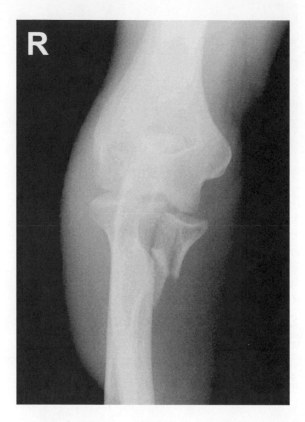

_____

_____

_____

304. The AP projection in Figure 4-74 demonstrates a distal ulnar fracture that prevented the patient from internally rotating the arm the needed amount to obtain an accurate AP elbow projection. How should the central ray and IR be adjusted to obtain an optimal projection?

Figure 4-74

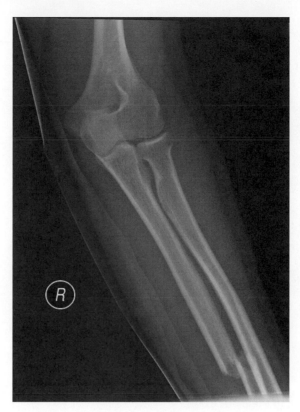

_____

_____

_____

Elbow: Anteroposterior Oblique Projections (Internal and External Rotation)

305. Identify the labeled anatomy in Figure 4-75.

Figure 4-75

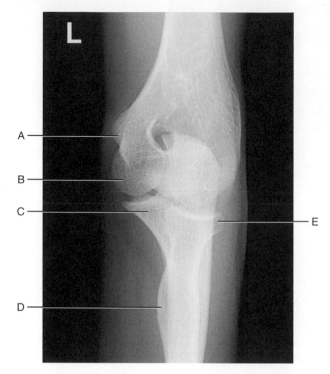

A. _____

B. _____

C. _____

D. _____

E. _____

306. Identify the labeled anatomy in Figure 4-76.

Figure 4-76

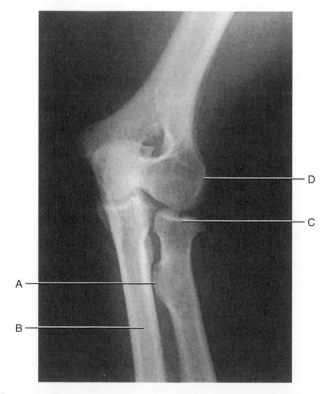

A. _____

B. _____

C. _____

D. _____

307. Complete the statements below, referring to AP oblique elbow projection analysis criteria.

> **Anteroposterior Oblique Elbow Projection Analysis Criteria**
>
> - External oblique: Capitulum-radial joint is open, and the radial head articulating surface is not demonstrated.
> - External oblique: The _____ (A) and _____ (B) are seen in profile; the _____ (C) is demonstrated without radial head, neck, and tuberosity superimposition; and the radioulnar articulation is open.
> - Internal oblique: The trochlear-coronoid process joint is open, and the coronoid process articulating surface is not demonstrated.
> - Internal oblique: The _____ (D), the trochlear notch, and the medial aspect of the trochlea are seen in profile. The trochlear-coronoid process articulation is open, and the radial head and neck superimpose the ulna.
> - The _____ (E) is at the center of the exposure field.

308. An AP oblique elbow projection with poor positioning demonstrates a closed capitulum-radial joint space. List two possible positioning problems that might have resulted in this projection.

A. _____

B. _____

309. Describe the anatomic changes that will occur between the olecranon fossa and the olecranon when the elbow is flexed. _____

_____

310. State whether the forearm or humerus should be placed parallel with the IR to best demonstrate the anatomy listed below in a patient whose arm will not fully extend.

A. Coronoid: _____

B. Radial head: _____

C. Medial trochlea: _____

D. Capitulum: _____

E. Capitulum-radial joint: _____

311. What is the degree of elbow rotation used for AP oblique projections?

_____

312. In which direction is the elbow rotated from the AP projection to obtain an AP oblique projection that demonstrates the radial head and ulna without superimposition? _____

313. Accurate central ray centering on an AP oblique elbow projection is accomplished by centering a _____ (A) central ray to the elbow joint located at a level _____ (B) distal to the _____ (C).

314. Which anatomic structures are included on an AP oblique elbow projection with accurate positioning?

_____

_____

For the following descriptions of AP oblique elbow projections with poor positioning, state how the patient would have been mispositioned for such a projection to be obtained.

315. The externally rotated AP oblique projection demonstrates a closed capitulum-radial joint space. The olecranon is positioned outside the olecranon fossa, and the radial articulating surface is demonstrated.

_____

316. On the internally rotated AP oblique projection, the radial head is demonstrated lateral to the coronoid process, without complete superimposition of the ulna, and the proximal aspect of the olecranon is not demonstrated in profile.

_____

317. On the internally rotated AP oblique projection, a portion of the radial head is demonstrated anterior to the coronoid process, without complete superimposition of the ulna.

_____

318. On the external rotated AP oblique projection, a portion of the radial head and tuberosity is superimposed over the ulna.

_____

319. On the externally rotated AP oblique projection, the coronoid is superimposed over a portion of the radial neck, and the radial head is free of superimposition. The radial tuberosity is not demonstrated in profile.

_____

For the following AP oblique elbow projections with poor positioning, state which anatomic structures are misaligned and how the patient should be repositioned for an optimal projection to be obtained.

Figure 4-77

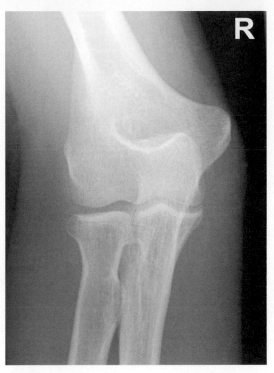

320. Figure 4-77 (external rotation): _____

_____

_____

_____

Figure 4-78

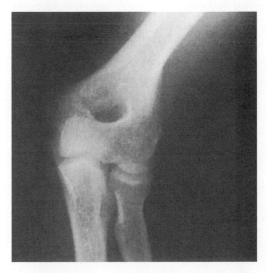

321. Figure 4-78 (external rotation):_____

_____

_____

_____

Figure 4-79

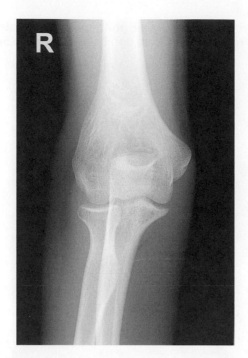

322. Figure 4-79 (internal rotation):_____

_____

_____

_____

Figure 4-80

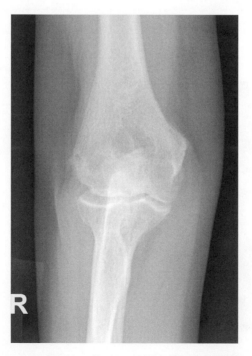

323. Figure 4-80 (internal rotation):_____

_____

_____

_____

Elbow: Lateral Projection (Lateromedial)

324. Identify the labeled anatomy in Figure 4-81.

Figure 4-81

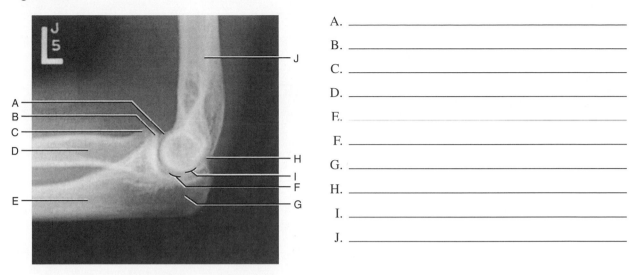

A. _____

B. _____

C. _____

D. _____

E. _____

F. _____

G. _____

H. _____

I. _____

J. _____

325. Complete the statements below, referring to lateral elbow projection analysis criteria.

Lateral Elbow Projection Analysis Criteria
• Contrast and density are adequate to demonstrate the anterior, posterior, and _____ (A) fat pads.
• The elbow is flexed 90 degrees.
• The distal humerus demonstrates three concentric arcs, which are formed by the _____ (B), capitulum, and medial trochlea. The elbow joint is open, and the distal and _____ (C) surfaces of the radial head and the coronoid process are aligned.
• The radial tuberosity is not demonstrated in _____ (D).
• The _____ (E) is at the center of the exposure field.

326. List the three soft tissue fat pads that may be demonstrated on a lateral elbow projection, and describe their locations.

A. _____

B. _____

C. _____

Displacement of these pads may indicate what to the reviewer?

D. _____

327. Why is it important to flex the elbow 90 degrees for a lateral elbow projection? _____

_____

328. What three anatomic structures form the three concentric arcs on a lateral elbow projection with accurate positioning?

A. _____

B. _____

C. _____

Which of these arcs is the smallest?

D. _____

Which is the largest?

E. _____

How will improper alignment of these arcs affect the elbow joint space?

F. _____

329. A lateral elbow projection with poor positioning demonstrates the radial head positioned posterior on the coronoid process. How would the capitulum and medial trochlea be misaligned on this projection?

_____

330. The distal forearm was positioned too low for a lateral elbow projection. What will be the relationship between the radial head and coronoid and the capitulum and medial trochlea on the resulting projection?

_____

331. A lateral elbow projection with poor positioning demonstrates the capitulum too far posterior to the medial trochlea. How will the radial head and coronoid be aligned on this projection?

_____

332. The proximal humerus was positioned lower than the distal humerus on a lateral elbow projection. What will be the relationship between the radial head and coronoid and the capitulum and medial trochlea on the resulting projection?

_____

333. The position of the radial tuberosity on a lateral elbow projection is determined by the position of the patient's hand and wrist. For the following hand positions, describe the position of the radial tuberosity.

A. Lateral hand and wrist: _____

B. Supinated hand and wrist: _____

C. Pronated hand and wrist: _____

Which of the radial tuberosity positions above is the desired position for an accurate lateral elbow projection?

D. _____

334. Accurate central ray centering on a lateral elbow projection is accomplished by centering a _____

(A) central ray to the elbow joint located _____ (B) inch _____ (C) to the lateral humeral epicondyle.

335. Which anatomic structures are included on a lateral elbow projection with accurate positioning? _____

_____

For the following descriptions of lateral elbow projections with poor positioning, state how the patient would have been mispositioned for such a projection to be obtained.

336. The olecranon is positioned within the olecranon fossa, and the posterior fat pad is demonstrated proximal to the olecranon process.

_____

337. The radial tuberosity is positioned in profile anteriorly.

_____

338. The radial head is positioned posterior on the coronoid process, and the distal surface of the capitulum is demonstrated distal to the distal surface of the medial trochlea.

_____

339. The radial head is positioned anterior on the coronoid process, and the distal surface of the capitulum is proximal to the distal surface of the medial trochlea.

_____

340. The radial head is distal to the coronoid process, and the capitulum appears anterior to the medial trochlea.

_____

341. The radial head is proximal to the coronoid process, and the capitulum appears posterior to the medial trochlea.

_____

For the following lateral elbow projections with poor positioning, state which anatomic structures are misaligned and how the patient should be repositioned for an optimal projection to be obtained.

Figure 4-82

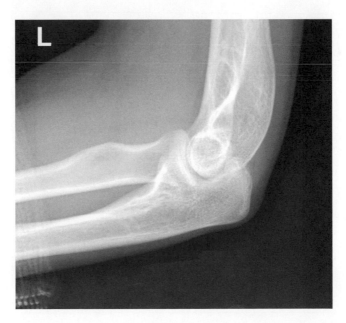

342. Figure 4-82: _____

_____

_____

_____

Figure 4-83

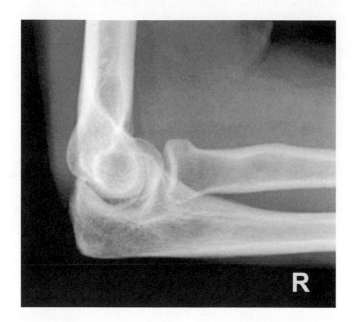

343. Figure 4-83: _____

_____

_____

_____

Figure 4-84

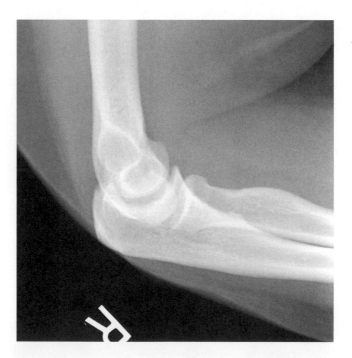

344. Figure 4-84: _____

_____

_____

_____

Figure 4-85

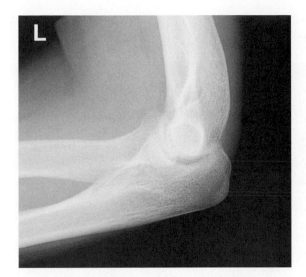

345. Figure 4-85: _____

_____

_____

_____

Figure 4-86

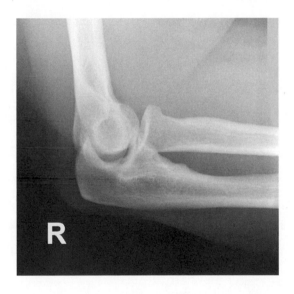

346. Figure 4-86: _____

_____

_____

_____

347. If the patient is unable to move the arm to adjust for the poor positioning demonstrated in Figure 4-83, how should the central ray and IR be adjusted for an optimal lateral elbow projection to be obtained?

_____

_____

_____

_____

348. Figure 4-87: The patient is unable to adjust positioning. How should the central ray and IR be adjusted for an optimal lateral elbow projection to be obtained?

Figure 4-87

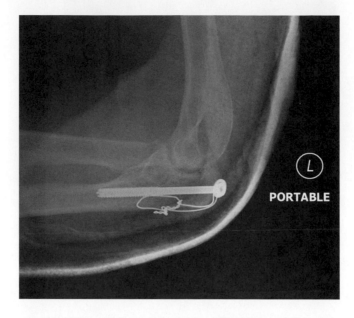

_____

_____

_____

Elbow: Axiolateral Projection (Coyle Method)

349. Identify the labeled anatomy in Figure 4-88.

Figure 4-88

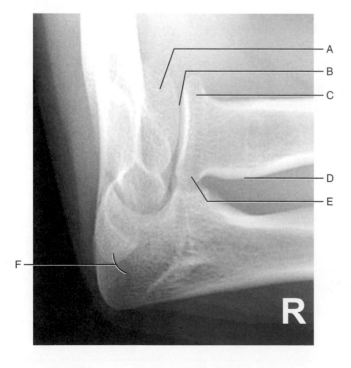

A. _____

B. _____

C. _____

D. _____

E. _____

F. _____

350. Complete the statements below, referring to axiolateral elbow projection analysis criteria.

Axiolateral Elbow Projection Analysis Criteria
• The elbow is flexed 90 degrees.
• The capitulum and _____ (A) are demonstrated without superimposition, and the radial head is superimposed on only the anterior tip of the coronoid process.
• The capitulum-radial joint is _____ (B) and the proximal radial head and coronoid process are aligned.
• The radial head surface of interest is demonstrated in profile.
• The _____ (C) is at the center of the exposure field.

351. In what position is the elbow placed to obtain the axiolateral projection of the elbow?

_____

352. The position of the distal forearm for an axiolateral projection affects the relationship of which anatomic elbow structures?

_____

_____

353. How can one determine from the projection if the forearm was elevated too high for the axiolateral elbow projection?

_____

_____

354. An axiolateral elbow projection with poor positioning demonstrates the radial head distal to the coronoid process. What is the relationship of the capitulum and medial trochlea on such a projection?

_____

_____

355. To separate the arcs of the distal humerus accurately, an imaginary line connecting the humeral epicondyles is positioned _____ (A) to the IR and a _____ -degree (B) central ray angulation is directed _____ (C). Will this angle cause the radial head or coronoid to project farther proximally _____ (D)? Will this angle cause the medial trochlea or capitulum to project farther proximally _____ (E)?

356. Which anatomic structure can be used to determine the portion of the radial head that is positioned in profile on an axiolateral elbow projection?

_____

357. For each of the following wrist projections, list the location of the radial tuberosity and the aspect of the radial head surface that are demonstrated in profile.

A. PA wrist: _____

_____

B. Lateral wrist: _____

223

358. State which aspects of the radial head surface are demonstrated in profile on the projection in Figure 4-89.

Figure 4-89

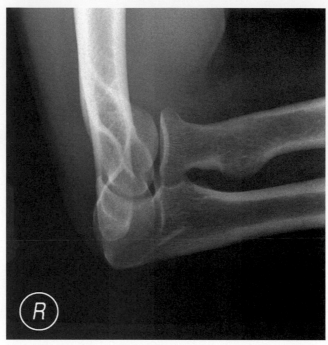

A. Anterior: _____

B. Posterior: _____

359. Accurate central ray centering on an axiolateral elbow projection is accomplished by centering the central ray to the

_____

360. Which anatomic structures are included on an axiolateral elbow projection with accurate positioning?

_____

For the following descriptions of axiolateral elbow projections with poor positioning, state how the patient would have been mispositioned for such a projection to be obtained.

361. The capitulum-radial joint space is closed, the radial head is demonstrated distal to the coronoid process, and the capitulum is demonstrated too far anterior to the medial trochlea.

_____

362. The capitulum-radial joint space is closed, the radial head is demonstrated proximal to the coronoid process, and the capitulum is demonstrated too far posterior to the medial trochlea.

_____

For the following axiolateral elbow projections with poor positioning, state which anatomic structures are misaligned and how the patient should be repositioned for an optimal projection to be obtained.

Figure 4-90

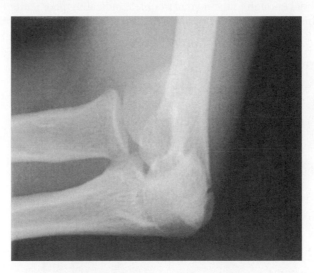

363. Figure 4-90: _____

_____

_____

_____

Figure 4-91

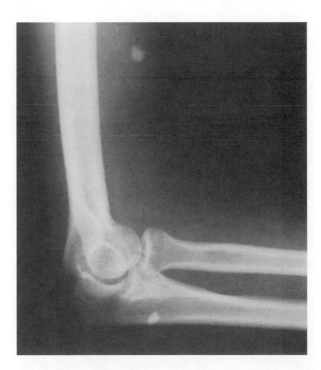

364. Figure 4-91: _____

_____

_____

_____

365. The axiolateral elbow projection in Figure 4-92 demonstrates a radial head and capitulum fracture. Even though the projection was obtained with a 45-degree central ray angle, the radial head is not anterior enough to the coronoid, nor is the capitulum proximal enough to the medial trochlea, indicating poor patient positioning. If the patient could not move the arm from this position, how should the central ray be adjusted to obtain an optimal capitulum-radial head projection?

Figure 4-92

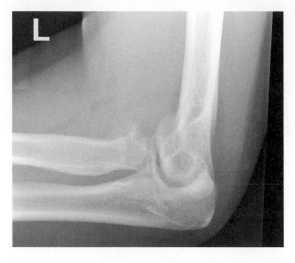

366. The patient was accurately positioned for the axiolateral elbow projection in Figure 4-93 but the central ray was poorly aligned with the elbow, causing less than optimal anatomic relationships. Describe how the central ray was aligned with the elbow to cause these results.

Figure 4-93

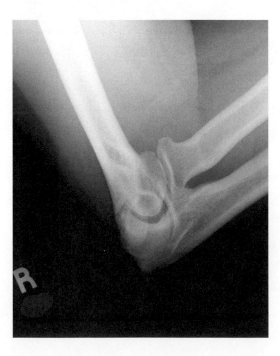

Humerus: Anteroposterior Projection

367. Identify the labeled anatomy in Figure 4-94.

Figure 4-94

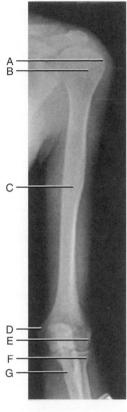

A. _____

B. _____

C. _____

D. _____

E. _____

F. _____

G. _____

368. Humeral projections can be taken without a grid and still display high projection contrast as long as the thickness measurement is below _____ (A) cm. When a grid is used for humeral projections, the kilovoltage peak (kVp) should be raised above _____ (B).

369. To take advantage of the anode heel effect, state how the humerus is positioned with respect to the x-ray tube.

_____

370. An AP projection of the distal humerus has been obtained when the radial head and tuberosity are superimposed over the ulna by approximately _____ (A) inch and the _____ (B) are demonstrated in profile.

371. On an AP proximal humeral projection with accurate positioning, the _____ (A) tubercle is demonstrated laterally in profile, the _____ (B) is demonstrated medially in profile, and the

_____ (C) will be visible approximately halfway between the greater tubercle and the humeral head.

372. When the patient is positioned for an AP humeral projection, the patient's _____ (A) is externally rotated until an imaginary line connecting the _____ (B) is positioned parallel with the IR.

373. If an AP humeral projection is ordered for a patient with a suspected proximal humeral fracture, why is it important not to rotate the patient's arm externally?

A. _____

How can the ordered procedure still be performed without adjusting the patient's arm position?

B. _____

_____

374. An AP humeral projection is ordered for a patient with a humerus that is longer than 17 inches (43 cm). How should the patient's arm be aligned with the IR to include the entire humerus on the same projection?

_____

_____

375. Why is it necessary to have the IR extend at least 1 inch (2.5 cm) beyond the shoulder and elbow joints when imaging the humerus in the AP projection?

_____

_____

_____

376. Describe how the shoulder and elbow joints can be located to ensure that the IR extends beyond each for an AP humeral projection.

A. Shoulder: _____

B. Elbow: _____

377. On an AP humeral projection with accurate positioning, the _____ is centered within the collimated field.

378. Which anatomic structures are included on an AP humeral projection with accurate positioning?

_____

_____

For the following descriptions of AP humeral projections with poor positioning, state how the patient would have been mispositioned for such a projection to be obtained.

379. The projection demonstrates the ulna without radial head superimposition.

_____

380. The projection demonstrates the radial head and tuberosity superimposed over more than 0.25 inch (0.6 cm) of the ulna.

_____

For the following AP humeral projections with poor positioning, state which anatomic structures are misaligned and how the patient should be repositioned for an optimal projection to be obtained.

Figure 4-95

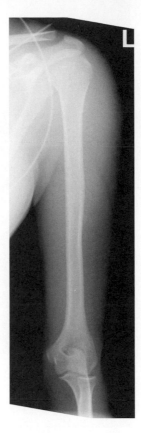

381. Figure 4-95: _____

_____

_____

_____

Figure 4-96

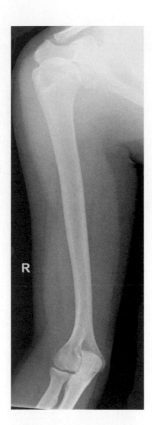

382. Figure 4-96: _____

_____

_____

_____

Humerus: Lateral Projection

383. Is the projection shown in Figure 4-97 a mediolateral or lateromedial projection?

_____

Figure 4-97

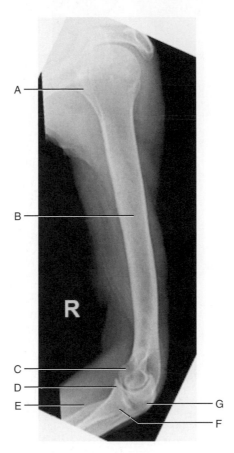

384. Identify the labeled anatomy in Figure 4-97.

A. _____

B. _____

C. _____

D. _____

E. _____

F. _____

G. _____

385. Is the projection demonstrated in Figure 4-98 a mediolateral or lateromedial projection?

_____

Figure 4-98

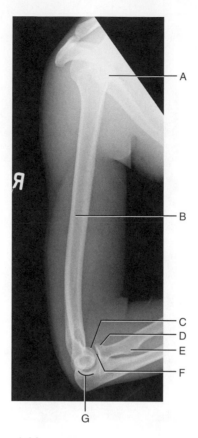

386. Identify the labeled anatomy in Figure 4-98.

A. _____

B. _____

C. _____

D. _____

E. _____

F. _____

G. _____

387. Will a mediolateral or lateromedial projection of the humerus allow the humerus to be positioned closer to the IR when it is in a lateral projection?

_____

388. A proximal lateral humeral projection with accurate positioning demonstrates the _____

(A) tubercle in profile _____ (medially/laterally) (B).

Which projection of the humerus demonstrates the capitulum distal to the medial trochlea and superimposition of

the radial head and coronoid process? _____

389. Which projection of the humerus demonstrates the radial head anterior to the coronoid and the capitulum proximal to the medial trochlea?

_____

390. What causes the anatomic structures of the distal humerus to align differently on the two lateral projections of the humerus?

_____

391. When positioning the patient for a lateral humeral projection, the _____ (A) should be internally rotated

until an imaginary line connecting the _____ (B) is positioned perpendicular to the IR.

392. List two alternative projections that can be used to image the humerus in the lateral projection on a patient with a suspected fractured proximal humerus.

A. _____

B. _____

393. When imaging the proximal humerus, how can one determine if the humeral epicondyles have been accurately positioned for a lateral humeral projection?

_____

_____

394. If the patient's humerus is aligned diagonally on the IR and the collimator head or tube column cannot be rotated, a flat contact shield may be used to protect the patient's thorax. Why is it important that these shields be positioned at least 2 inches (5 cm) away from the humeral head?

_____

395. On a lateral humeral projection with accurate positioning, the _____ is centered within the collimated field.

396. Which anatomic structures are included on a lateral humeral projection with accurate positioning?

_____

For the following description of a lateral humeral projection with poor positioning, state how the patient would have been mispositioned for such a projection to be obtained.

397. The mediolateral projection demonstrates a decrease in projection density at the proximal humerus, and the distal humerus displays adequate density.

_____

For the following lateral humeral projections with poor positioning, state which anatomic structures are misaligned and how the patient should be repositioned for an optimal projection to be obtained.

Figure 4-99

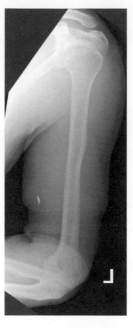

398. Figure 4-99: _____

_____

_____

_____

Figure 4-100

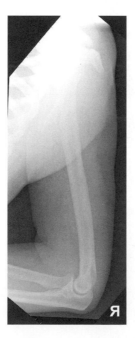

399. Figure 4-100: _____

_____

_____

_____

5 | Shoulder

STUDY QUESTIONS

1. Describe how the following shoulder projections should be displayed on a view box or digital monitor.

   A. Inferosuperior axial shoulder: _____

   B. Left AP axial clavicle: _____

   C. Right PA oblique (scapular Y) shoulder: _____

2. List anatomic structures that are demonstrated on shoulder projections if proper projection density and penetration were demonstrated. _____

3. Routine shoulder projections are obtained using _____ (A) kVp (kilovoltage peak) and

   _____ (B) SID (source–image receptor distance).

4. When an exposure is set for shoulder projections that adequately demonstrates the glenohumeral joint, the acromion process and lateral clavicular end are often overexposed. How can the technologist provide a projection that adequately demonstrates all of these structures?

   _____

5. When should a grid be used for the inferosuperior axial projection?

   _____

Shoulder: Anteroposterior Projection

6. Identify the labeled anatomy on Figure 5-1.

Figure 5-1

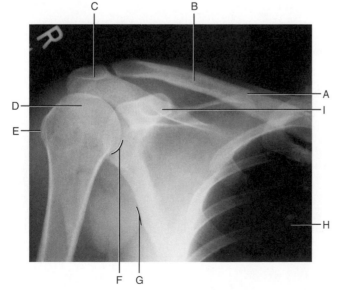

A. _____

B. _____

C. _____

D. _____

E. _____

F. _____

G. _____

H. _____

I. _____

7. Complete the statements below referring to AP shoulder projection analysis criteria.

> **Anteroposterior Shoulder Projection Analysis Criteria**
>
> - The superolateral border of the scapula is visible without _____ (A) superimposition.
> - The clavicle is demonstrated horizontally, with the medial end positioned adjacent to the _____ (B).
> - The superior scapular angle is superimposed by _____ (C).
> - The humerus is aligned parallel with the body and the glenoid cavity is partially visualized, facing laterally.
> - Neutral humerus: The _____ (D) tubercle is partially seen in profile laterally and the humeral head is partially seen in profile _____ (E).
> - Externally rotated humerus: The greater tubercle is in profile _____ (F) and the humeral head is in profile _____ (G).
> - Internally rotated humerus: The _____ (H) tubercle is in profile medially and the humeral head is superimposed by the greater tubercle.
> - The glenohumeral joint and coracoid processes are at the center of the exposure field.

8. Define the following terms.

   A. Overexposed: _____

   B. Shoulder retraction: _____

   C. Shoulder dislocation: _____

9. If an arrow marker is used to indicate internal and external humeral rotation on an AP shoulder projection, how is it positioned on the image receptor (IR) for each of the following projections?

   A. Internal rotation: _____

   B. External rotation: _____

10. How can the technologist position the patient to prevent rotation on an AP shoulder projection?

   _____

11. What is the degree of scapular obliquity on an AP shoulder projection?

   A. _____

   What portion of the scapula is situated anteriorly?

   B. _____

12. A nondislocated shoulder demonstrates slight superimposition of the humeral head and _____.

13. Which shoulder dislocation is more common? _____ (anterior/posterior)

14. How is the patient positioned to demonstrate the scapular body without longitudinal foreshortening on an AP shoulder projection? _____

15. If the scapula is longitudinally foreshortened, the superior scapular angle is projected inferiorly or superiorly to the

_____.

16. How can longitudinal scapular foreshortening be avoided when obtaining an AP shoulder projection in a kyphotic patient? _____

_____

17. When the shoulder is demonstrated without humeral abduction, the glenoid cavity faces _____ (A), whereas on humeral abduction the glenoid cavity shifts _____ (B).

18. The lateral humeral epicondyle is aligned with the _____ (A) and the medial epicondyle is aligned with the _____ (B) of the proximal humerus.

19. State how the humeral epicondyles are positioned in reference to the IR to place the anatomic structures as described on the following AP shoulder projections.

    A. Greater tubercle is partially in profile laterally: _____

    B. Lesser tubercle is in profile medially: _____

    C. Greater tubercle is in profile laterally: _____

    D. Humeral head is in profile medially: _____

20. How is the patient's arm positioned for an AP shoulder projection if a shoulder dislocation or humeral fracture is suspected? _____

_____

21. Accurate central ray centering on an AP shoulder projection is accomplished by centering a _____ (A) central ray 1 inch (2.5 cm) _____ (B).

22. Which anatomic structures are demonstrated within the collimated field on an AP shoulder projection with accurate positioning? _____

_____

23. Describe the location of the palpable coracoid process. _____

_____

For the following descriptions of AP shoulder projections with poor positioning, state how the patient would have been mispositioned for such a projection to be obtained.

24. The glenoid cavity is almost in profile, with only a small amount of the articulating surface demonstrated, the superolateral border of the scapula is superimposed by the thorax, and the medial clavicular end has been rolled away from the vertebral column.

_____

25. The scapular body is drawn from beneath the thorax and is transversely foreshortened, the glenoid cavity is demonstrated on end, and the medial clavicular end is superimposed over the vertebral column.

_____

26. The superior scapular angle is demonstrated superior to the clavicle, and the acromion process and humeral head demonstrate no superimposition.

_____

27. A neutral shoulder projection demonstrates the greater tubercle in profile laterally and the humeral head in profile medially.

_____

_____

28. A neutral shoulder projection demonstrates the lesser tubercle in profile medially.

_____

_____

For the following AP shoulder projections with poor positioning, state which anatomic structures are misaligned and how the patient should be repositioned for an optimal projection to be obtained.

Figure 5-2

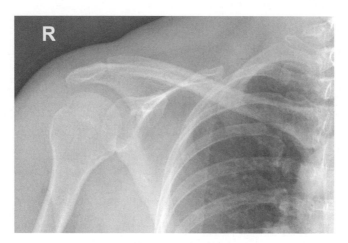

29. Figure 5-2: _____

_____

_____

Figure 5-3

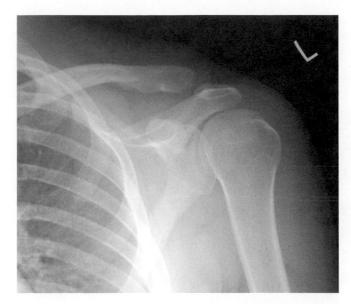

30. Figure 5-3: _____

_____

_____

Figure 5-4

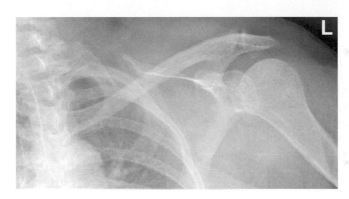

31. Figure 5-4: _____

_____

_____

Shoulder: Inferosuperior Axial Projection

32. Identify the labeled anatomy in Figure 5-5.

Figure 5-5

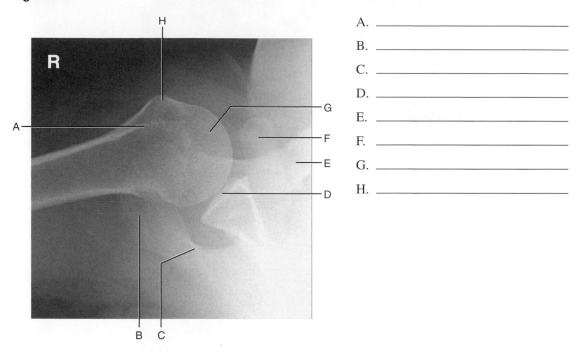

A. _____

B. _____

C. _____

D. _____

E. _____

F. _____

G. _____

H. _____

33. Complete the statements below referring to inferosuperior axial shoulder projection analysis criteria.

Inferosuperior Axial Shoulder Projection Analysis Criteria

- The inferior and superior margins of the _____ (A) are almost superimposed, with only a small amount of humeral head superimposition.

- The lateral edge of the coracoid process base is aligned with the _____ (B) glenoid cavity margin.

- The proximal humerus is seen without distortion, and the long axis of the humeral shaft is seen with minimal foreshortening

- The epicondyles are _____ (C) with the floor, with the lesser tubercle in profile anteriorly.

- The epicondyles are at a _____ (D) with the floor, with the lesser tubercle in partial profile anteriorly and the posterolateral aspect of the humeral head in profile posteriorly.

- The entire coracoid process is demonstrated in profile.

- The humeral head is at the center of the exposure field.

34. Humeral abduction of the arm is obtained by combined movements of the _____ (A) and _____ (B).

35. On a patient who has no trouble abducting the humerus to a 90-degree angle with the body, the glenoid cavity is placed at a _____ angle with the lateral body surface.

36. Describe how and at what angle to the body's lateral surface the central ray should be aligned on a patient who is able to abduct the humerus to a 90-degree angle with the body for an inferosuperior axial shoulder projection.

_____

_____

37. How should the angle between the lateral body surface and the central ray be adjusted if the patient can abduct the humerus to only a 45-degree angle with the body?

A. _____

Why is this change required?

B. _____

38. How is the IR positioned for an axial shoulder projection? _____

_____

_____

39. When is the humeral shaft foreshortened on an inferosuperior axial shoulder projection?

_____

40. Describe the anatomic structures of the proximal humerus that are demonstrated anteriorly and posteriorly in profile on an inferosuperior axial shoulder projection when the humerus is positioned as stated below.

A. Arm externally rotated until the humeral epicondyles are at a 45-degree angle with the floor:

_____

_____

B. Arm externally rotated until the humeral epicondyles are perpendicular to the floor:

_____

_____

C. Arm externally rotated until the humeral epicondyles are parallel with the floor:

_____

_____

41. What is the name of the proximal humerus compression fracture that is better demonstrated on an inferosuperior axial shoulder projection when the patient's arm is placed in exaggerated external rotation?

A. _____

How must the humeral epicondyles be positioned to demonstrate this fracture on an inferosuperior axial shoulder projection?

B. _____

42. Accurate central ray centering on an inferosuperior axial shoulder projection is accomplished by centering a _____ (A) central ray to the midaxillary region at the same transverse level as the _____ (B).

43. Which anatomic structures are included on an inferosuperior axial shoulder projection with accurate positioning?

_____

_____

44. For an inferosuperior axial shoulder projection, elevation of the shoulder on a sponge or washcloth prevents clipping of the _____ aspect of the humerus and shoulder.

45. Turning and tilting the patient's head away from the affected shoulder prevents clipping of the

(A) _____, (B) _____, and (C) _____.

46. How were the humeral epicondyles positioned for the inferosuperior axial shoulder projection in Figure 5-6?

Figure 5-6

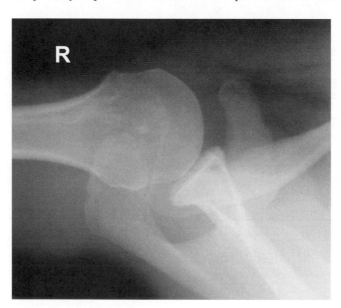

A. _____

How were the humeral epicondyles positioned for the inferosuperior axial shoulder projection in Figure 5-7?

Figure 5-7

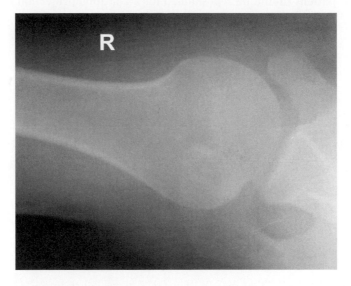

B. _____

For the following descriptions of inferosuperior axial shoulder projections with poor positioning, state how the patient would have been mispositioned or the central ray aligned for such a projection to be obtained.

47. The glenohumeral joint space is obscured, and the inferior glenoid cavity is demonstrated lateral to the coracoid process base.

_____

48. The glenohumeral joint space is obscured, and the inferior glenoid cavity is demonstrated medial to the lateral edge of the coracoid process base.

_____

49. The greater tubercle is demonstrated in profile posteriorly.

_____

50. The acromion process, scapular spine, and posterior aspect of the proximal humerus were not included on the projection.

_____

For the following inferosuperior axial shoulder projections with poor positioning, state which anatomic structures are misaligned and how the patient should be repositioned for an optimal projection to be obtained.

Figure 5-8

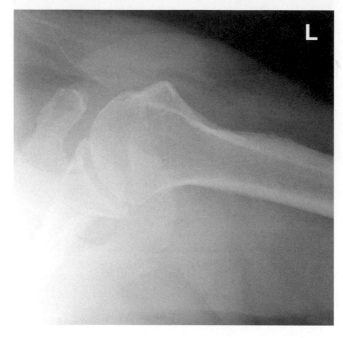

51. Figure 5-8: _____

_____

_____

Figure 5-9

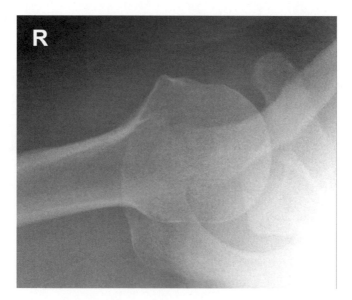

52. Figure 5-9: _____

_____

_____

Figure 5-10

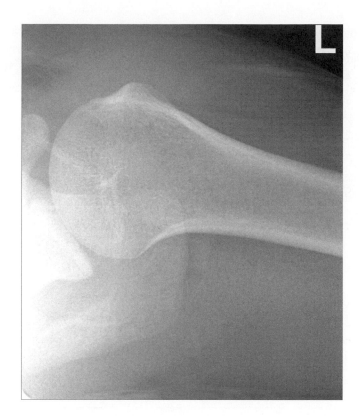

53. Figure 5-10: _____

_____

_____

Shoulder: Anteroposterior Oblique Projection (Grashey Method)

54. Identify the labeled anatomy in Figure 5-11.

Figure 5-11

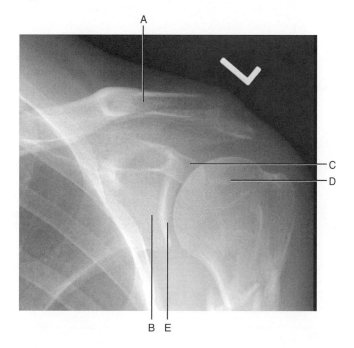

A. _____

B. _____

C. _____

D. _____

E. _____

55. Complete the statements below referring to AP oblique shoulder projection analysis criteria.

Anteroposterior Oblique Projection (Grashey Method) Analysis Criteria
• The glenoid cavity is in _____ (A) with the open glenohumeral joint space.
• The lateral coracoid process is superimposing the humeral head by about _____ (B).
• The _____ (C) is at the center of the exposure field.

56. Define shoulder protraction. _____

57. The _____ (A) and _____ (B) joints function cooperatively to allow the shoulder to be protracted.

58. The scapular body is positioned parallel with the IR for the AP oblique shoulder projection by aligning an imaginary

line connecting the _____ (A) and _____ (B) perpendicular to the IR.

59. A 45-degree oblique is routinely used for the AP oblique shoulder projection. List three situations in which the patient requires more than 45 degrees of obliquity to obtain an AP oblique shoulder projection with accurate positioning.

A. _____

B. _____

C. _____

60. Where is the coracoid process positioned with reference to the humeral head on an AP oblique shoulder projection with accurate rotation?

A. _____

_____

How will this relationship change if the patient is overrotated for the AP oblique shoulder projection?

B. _____

Underrotated?

C. _____

61. How is the clavicle positioned on an AP oblique shoulder projection with accurate rotation that was exposed with

the patient recumbent? _____

62. Accurate central ray centering on an AP oblique shoulder projection is accomplished by centering a

_____ (A) central ray 1 inch (2.5 cm) _____ (B) and _____ (C) to

the _____ (D).

63. Which anatomic structures are demonstrated within the collimated field on an AP oblique shoulder projection with accurate positioning?

_____

_____

For the following descriptions of AP oblique shoulder projections with poor positioning, state how the patient would have been mispositioned for such a projection to be obtained.

64. The glenohumeral joint space is closed, approximately 0.5 inch (1.25 cm) of the coracoid process is superimposed over the humeral head, and the clavicle demonstrates excessive transverse foreshortening.

_____

65. The glenohumeral joint space is closed, the lateral tip of the coracoid process is not superimposed over the humeral head, and the clavicle demonstrates little foreshortening.

_____

66. Recumbent patient: The glenohumeral joint is closed, and the clavicle is superimposed over the scapular neck.

_____

For the following AP oblique shoulder projections with poor positioning, state which anatomic structures are misaligned and how the patient should be repositioned for an optimal projection to be obtained.

Figure 5-12

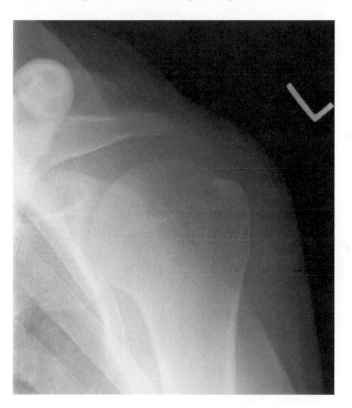

67. Figure 5-12: _____

_____

_____

Figure 5-13

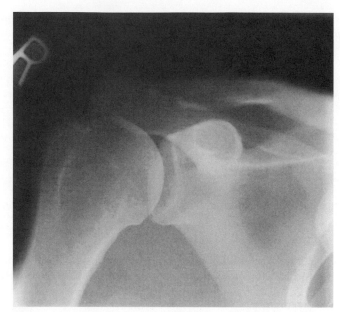

68. Figure 5-13: _____

_____

_____

Shoulder: Posteroanterior Oblique Projection (Scapular Y)

69. Identify the labeled anatomy in Figure 5-14.

Figure 5-14

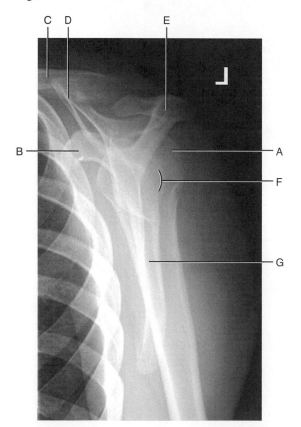

A. _____

B. _____

C. _____

D. _____

E. _____

F. _____

G. _____

70. Complete the statements below referring to PA oblique (scapular Y) shoulder projection analysis criteria.

Posteroanterior Oblique (Scapular Y) Shoulder Projection Analysis Criteria
• The scapula demonstrates the least possible magnification.
• The lateral and vertebral scapular borders are _____ (A).
• The scapular body and the _____ (B) and _____ (C) form a Y.
• The relationship between humeral head and glenoid cavity is demonstrated.
• The superior scapular angle is superimposed over the _____ (D).
• The _____ (E) is at the center of the exposure field.

71. Why is a PA oblique projection chosen over an AP oblique projection when obtaining a scapular Y shoulder image?

   A. _____

   B. _____

72. Which anatomic structures make up the arms of the Y formation demonstrated on a PA oblique shoulder projection?

   A. _____

   B. _____

   Which anatomic structure makes up the leg of the Y formation?

   C. _____

   Which anatomic structure is located at the converging point of the arms and leg of the Y?

   D. _____

73. Allowing the arm to dangle freely for the PA oblique shoulder projection places which border of the scapula parallel with the IR when the patient is accurately positioned?

   _____

74. The scapular body is placed in a lateral projection for the PA oblique shoulder projection by rotating the patient until

   an imaginary line is drawn between the _____ (A) and _____ (B) is aligned parallel with the IR.

75. List two indications for the PA oblique (scapular Y) projection.

   A. _____

   B. _____

76. For a PA oblique (scapular Y) shoulder projection the patient is rotated toward the _____ (affected/unaffected) (A) shoulder. For an AP oblique (scapular Y) shoulder projection the patient is rotated toward the

   _____ (affected/unaffected) (B) shoulder.

77. How can one distinguish the medial and lateral scapular borders from each other on a PA oblique shoulder projection with poor positioning?

   _____

78. If the patient is overrotated or underrotated for a PA oblique shoulder projection, how can one determine from the projection how the patient should be repositioned?

_____

79. Where are the humeral head and shaft positioned on a nondislocated PA oblique shoulder projection?

_____

_____

80. If the patient's shoulder is dislocated, should the Y formation desired on the PA oblique shoulder projection be visualized? _____ (Yes/No)

81. Where is the humeral head positioned on the AP oblique shoulder projection if the shoulder is dislocated anteriorly?

A. _____

If the shoulder is dislocated posteriorly?

B. _____

82. How can the patient be positioned to prevent longitudinal foreshortening of the scapula on a PA oblique shoulder projection?

_____

83. What spinal condition results in longitudinal scapular foreshortening on a PA oblique shoulder projection?

A. _____

How can the central ray be adjusted to offset this foreshortening when obtaining a PA oblique projection?

B. _____

How can the central ray be adjusted to offset this foreshortening when obtaining an AP oblique projection?

C. _____

84. Accurate central ray centering on a PA oblique shoulder projection is accomplished by centering a _____ (A) central ray to the _____ (B) border of the scapula halfway between the _____ (C) and _____ (D).

85. Which anatomic structures are demonstrated on a PA oblique shoulder projection with accurate positioning?

_____

For the following descriptions of PA oblique (scapular Y) shoulder projections with poor positioning, state how the patient would have been mispositioned for such a projection to be obtained.

86. The vertebral and lateral borders of the scapular body are demonstrated without superimposition, the lateral scapular border is demonstrated next to the ribs, and the medial border appears laterally.

_____

87. The lateral and medial borders of the scapula are demonstrated without superimposition, the thicker scapular border is demonstrated laterally, and the thinner scapular border is demonstrated next to the ribs.

_____

88. The scapular body, acromion process, and coracoid process demonstrate a Y formation, but the superior scapular angle is demonstrated superior to the coracoid process and the scapular spine is demonstrated superior to the clavicle.

For the following AP oblique (scapular Y) shoulder projections with poor positioning, state which anatomic structures are misaligned and how the patient should be repositioned for an optimal projection to be obtained.

Figure 5-15

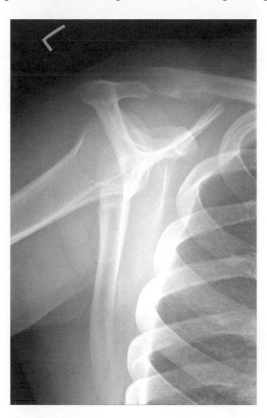

89. Figure 5-15: _____

_____

_____

Figure 5-16

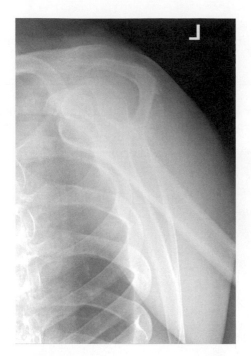

90. Figure 5-16: _____

_____

_____

Figure 5-17

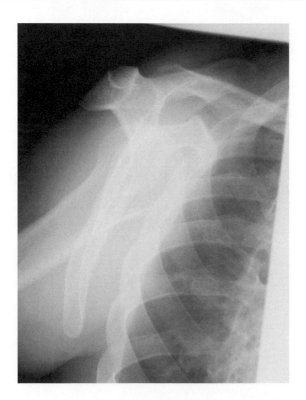

91. Figure 5-17: _____

_____

_____

Figure 5-18

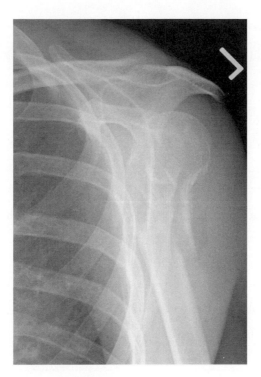

92. Figure 5-18 (trauma): _____

_____

_____

Proximal Humerus: Anteroposterior Axial Projection (Stryker "Notch" Method)

93. Identify the labeled anatomy in Figure 5-19.

Figure 5-19

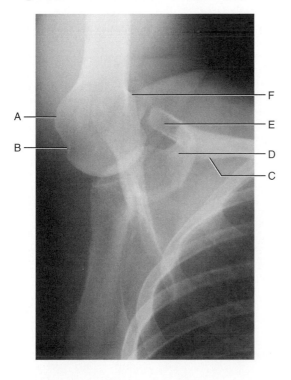

A. _____

B. _____

C. _____

D. _____

E. _____

F. _____

94. Complete the statements below referring to AP axial shoulder projection analysis criteria.

Anteroposterior Axial Shoulder Projection (Stryker Notch Method) Analysis Criteria
• The coracoid process is situated directly lateral to the _____ (A) of the clavicle.
• The _____ (B) aspect of the humeral head is in profile laterally, and the greater and lesser tubercles are seen in partial profile.
• The _____ (C) is superimposed over the lateral clavicle.
• The _____ (D) is at the center of the exposure field.

95. The AP axial shoulder projection is performed to diagnose the presence of the _____ (A) defect of the shoulder. When present, the defect is demonstrated on the _____ (B) aspect of the humeral head.

96. For the AP axial shoulder projection, the affected arm is elevated until the humerus is _____ (A), and then the elbow is flexed and the palm of the hand is placed _____ (B).

97. Accurate central ray centering on an AP axial projection is accomplished when the central ray is centered to the _____.

98. Which anatomic structures are demonstrated on an AP axial projection with accurate positioning?

_____

For the following descriptions of AP axial shoulder projections (Stryker Notch Method) with poor positioning, state how the patient would have been mispositioned for such a projection to be obtained.

99. The coracoid process is seen inferior to the clavicle, and the humeral shaft demonstrates increased foreshortening.

_____

100. The lesser tubercle is seen in profile medially, but the greater tubercle and posterolateral humeral head are obscured.

_____

101. The posterolateral humeral head is obscured, and the humeral shaft demonstrates increased foreshortening.

_____

For the following AP axial shoulder projections (Stryker Notch Method) with poor positioning, state which anatomic structures are misaligned and how the patient should be repositioned for an optimal projection to be obtained.

Figure 5-20

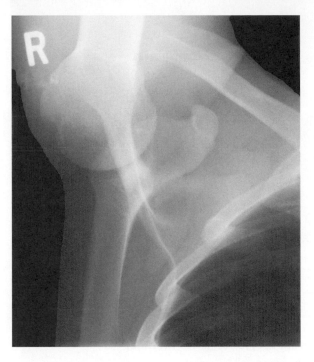

102. Figure 5-20: _____

_____

_____

Figure 5-21

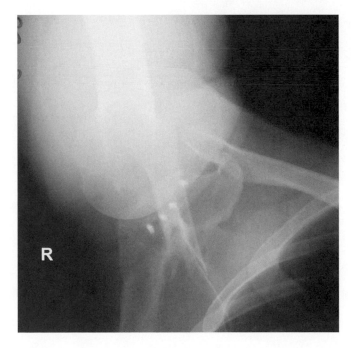

103. Figure 5-21: _____

_____

_____

Figure 5-22

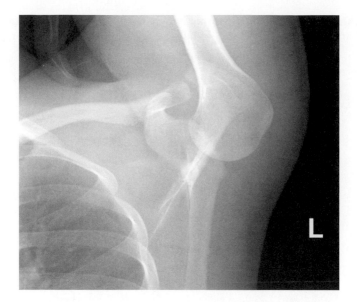

104. Figure 5-22: _____

_____

_____

Supraspinatus "Outlet": Tangential Projection (Neer Method)

105. Identify the labeled anatomy in Figure 5-23.

Figure 5-23

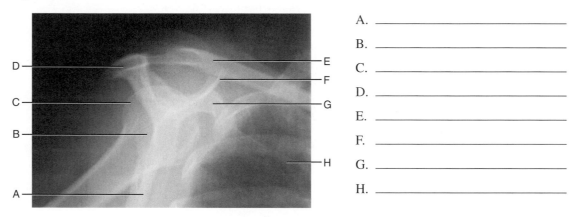

A. _____

B. _____

C. _____

D. _____

E. _____

F. _____

G. _____

H. _____

106. Complete the statements below referring to tangential supraspinatus outlet projection analysis criteria.

> **Tangential Supraspinatus Outlet Projection (Neer Method) Analysis Criteria**
>
> - The lateral and vertebral scapular borders are _____ (A).
> - The _____ (B), _____ (C), and _____ (D) form
>   a Y, with the glenoid cavity demonstrated on end.
> - The lateral clavicle and acromion process form a smooth continuous arch, the superior scapular angle is
>   at the level of the _____ (E) and is positioned about 0.5 inch (1.25 cm) inferior to the
>   _____ (F).
> - The _____ (G) is at the center of the exposure field.

107. Should the patient be placed in an AP or PA oblique projection to obtain a tangential outlet projection with the least scapular magnification and the greatest scapular detail?

_____

108. Allowing the arm to dangle freely for the tangential outlet projection places which border of the scapula parallel with the IR when the patient is accurately positioned?

A. _____

How much should the patient be rotated when the arm is in this position?

B. _____

109. How can one distinguish the medial and lateral scapular borders from each other on a tangential outlet shoulder projection with poor positioning?

_____

_____

110. The tangential outlet projection is taken to identify osteophyte formation on the _____ surfaces of the lateral clavicle and acromion angle.

111. Accurate central ray centering on a tangential outlet shoulder projection is accomplished when the _____ (A) plane is vertical and the central ray is angled _____ (B).

112. Which anatomic structures should be included within the collimated field?

_____

_____

For the following descriptions of tangential outlet shoulder projections (Neer Method) with poor positioning, state how the patient would have been mispositioned for such a projection to be obtained.

113. The vertebral and lateral borders of the scapular body are demonstrated without superimposition, the lateral scapular border is demonstrated next to the ribs, and the medial border appears laterally.

_____

114. The lateral clavicle and acromion process are demonstrated less than 0.5 inch (1.25 cm) superior to the humeral head and supraspinous fossa, and the superior scapular spine appears superior to the clavicle.

_____

For the following tangential outlet shoulder projections (Neer Method) with poor positioning, state which anatomic structures are misaligned and how the patient should be repositioned for an optimal projection to be obtained.

Figure 5-24

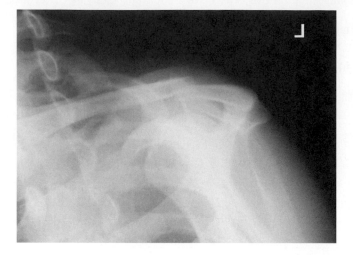

115. Figure 5-24: _____

_____

_____

Figure 5-25

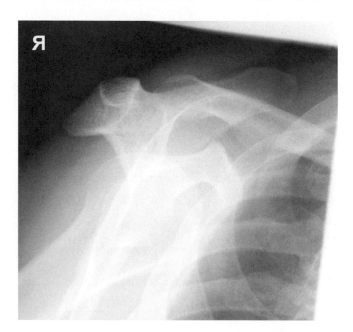

116. Figure 5-25: _____

_____

_____

Clavicle: Anteroposterior Projection

117. Identify the labeled anatomy in Figure 5-26

Figure 5-26

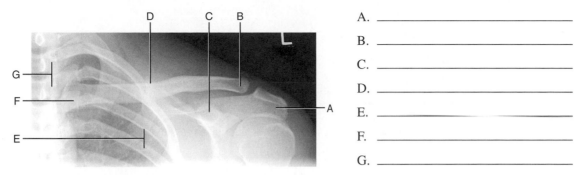

A. _____

B. _____

C. _____

D. _____

E. _____

F. _____

G. _____

118. Complete the statements below referring to AP clavicle projection analysis criteria.

Anteroposterior Clavicle Projection Analysis Criteria
• The medial clavicular end lies next to the _____ (A) of the vertebral column.
• The midclavicle is superimposed on the _____ (B).
• The _____ (C) is at the center of the exposure field.

119. Where is the compensating filter positioned for an AP clavicular projection to demonstrate uniform density of the clavicle?

_____

120. Which projection demonstrates the clavicle with the least magnification?

A. _____

Why is it uncommon for this projection to be used?

B. _____

121. How can the technologist position the patient to prevent rotation on an AP clavicular projection?

_____

122. What patient mispositioning causes inferosuperior clavicular foreshortening on an AP clavicular projection?

_____

123. Accurate central ray centering on an AP clavicular is accomplished by centering a _____ (A) central ray halfway between the _____ (B) and _____ (C) ends of the clavicle.

124. Which anatomic structures are demonstrated on an AP clavicular projection with accurate positioning?

_____

_____

For the following descriptions of AP clavicular projections with poor positioning, state how the patient would have been mispositioned for such a projection to be obtained.

125. The medial clavicular end is superimposed over the vertebral column, and the vertebral border of the scapula is positioned away from the thoracic cavity.

_____

126. The medial clavicular end is placed 1 inch (2.5 cm) away from the vertebral column, and the lateral border of the scapula is mostly superimposed by the thoracic cavity.

_____

127. The lateral clavicular end is superimposed over the scapular spine, and the superior scapular angle is projected above the midclavicle.

_____

For the following AP clavicular projections with poor positioning, state which anatomic structures are misaligned and how the patient should be repositioned for an optimal projection to be obtained.

Figure 5-27

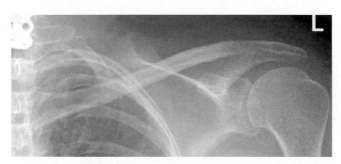

128. Figure 5-27: _____

_____

_____

Figure 5-28

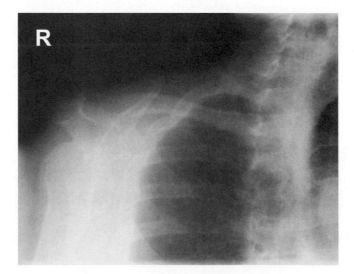

129. Figure 5-28: _____

_____

_____

Clavicle: Anteroposterior Axial Projection (Lordotic Position)

130. Identify the labeled anatomy in Figure 5-29.

Figure 5-29

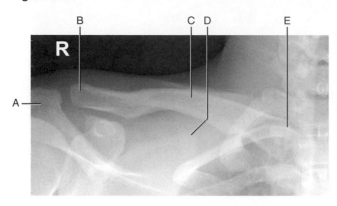

A. _____

B. _____

C. _____

D. _____

E. _____

131. Complete the statements below, referring to AP axial clavicle projection analysis criteria.

Anteroposterior Axial Clavicle Projection Analysis Criteria
• The _____ (A) of the clavicle lies next to the lateral edge of the vertebral column.
• The medial end of the clavicle is superimposed over the _____ (B) rib.
• The middle and lateral thirds of clavicle are seen superior to the _____ (C) and the clavicle bows upwardly.
• The _____ (D) is at the center of the exposure field.

132. What are the degree and direction of central ray angulation used for the AP axial clavicular projection?

_____

133. Where do most fractures of the clavicle occur? _____

134. Accurate central ray centering on an AP axial clavicular projection is accomplished by centering the central ray

halfway between the _____ (A) and _____ (B) ends of the clavicle.

135. Which anatomic structures are demonstrated on an AP axial clavicular projection with accurate positioning?

_____

For the following descriptions of AP axial clavicular projections with poor positioning, state how the patient would have been mispositioned or the central ray aligned for such a projection to be obtained.

136. The medial clavicular end is drawn away from the vertebral column, the vertebral and lateral borders of the scapula are superimposed by the thoracic cavity, and the clavicle is longitudinally foreshortened.

_____

137. The lateral and middle thirds of the clavicle are superimposed over the scapula.

_____

For the following AP axial clavicular projection with poor positioning, state which anatomic structures are misaligned and how the patient should be repositioned for an optimal projection to be obtained.

Figure 5-30

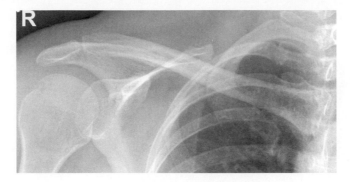

138. Figure 5-30: _____

_____

_____

Acromioclavicular Joint: Anteroposterior Projection

139. Identify the labeled anatomy in Figure 5-31.

Figure 5-31

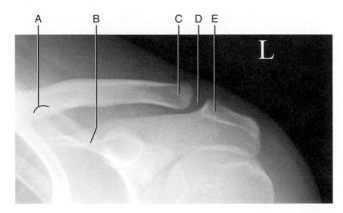

A. _____

B. _____

C. _____

D. _____

E. _____

140. Complete the statements below referring to AP acromioclavicular (AC) joint projection analysis criteria.

Anteroposterior Acromioclavicular Joint Projection Analysis Criteria
• The weight-bearing projection displays a _____ (A) marker to indicate that it is the weight-bearing projection.
• The lateral clavicle is almost _____ (B), and about 0.125 inch (0.3 cm) of space is present between the lateral clavicle and acromial apex.
• The lateral clavicle demonstrates minimal _____ (C) superimposition, and the midclavicle is superimposed over the _____ (D).
• The _____ (E) is at the center of the exposure field.

141. Define the following terms.

   A. Weight-bearing: _____

   B. Unilateral: _____

   C. Bilateral: _____

142. Why is it necessary to use an "arrow" or "word" marker on the weight-bearing AC joint projection?

   A. _____

   How is the arrow marker placed on the IR?

   B. _____

143. How is the patient positioned to ensure that an AP AC joint projection is obtained?

   _____

   _____

144. Why are weight- and non–weight-bearing AP AC joint projections often requested?

   _____

   _____

145. How is an AC ligament injury identified on an AP AC joint projection?

   _____

   _____

146. How much weight does the patient hold in each arm for the weight-bearing AC joint projection?

   _____

147. What mispositioning causes inferosuperior clavicular foreshortening on an AP AC joint projection?

   A. _____

   How can this foreshortening be identified on an AP AC joint projection?

   B. _____

148. Accurate central ray centering on a unilateral AP AC joint is accomplished by centering the central ray 0.5 inch (1 cm) _____ (A) to the _____ (B).

149. Which anatomic structures are demonstrated on an AP AC joint projection with accurate positioning?

   _____

150. Why is it necessary to place the central ray at the same area when weight- and non–weight-bearing projections are requested?

   _____

   _____

For the following description of an AP AC joint projection with poor positioning, state how the patient would have been mispositioned for such a projection to be obtained.

151. The left AC joint is closed, and the scapular body demonstrates an increased amount of thoracic superimposition.

_____

For the following AC joint projection with poor positioning, state which anatomic structures are misaligned and how the patient should be repositioned for an optimal projection to be obtained.

Figure 5-32

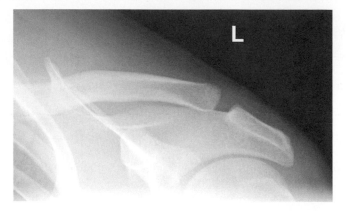

152. Figure 5-32: _____

_____

_____

Scapula: Anteroposterior Projection

153. Identify the labeled anatomy in Figure 5-33.

Figure 5-33

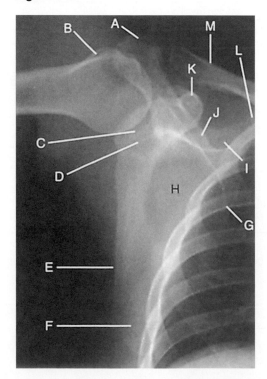

A. _____

B. _____

C. _____

D. _____

E. _____

F. _____

G. _____

H. _____

I. _____

J. _____

K. _____

L. _____

M. _____

154. Complete the statements below referring to AP scapula projection analysis criteria.

> **Anteroposterior Scapula Projection Analysis Criteria**
>
> - The anterior and posterior margins of the _____ (A) are almost superimposed.
> - The superior scapular angle is about 0.25 inch (0.6 cm) inferior to the _____ (B).
> - The lateral border of scapula is seen without _____ (C) superimposition, and the supraspinatus fossa and superior angle of the scapular are seen without superimposition of the clavicle.
> - The thoracic cavity is superimposed over the vertebral border of the scapula.
> - The humeral shaft demonstrates 90 degrees of abduction.
> - The _____ (D) is at the center of the exposure field.

155. Even though the AP thickness is approximately the same across the scapula, why is the projection density not uniform over all parts of the scapula?

_____

_____

156. If a breathing technique cannot be used for the AP scapular projection, what respiration should be used?

_____

157. List the two dimensions that are foreshortened on a scapular projection with poor positioning.

A. _____

B. _____

158. What degree of scapular rotation is demonstrated when the patient is positioned in an AP projection with the humerus resting against the side?

A. _____

Which scapular dimension is foreshortened in this position?

B. _____

159. How is the patient positioned for an AP projection of the scapula to be obtained?

A. _____

_____

What effect does the position you described in A have on the shoulder when the projection is obtained with the patient in a supine position?

B. _____

What effect does the position have on the visualization of the glenoid cavity on an AP scapular projection?

C. _____

160. What scapular dimension is foreshortened when the patient's midcoronal plane is poorly positioned?

_____

161. Accurate central ray centering on an AP scapular projection is accomplished by centering a _____

   (A) central ray _____ (B) inches _____ (C) to the palpable coracoid process.

162. Which anatomic structures are included on an AP scapular projection with accurate positioning?

   _____

   _____

For the following descriptions of AP scapular projections with poor positioning, state how the patient would have been mispositioned for such a projection to be obtained.

163. The glenoid cavity is not in profile, and approximately 0.5 inch (1 cm) of it is demonstrated.

   _____

   _____

164. A projection of a patient who was very mobile demonstrates the inferior scapular angle and inferolateral scapular border with thoracic cavity superimposition.

   _____

   _____

For the following AP scapular projections with poor positioning, state which anatomic structures are misaligned and how the patient should be repositioned for an optimal projection to be obtained.

Figure 5-34

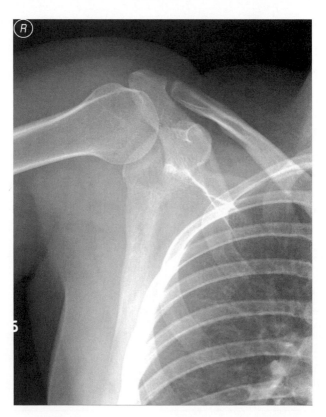

165. Figure 5-34: _____

   _____

   _____

Figure 5-35

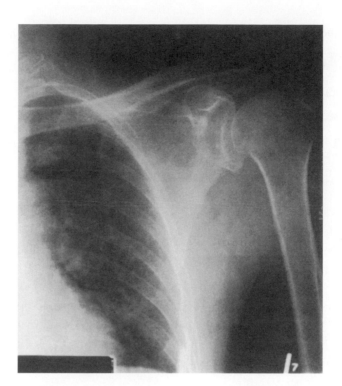

166. Figure 5-35: _____

_____

_____

Scapula: Lateral Projection (Lateromedial or Mediolateral)

167. Identify the labeled anatomy in Figure 5-36.

Figure 5-36

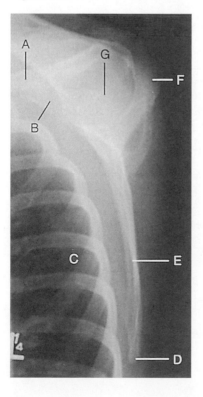

A. _____

B. _____

C. _____

D. _____

E. _____

F. _____

G. _____

168. Complete the statements below referring to lateral scapula projection analysis criteria.

> **Lateral Scapula Projection Analysis Criteria**
>
> - The lateral and vertebral scapular borders are _____ (A).
> - The scapular body is seen without superimposing the thoracic cavity.
> - The humerus is drawn away from the superior scapular body, and the _____ (B) is superimposed over the coracoid process base.
> - The _____ (C) is at the center of the exposure field.

169. The lateral scapula is projectioned with the patient placed in an AP or a PA oblique projection. For the AP oblique projection, the patient is rotated _____ (toward/away from) (A) the affected scapula. In the PA oblique projection, the patient is rotated _____ (toward/away from) (B) the affected scapula.

170. What patient positioning procedure determines the degree of obliquity needed to place the scapula in a lateral projection?

_____

171. Which border of the scapula has a thick, rough-appearing cortical outline? _____

172. How is rotation identified on a lateral scapular projection with poor positioning?

_____

173. Most scapular fractures occur at the _____ (A) and _____ (B) of the scapula.

174. What humeral position with respect to the body places the long axis of the scapula parallel with the IR for a lateral scapular projection?

_____

175. What humeral position with respect to the body places the lateral border of the scapula parallel with the IR for a lateral scapular projection?

_____

176. The higher the humerus is elevated for a lateral scapular projection, the _____ (more/less) (A) the patient needs to be rotated to obtain accurate positioning. Why? (B) _____

_____

_____

177. Accurate central ray centering on a lateral scapular projection is accomplished by centering a _____ (A) central ray 1 inch (2.5 cm) _____ (B) to the vertebral border halfway between the _____ (C) angle and _____ (D).

178. Which anatomic structures are included on a lateral scapular projection with accurate positioning?

_____

_____

For the following descriptions of lateral scapular projections with poor positioning, state how the patient would have been mispositioned for such a projection to be obtained.

179. The lateral and vertebral borders of the scapula are demonstrated without superimposition, the thick border is next to the ribs, and the thin border is demonstrated laterally.

_____

180. The lateral and vertebral borders of the scapula are demonstrated without superimposition, the lateral border is demonstrated laterally, and the vertebral border appears next to the ribs.

_____

For the following lateral scapular projections with poor positioning, state which anatomic structures are misaligned and how the patient should be repositioned for an optimal projection to be obtained.

Figure 5-37

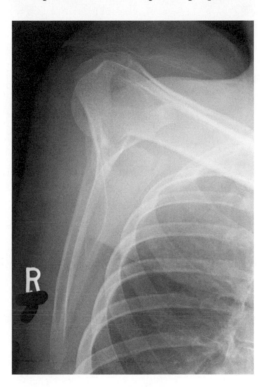

181. Figure 5-37: _____

_____

_____

Figure 5-38

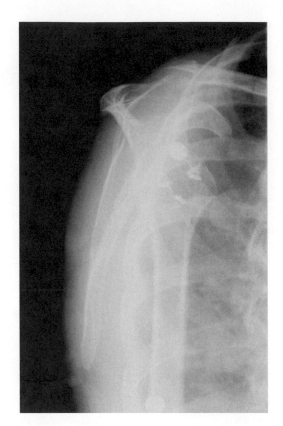

182. Figure 5-38: _____

_____

_____

6 Lower Extremity

STUDY QUESTIONS

1. Describe how the following lower extremity projections should be displayed on a view box or digital monitor.

   A. AP toe: _____

   B. Lateral ankle: _____

   C. AP oblique ankle: _____

   D. Lateral knee: _____

2. State the kilovoltage (kVp) range for the following projections.

   A. Lateral ankle: _____

   B. Grid, AP knee: _____

   C. AP femur: _____

3. Match the term with its definition.

   _____ A. Abductor tubercle
   _____ B. Dorsiflex
   _____ C. Intermalleolar line
   _____ D. Lateral mortise
   _____ E. Plantar
   _____ F. Plantar-flex
   _____ G. Subluxation
   _____ H. Tarsal sinus
   _____ I. Valgus deformity
   _____ J. Varus deformity

   1. Partial dislocation
   2. Sole of foot
   3. Located posteriorly on medial femoral condyle
   4. Act of moving toes and forefoot downward
   5. Lateral side of knee joint is narrower
   6. Opening between the calcaneus and talus
   7. Line connecting medial and lateral malleoli
   8. Medial side of knee joint narrower
   9. Act of moving toes and forefoot upward
   10. Tibiofibular joint

Toe: Anteroposterior Axial Projection

4. Identify the labeled anatomy in Figure 6-1.

Figure 6-1

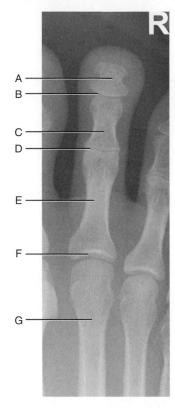

A. _____

B. _____

C. _____

D. _____

E. _____

F. _____

G. _____

5. Complete the statements below referring to AP axial toe projection analysis criteria.

Anteroposterior Axial Toe(s) Projection Analysis Criteria

- The soft tissue width and midshaft concavity are equal on both sides of phalanges.

- The _____ (A) and _____ (B) joints are open and the phalanges are seen without foreshortening.

- No soft tissue or bony overlap from adjacent digits is present.

- The _____ (C) joint is at the center of the exposure field for a toe projection and

  the _____ (D) MTP joint is at the center when all toes are projectioned.

MTP, Metatarsophalangeal.

6. For an AP axial toe projection, equal pressure is placed on the _____ (A) foot surface and the

   _____ (B), _____ (C), and _____ (D) should remain aligned.

7. If the toe is medially rotated for a right AP axial toe projection, which side of the toe demonstrates the greatest soft tissue width?

   A. _____(lateral/medial)

The greatest phalangeal midshaft concavity?

B. _____ (lateral/medial)

8. When the toenail is visualized on an AP toe projection, it can be used to identify the direction of patient rotation. If the first toenail is rotated medially, in what direction was the patient's foot rotated?

_____

9. To obtain open joint spaces on an AP axial toe projection, align the central ray _____ (A) to the joint space and align the joint space _____ (B) to the image receptor (IR).

10. The long axis of the affected toe is aligned with the long axis of the _____ for toe projections to obtain tight collimation.

11. How is the patient positioned for an AP axial toe projection to prevent soft tissue overlap of adjacent toes onto the affected toe?

_____

12. On an AP axial toe projection with accurate positioning, the _____ is centered within the collimated field.

13. Which anatomic structures are included on an AP axial toe projection with accurate positioning?

_____

For the following descriptions of AP axial toe projections with poor positioning, state how the patient would have been mispositioned for such a projection to be obtained.

14. The phalanges demonstrate more soft tissue width on the medial toe surface, and the outline of the toenail is visualized toward the lateral toe surface.

_____

15. The phalanges demonstrate more midshaft concavity on the lateral surface of the toe than the medial surface.

_____

16. The interphalangeal (IP) and metatarsophalangeal (MTP) joint spaces are closed, and the phalanges are foreshortened.

_____

For the following AP axial toe projections with poor positioning, state which anatomic structures are misaligned and how the patient should be repositioned for an optimal projection to be obtained.

Figure 6-2

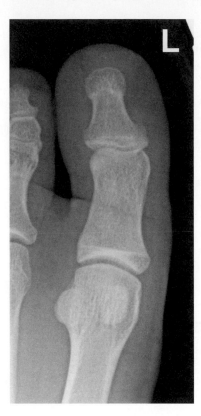

17. Figure 6-2: _____

_____

_____

_____

Toe: Anteroposterior Oblique Projection

18. Identify the labeled anatomy in Figure 6-3.

Figure 6-3

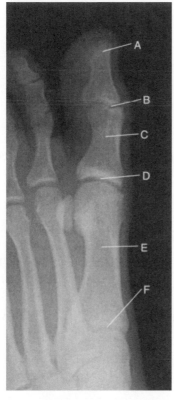

A. _____

B. _____

C. _____

D. _____

E. _____

F. _____

19. Complete the statements below referring to AP oblique toe projection analysis criteria.

Anteroposterior Oblique Toe(s) Projection Analysis Criteria
• _____ (A) as much soft tissue width and more phalangeal and metatarsal concavity are present on the side of the digit rotated _____ (B) the IR.
• The _____ (C) and _____ (D) joint(s) are open and the phalanges are demonstrated without foreshortening.
• No soft tissue or bony overlap from adjacent digits.
• The _____ (E) joint is at the center of the exposure field for a toe projection and third MTP joint is at the center when all toes are projectioned.

IR, Image receptor; *MTP*, metatarsophalangeal.

20. What degree of patient toe obliquity is used for an AP oblique toe projection?

A. _____

How is the accuracy of the degree of toe obliquity identified on an AP oblique toe projection?

B. _____

21. In what direction are the foot and toe rotated for a first through third AP oblique toe projection?

A. _____

For a fourth through fifth AP oblique toe projection?

B. _____

Why are the patient's foot and toe rotated differently for these examinations?

C. _____

22. The patient was unable to extend the toe fully for an AP oblique toe projection. What will the resulting projection demonstrate if a perpendicular central ray was used for this patient?

_____

23. The _____ is at the center of the collimated field on an AP oblique toe projection with accurate positioning.

24. Which anatomic structures are included on an AP oblique toe projection with accurate positioning?

_____

25. To ensure that half of the affected toe's metatarsal is included on an AP oblique toe projection, the longitudinally collimated field should extend 2 inches (5 cm) proximal to the _____.

For the following descriptions of AP oblique toe projections with poor positioning, state how the patient would have been mispositioned for such a projection to be obtained.

26. The soft tissue width demonstrated on each side of the phalanges is almost equal.

_____

27. The proximal phalanx demonstrates more concavity on the posterior aspect than on the anterior aspect.

_____

28. The IP and MTP joint spaces are obscured and the phalanges foreshortened.

_____

For the following AP oblique toe projections with poor positioning, state which anatomic structures are misaligned and how the patient should be repositioned for such a projection to be obtained.

Figure 6-4

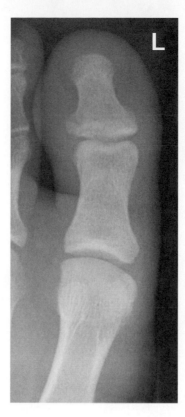

29. Figure 6-4: _____

_____

_____

_____

Figure 6-5

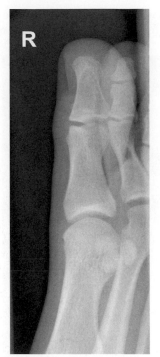

30. Figure 6-5: _____

_____

_____

_____

Figure 6-6

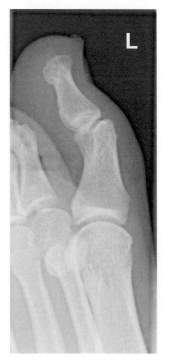

31. Figure 6-6: _____

_____

_____

Toe: Lateral Projection

32. Identify the labeled anatomy in Figure 6-7.

Figure 6-7

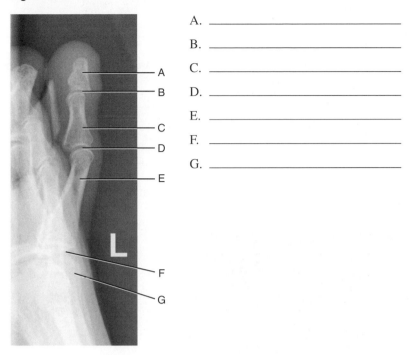

A. _____

B. _____

C. _____

D. _____

E. _____

F. _____

G. _____

33. Complete the statements below referring to lateral toe projection analysis criteria.

Lateral Toe Projection Analysis Criteria
• The _____ (A) surface of the proximal phalanx demonstrates more concavity than the _____ (B) surface, and the condyles of the proximal phalanx are superimposed.
• There is no soft tissue or bony overlap from adjacent toes.
• The _____ (C) joint is at the center of the exposure field.

34. To position the toe in a lateral projection, the foot is rotated _____ (medially/laterally) (A) when the first, second, and third toes are imaged and _____ (medially/laterally) (B) when the fourth and fifth toes are imaged.

35. Where is the toenail demonstrated on a lateral toe projection with accurate positioning? _____

36. Accurate central ray centering on a lateral toe projection is accomplished by centering a _____ (A) central ray to the _____ (B).

37. Which anatomic structures are included on a lateral toe projection with accurate positioning?

_____

For the following descriptions of lateral toe projections with poor positioning, state how the patient would have been mispositioned for such a projection to be obtained.

38. The proximal phalanx demonstrates almost equal midshaft concavity, the condyles appear without superimposition, and the metatarsal heads appear without superimposition.

_____

39. The proximal phalanx demonstrates almost equal midshaft concavity, the condyles are shown without superimposition, and the metatarsal heads are slightly superimposed.

_____

40. Soft tissue and bony overlap of unaffected digits onto the affected digit are present.

_____

For the following lateral toe projections with poor positioning, state which anatomic structures are misaligned and how the patient should be repositioned for an optimal projection to be obtained.

Figure 6-8

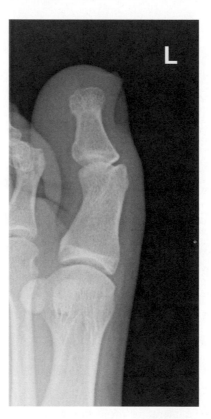

41. Figure 6-8: _____

_____

_____

_____

Figure 6-9

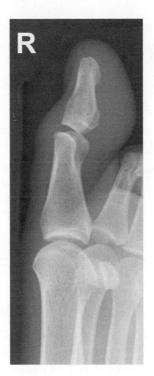

42. Figure 6-9: _____

_____

_____

_____

Foot: Anteroposterior Axial Projection (Dorsoplantar Projection)

43. Identify the labeled anatomy in Figure 6-10.

Figure 6-10

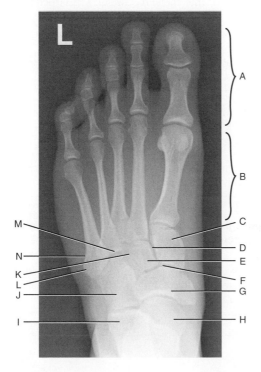

A. _____

B. _____

C. _____

D. _____

E. _____

F. _____

G. _____

H. _____

I. _____

J. _____

K. _____

L. _____

M. _____

N. _____

44. Complete the statements below referring to AP axial foot projection analysis criteria.

> **Anteroposterior Axial Foot Projection Analysis Criteria**
>
> - The foot demonstrates uniform density across the phalanges, metatarsals, and tarsals.
> - The joint space between the _____ (A) and _____ (B) cuneiforms is open, about _____ inch (C) of the calcaneus is demonstrated without talar superimposition, and concavity on both sides of the first metatarsal midshaft is equal.
> - The _____ (D) and navicular-cuneiform joint spaces are open.
> - The _____ (E) metatarsal base is at the center of the exposure field.

45. When an exposure is set that adequately demonstrates the proximal metatarsals and tarsals, the distal metatarsals and phalanges are overexposed. Why does this density variation exist?

   A. _____

   How can the positioning setup be adjusted to obtain uniform projection density over the entire foot?

   B. _____

46. The MTP joints of the foot are located _____ (A) inch _____ (B) to the toe interconnecting tissue.

47. For an AP axial foot projection, equal pressure is placed on the _____ (A) foot surface and the _____ (B), _____ (C), and _____ (D) should remain aligned.

48. Should the navicular tuberosity be demonstrated on an AP axial foot projection with accurate positioning? _____ (Yes/No)

49. Will medial or lateral foot rotation result in the talus moving away from the calcaneus? _____ (medial/lateral)

50. Will medial or lateral foot rotation result in increased superimposition of the metatarsal bases? _____ (medial/lateral)

51. A _____ (A) degree proximal angulation is required for an AP axial foot projection to demonstrate open joint spaces, with _____ (B) degrees needed in a patient with a low longitudinal arch and _____ (C) degrees needed for a high longitudinal arch.

52. Accurate central ray centering is demonstrated on an AP axial foot projection when the central ray is centered to the midline of the foot at a level _____ (A) inch distal to the _____ (B).

53. Which anatomic structures are included on an AP axial foot projection with accurate positioning?

   _____

For the following descriptions of AP axial foot projections with poor positioning, state how the patient or central ray would have been mispositioned for such a projection to be obtained.

54. The joint space between the medial and intermediate cuneiforms is closed, the navicular bone is demonstrated in profile, and less than 0.75 inch (2 cm) of the calcaneus is demonstrated without talar superimposition.

   _____

55. The joint space between the medial and intermediate cuneiforms is closed, the calcaneus is demonstrated without talar superimposition, and the metatarsal bases demonstrate decreased superimposition.

_____

56. The tarsometatarsal and navicular-cuneiform joint spaces are obscured.

_____

For the following AP axial foot projections with poor positioning, state which anatomic structures are misaligned and how the patient should be repositioned for an optimal projection to be obtained.

Figure 6-11

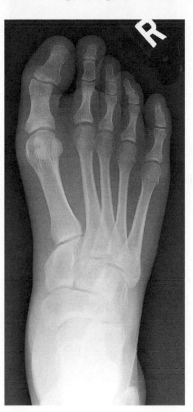

57. Figure 6-11: _____

_____

_____

_____

Figure 6-12

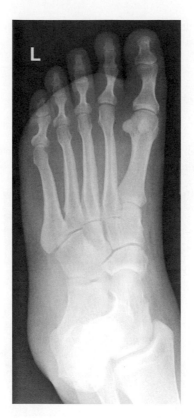

58. Figure 6-12: _____

_____

_____

_____

Foot: Anteroposterior Oblique Projection (Medial Rotation)

59. Identify the labeled anatomy in Figure 6-13.

Figure 6-13

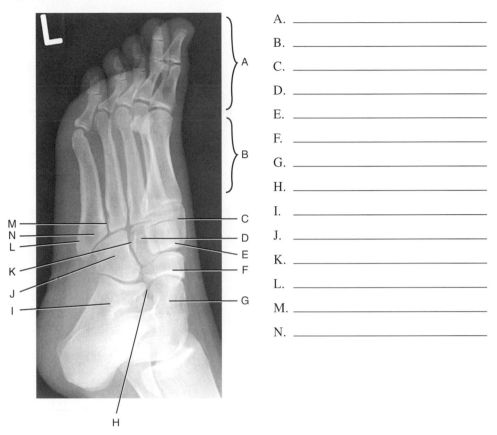

A. _____

B. _____

C. _____

D. _____

E. _____

F. _____

G. _____

H. _____

I. _____

J. _____

K. _____

L. _____

M. _____

N. _____

60. Complete the statements below referring to AP oblique foot projection analysis criteria.

Anteroposterior Oblique Foot Projection Analysis Criteria
• The foot demonstrates uniform density across the phalanges, metatarsals, and tarsals.
• The _____ (A) and _____ (B) intermetatarsal joint spaces are open.
• The tarsal sinus and _____ (C) metatarsal tuberosity are visualized.
• The _____ (D) base is at the center of the exposure field.

61. Which of the joint spaces that surround the cuboid is the first to close if the patient's foot is not adequately rotated?

_____

62. An AP oblique foot projection is obtained by rotating the patient 30 to 60 degrees _____ (medially/laterally).

63. The degree of foot obliquity needed for an AP oblique foot projection varies according to the height of the patient's longitudinal arch. What degree of obliquity is used in a patient with a high longitudinal arch?

A. _____

In a patient with a low longitudinal arch?

B. _____

On a patient with an average longitudinal arch?

C. _____

64. View the AP oblique foot projection in Figure 6-14. State whether the patient has a high or low longitudinal arch.

A. _____

How did you determine this?

B. _____

_____

65. View the lateral foot projections in Figures 6-15 and 6-17. State which projection was obtained from the patient with the higher longitudinal arch.

A. _____

How did you determine this difference?

B. _____

_____

66. As a patient's foot is rotated medially from an AP projection, the _____ (A) metatarsal base rotates beneath the _____ (B) metatarsal base and the second through third metatarsal heads move _____ (closer to/farther away from) (C) one another.

67. Is the fourth metatarsal tubercle or the fifth metatarsal located more posteriorly when the patient's foot is overrotated for an AP oblique foot projection?

A. _____

When the foot is medially rotated more than needed for an AP oblique foot projection, will the fourth metatarsal tubercle be superimposed over the fifth metatarsal or will the fifth metatarsal be superimposed over the fourth metatarsal?

B. _____

_____

68. Accurate central ray centering on an AP oblique foot projection is accomplished by centering a _____ (A) central ray to the _____ (B) of the foot at the level of the _____ (C).

69. Which anatomic structures are demonstrated within the collimated field on an AP oblique foot projection with accurate positioning? _____

_____

For the following descriptions of AP oblique foot projections with poor positioning, state how the patient would have been mispositioned for such a projection to be obtained.

70. The lateral cuneiform-cuboid, navicular-cuboid, and third through fifth intermetatarsal spaces are closed, and the fourth metatarsal tubercle is demonstrated without fifth metatarsal superimposition.

_____

71. The lateral cuneiform-cuboid, navicular-cuboid, and intermetatarsal joint spaces are closed, and the fifth metatarsal is superimposed over the fourth metatarsal tubercle.

_____

For the following AP oblique foot projection with poor positioning, state which anatomic structures are misaligned and how the patient should be repositioned for an optimal projection to be obtained.

Figure 6-14

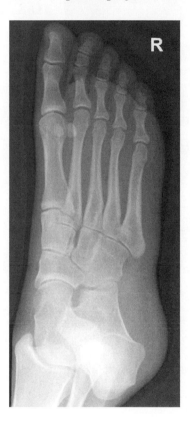

72. Figure 6-14: _____

_____

_____

_____

Foot: Lateral Projection (Mediolateral and Lateromedial)

73. Identify the labeled anatomy in Figure 6-15.

Figure 6-15

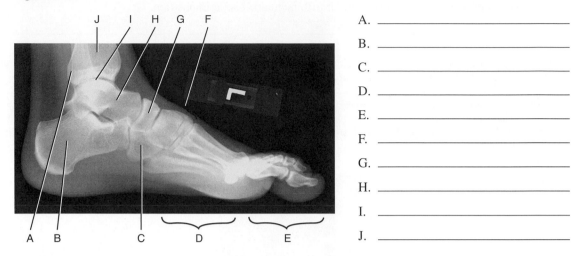

A. _____

B. _____

C. _____

D. _____

E. _____

F. _____

G. _____

H. _____

I. _____

J. _____

74. Complete the statements below referring to lateral foot projection analysis criteria.

Lateral Foot Projection Analysis Criteria
• Contrast and density are adequate to demonstrate the _____ (A) and _____ (B) fat pads.
• The talar domes are superimposed, the _____ (C) joint is open, and the distal fibula is superimposed by the posterior half of the distal tibia.
• The long axis of the foot is positioned at a 90-degree angle with the lower leg.
• The _____ (D) are at the center of the exposure field.

75. Which surface of the foot is positioned against the IR for a mediolateral projection of the foot? _____

76. List the two soft tissue fat pads that should be demonstrated on a lateral foot projection, and describe their locations.

   A. _____

   B. _____

77. How is the patient's lower leg placed to obtain a lateral foot projection with accurate positioning?

   _____

78. How is the patient's foot positioned with the lower leg and IR to obtain a lateral foot projection with accurate positioning?

   A. Lower leg: _____

   B. IR: _____

79. A lateral foot projection was requested for a patient with a large upper thigh that prevented the lower leg from aligning parallel with the imaging table when the patient was positioned. If the projection was obtained with the patient positioned in this manner, how would this poor positioning be identified on the resulting projection?

A. _____

How is the positioning setup adjusted in this situation before the projection is obtained?

B. _____

80. The height of the longitudinal arch can be determined on a lateral foot projection with accurate positioning by measuring the amount of cuboid that appears _____ (A) to the _____ (B).

81. The average foot projection demonstrates approximately _____ inch of the cuboid posterior to the navicular bone.

82. In a patient with a low foot arch, _____ (more/less) (A) of the cuboid will be demonstrated posterior to the navicular bone and, in a patient with a high foot arch, _____ (more/less) (B) will be demonstrated.

83. The actual height of the foot arch on a lateral foot projection is accurate only when the _____ are superimposed.

84. Which anatomic structures form the talar domes?

_____

85. Misalignment of the talar domes can be caused by poor _____ (A) and/or _____ (B) positioning.

86. If the distal tibia is positioned farther from the imaging table than the proximal tibia for a lateral foot projection, the _____ (lateral/medial) (A) dome is demonstrated _____ (B) to the _____ (lateral/medial) (C) talar dome and the longitudinal foot arch appears _____ (higher/lower) (D) on the resulting projection.

87. If the proximal tibia is positioned farther from the imaging table than the distal tibia for a lateral foot projection, the _____ (A) dome is demonstrated _____ (B) to the _____ (C) talar dome and the longitudinal foot arch appears _____ (higher/lower) (D) on the resulting projection.

88. If a lateral foot projection with poor positioning demonstrates an obscured tibiotalar joint space, one talar dome proximal to the other, and the navicular bone superimposed over most of the cuboid, which dome is proximal?

_____

89. If the calcaneus is positioned too close to the IR and the forefoot is raised off the IR for a lateral foot projection, the _____ (A) talar dome is demonstrated _____ (B) to the _____ (C) talar dome and the fibula is demonstrated too far _____ (D) on the tibia.

90. If the forefoot is positioned too close to the IR and the calcaneus is elevated off the IR for a lateral foot projection, the _____ (A) talar dome is demonstrated _____ (B) to the _____ (C) talar dome and the fibula is demonstrated too far _____ (D) on the tibia.

91. Why is it important to dorsiflex the foot to a 90-degree angle with the lower leg?

A. _____

B. _____

C. _____

92. Against which aspect of the foot is the IR placed for a standing lateromedial projection of the foot?

A. _____

What surface (medial/lateral) of the foot is aligned parallel with the IR for a lateromedial projection of the foot with accurate positioning?

B. _____

93. If a standing lateromedial projection of the foot with poor positioning demonstrates one talar dome posterior to the other talar dome and the fibula is situated too far posterior on the tibia, how should the patient's position be adjusted for an optimal projection to be obtained?

_____

94. Accurate central ray centering on a lateral foot projection is accomplished by centering a _____ (A) central ray halfway between the distal toes and the _____ (B).

95. Which anatomic structures are included on a lateral foot projection with accurate positioning?

_____

_____

For the following descriptions of mediolateral foot projections with poor positioning, state how the patient would have been mispositioned for such a projection to be obtained.

96. The tibiotalar joint space is obscured, one talar dome is demonstrated proximal to the other dome, and the navicular bone is superimposed over most of the cuboid.

_____

97. The tibiotalar joint space is obscured, one talar dome is demonstrated proximal to the other dome, and more than 0.5 inch (1.25 cm) of the cuboid appears posterior to the navicular bone.

_____

98. The tibiotalar joint is obscured, one talar dome is demonstrated anterior to the other dome, and the fibula is demonstrated too posterior on the tibia.

_____

99. The tibiotalar joint is obscured, one talar dome is demonstrated anterior to the other dome, and the fibula is demonstrated too anterior on the tibia.

_____

For the following lateral foot projections with poor positioning, state which anatomic structures are misaligned and how the patient should be repositioned for an optimal projection to be obtained.

Figure 6-16

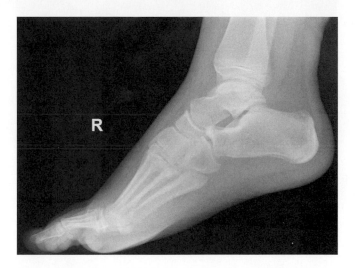

100. Figure 6-16: _____

_____

_____

_____

Figure 6-17

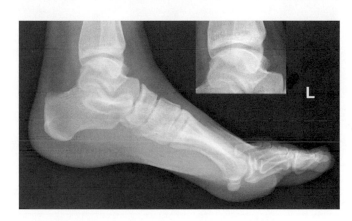

101. Figure 6-17: _____

_____

_____

_____

Figure 6-18

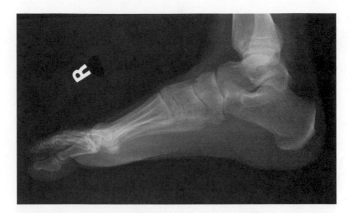

102. Figure 6-18 (lateromedial projection, average longitudinal arch): _____

_____

_____

_____

Figure 6-19

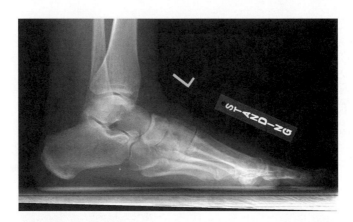

103. Figure 6-19 (lateromedial projection): _____

_____

_____

_____

Calcaneus: Axial Projection (Plantodorsal)

104. Identify the labeled anatomy in Figure 6-20.

Figure 6-20

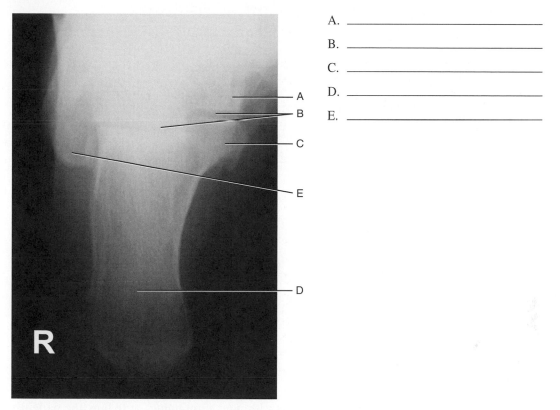

A. _____

B. _____

C. _____

D. _____

E. _____

105. Complete the statements below referring to axial calcaneus projection analysis criteria.

Axial Calcaneus Projection Analysis Criteria
• The _____ (A) joint is open and the calcaneal tuberosity is demonstrated without distortion.
• The second through fourth distal metatarsals are not demonstrated on the _____ (B) or _____ (C) aspect of the foot, respectively.
• The _____ (D) is at the center of the exposure field.

106. To obtain an axial calcaneal projection with accurate positioning, position the foot _____ (A) and direct a _____-degree (B) central ray angulation toward the _____ (C) foot surface.

107. When the central ray and foot are accurately aligned, the central ray is aligned _____ (A) to the talocalcaneal joint space and _____ (B) to the calcaneal tuberosity.

108. If an axial calcaneal projection is requested for a patient who is unable to dorsiflex the foot to a vertical position, how is the positioning setup adjusted before the projection is obtained?

A. _____

How is the setup changed if the patient dorsiflexed the foot beyond the vertical position?

B. _____

109. Which anatomic structures can be used to estimate the central ray angulation needed when the patient is unable to dorsiflex the foot into a vertical position?

_____

110. Describe where to palpate to locate the fifth metatarsal base.

_____

111. How is the patient positioned to prevent calcaneal tilting?

A. _____

How is calcaneal tilting identified on an axial calcaneal projection with poor positioning?

B. _____

112. Accurate central ray centering on an axial calcaneal projection is accomplished by centering the central ray to the midline of the foot at the level of the _____.

113. Which anatomic structures are included on an axial calcaneal projection with accurate positioning?

_____

For the following descriptions of axial calcaneal projections with poor positioning, state how the patient would have been mispositioned for such a projection to be obtained.

114. The talocalcaneal joint space is obscured, and the calcaneal tuberosity is elongated. The standard 40-degree angulation was used.

_____

115. The talocalcaneal joint space is obscured, and the calcaneal tuberosity is foreshortened. The standard 40-degree angulation was used.

_____

116. The first metatarsal is demonstrated medially.

_____

117. The fourth and fifth metatarsals are demonstrated laterally.

_____

For the following axial calcaneal projection with poor positioning, state which anatomic structures are misaligned and how the patient should be repositioned for an optimal projection to be obtained.

Figure 6-21

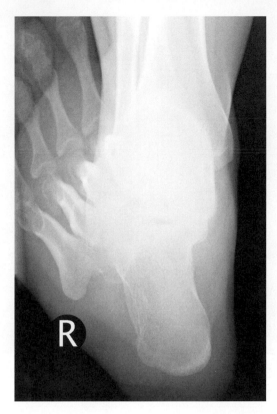

118. Figure 6-21: _____

_____

_____

_____

Figure 6-22

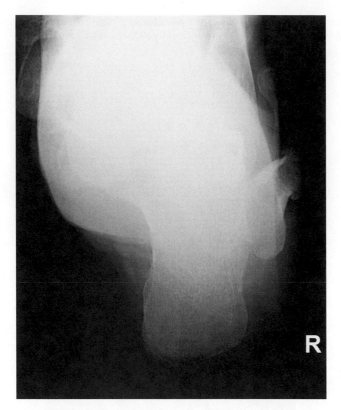

119. Figure 6-22: _____

_____

_____

_____

Figure 6-23

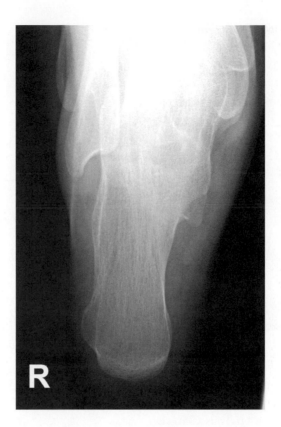

120. Figure 6-23: _____

_____

_____

_____

Calcaneus: Lateral Projection (Mediolateral)

121. Identify the labeled anatomy in Figure 6-24.

Figure 6-24

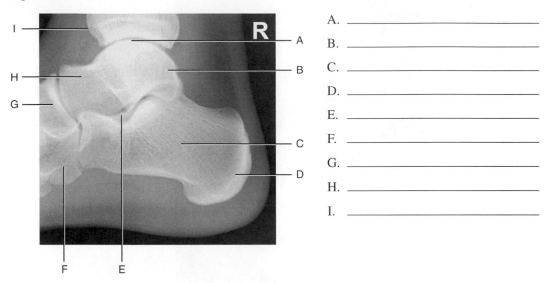

A. _____

B. _____

C. _____

D. _____

E. _____

F. _____

G. _____

H. _____

I. _____

122. Complete the statements below referring to lateral calcaneus projection analysis criteria.

Lateral Calcaneus Projection Analysis Criteria
• The talar domes are superimposed, the tibiotalar joint space is open, and the distal fibula is superimposed by the _____ (A) half of the distal tibia.   • The long axis of the foot is positioned at a 90-degree angle with the _____ (B).   • The _____ (C) is at the center of the exposure field.

123. How is the patient's lower leg positioned to obtain a lateral calcaneal projection with accurate positioning?

_____

124. How is the patient's foot positioned with the lower leg and IR to obtain a lateral calcaneal projection with accurate positioning?

A. Lower leg: _____.

B. IR: _____

125. A calcaneal foot projection was requested for a patient with a large upper thigh that prevented the lower leg from aligning parallel with the imaging table when the patient was positioned. If the projection was obtained with the patient positioned in this manner, how would this poor positioning be identified on the resulting projection?

_____

_____

126. The height of the longitudinal arch is determined on a lateral calcaneal projection with accurate positioning by measuring the amount of cuboid that appears _____ (A) to the _____ (B).

127. The average calcaneal projection demonstrates approximately _____ inch of the cuboid posterior to the navicular bone.

128. A projection from a patient with a low foot arch shows _____ (more/less) (A) of the cuboid posterior to the navicular bone, and a projection from a patient with a high foot arch shows _____ (more/less) (B).

129. The actual height of the foot arch on a lateral calcaneal projection is accurate only when the _____ are superimposed.

130. Which anatomic structures form the talar domes on a lateral calcaneal projection?

_____

131. Misalignment of the talar domes can be caused by poor _____ (A) and/or _____ (B) positioning.

132. If the distal tibia is positioned farther from the imaging table than the proximal tibia for a lateral calcaneal projection, the _____ (A) dome is demonstrated _____ (B) to the _____ (C) talar dome and the longitudinal foot arch appears _____ (higher/lower) (D) on the resulting projection.

133. If the proximal tibia is positioned farther from the imaging table than the distal tibia for a lateral calcaneal projection, the _____ (A) dome is demonstrated _____ (B) to the _____ (C) talar dome and the longitudinal foot arch appears _____ (higher/lower) (D) on the resulting projection.

134. If the calcaneus is positioned too close to the IR and the forefoot is raised off the IR for a lateral calcaneal projection, the _____ (A) talar dome is demonstrated _____ (B) to the _____ (C) talar dome and the fibula is demonstrated too far _____ (D) on the tibia.

135. If the forefoot is positioned too close to the IR and the calcaneus is raised off the IR for a lateral calcaneal projection, the _____ (A) talar dome is demonstrated _____ (B) to the _____ (C) talar dome and the fibula is demonstrated too far _____ (D) on the tibia.

136. Positioning the long axis of the foot at a 90-degree angle with the lower leg prevents _____ rotation.

137. Accurate central ray centering on a lateral calcaneal projection is accomplished by centering a _____ (A) central ray 1 inch (2.5 cm) _____ (B) to the _____ (C).

138. Which anatomic structures are included on a lateral calcaneal projection with accurate positioning?

_____

139. To ensure that the needed joint spaces are included on a lateral calcaneal projection, the longitudinal collimation is open to the level of the _____ (A) and transverse collimation extends 2 inches (5 cm) anterior to the _____ (B).

For the following descriptions of lateral calcaneal projections with poor positioning, state how the patient would have been mispositioned for such a projection to be obtained.

140. The tibiotalar joint space is obscured, one talar dome is demonstrated proximal to the other, and the navicular bone is superimposed over most of the cuboid.

_____

141. The tibiotalar joint space is obscured, one talar dome is demonstrated proximal to the other, and more than 0.5 inch (1.25 cm) of cuboid appears posterior to the navicular bone.

_____

142. The tibiotalar joint is obscured, one talar dome is demonstrated anterior to the other dome, and the fibula is demonstrated too posterior on the tibia.

_____

143. The tibiotalar joint is obscured, one talar dome is demonstrated anterior to the other dome, and the fibula is demonstrated too anterior on the tibia.

_____

For the following axial calcaneal projections with poor positioning, state which anatomic structures are misaligned and how the patient should be repositioned for an optimal projection to be obtained.

Figure 6-25

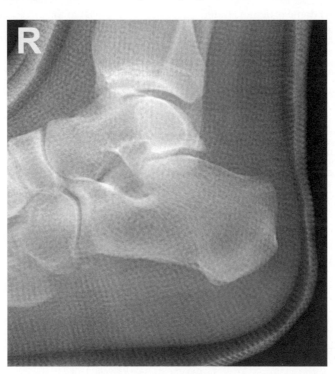

144. Figure 6-25: _____

_____

_____

_____

Figure 6-26

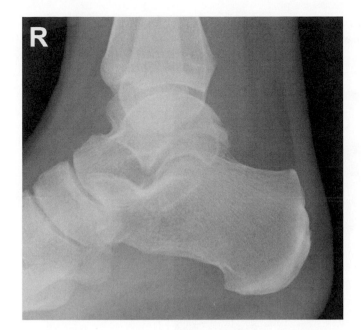

145. Figure 6-26: _____

_____

_____

_____

Figure 6-27

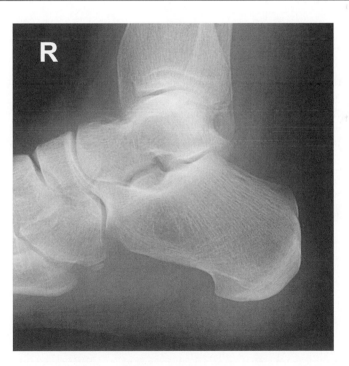

146. Figure 6-27: _____

_____

_____

_____

Ankle: Anteroposterior Projection

147. Identify the labeled anatomy in Figure 6-28.

Figure 6-28

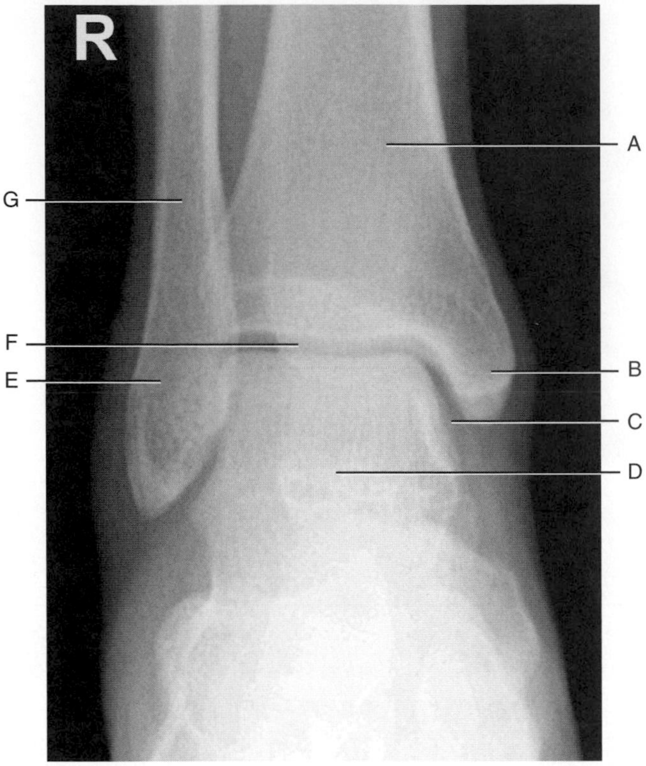

A. _____

B. _____

C. _____

D. _____

E. _____

F. _____

G. _____

148. Complete the statements below referring to AP ankle projection analysis criteria.

Anteroposterior Ankle Projection Analysis Criteria
• The medial mortise is open and the distal tibia and talus are superimposed over the _____ (A) by approximately ⅛ inch, closing the _____ (B) mortise.   • The tibiotalar joint space is open, and the tibia is demonstrated without foreshortening.   • The _____ (C) is at the center of the exposure field.

149. The ankle joint is located at the same level as what palpable anatomic structure? _____

150. Is the distal fibula superimposed by the tibia or is the tibia superimposed by the distal fibula on an AP ankle projection?

_____

151. The intermalleolar line is at what angle with the IR when the patient is accurately positioned for an AP ankle projection?

_____

152. The patient's leg was externally rotated for an AP ankle projection. How can this mispositioning be identified on an AP ankle projection?

_____

_____

153. How is the patient positioned for an AP ankle projection to obtain an open tibiotalar joint space?

_____

154. The central ray was centered proximal to the ankle joint space for an AP ankle projection. How is this mispositioning identified on an AP ankle projection? _____

_____

155. Accurate central ray centering on an AP ankle projection is accomplished by centering a _____

(A) central ray to the ankle midline at the level of the _____ (B).

156. Which anatomic structures are included on an AP ankle projection with accurate positioning?

_____

For the following descriptions of AP ankle projections with poor positioning, state how the patient would have been mispositioned for such a projection to be obtained.

157. The medial mortise is obscured, the tibia and talus demonstrate increased superimposition of the fibula, and the posterior aspect of the medial malleolus is situated medial to the anterior aspect.

_____

158. The medial mortise is closed, and the fibula demonstrates no talar superimposition.

_____

159. The tibiotalar joint is closed, and the anterior tibial margin has been projected into the joint space.

_____

For the following AP ankle projection with poor positioning, state which anatomic structures are misaligned and how the patient should be repositioned for an optimal projection to be obtained.

Figure 6-29

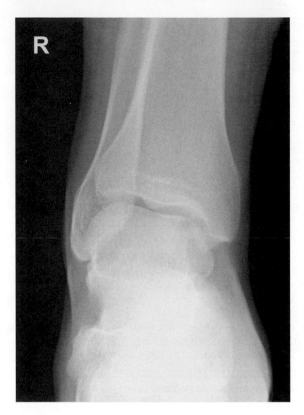

160. Figure 6-29: _____

_____

_____

_____

Figure 6-30

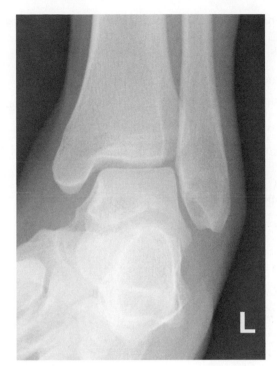

161. Figure 6-30: _____

_____

_____

_____

Ankle: Anteroposterior Oblique Projection (Medial Rotation)

162. Identify the labeled anatomy in Figure 6-31.

Figure 6-31

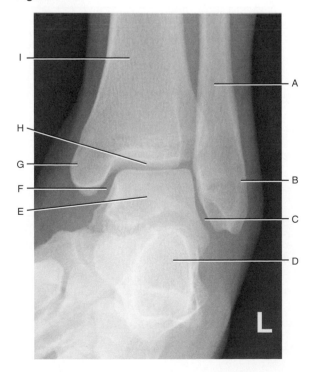

A. _____

B. _____

C. _____

D. _____

E. _____

F. _____

G. _____

H. _____

I. _____

163. Complete the statements below referring to AP oblique ankle projection analysis criteria.

> **Anteroposterior Oblique Ankle Projection Analysis Criteria**
>
> - Mortise (15-20 degree) oblique: The distal fibula is demonstrated without _____ (A) superimposition, demonstrating an open _____ (B) mortise, and the lateral and medial malleoli are in profile. The fibula demonstrates slight (0.125 inch [0.3 cm]) _____ (C) superimposition.
> - 45-degree oblique: The medial mortise is closed and the lateral mortise is partially closed, the fibula is seen without _____ (D) superimposition, and the tarsal sinus is demonstrated.
> - The tibiotalar joint space is open and the tibia is seen without foreshortening.
> - The calcaneus is visualized _____ (E) to the lateral mortise and fibula.
> - The _____ (F) is at the center of the exposure field.

164. Approximately how much ankle obliquity is needed for a mortise AP oblique ankle projection with accurate positioning?

   A. _____

   In which direction is the patient's leg rotated?

   B. _____

165. How is the patient positioned to obtain an open tibiotalar joint space on an AP oblique ankle projection with accurate positioning?

   _____

166. The central ray was centered distal to the ankle joint for an AP oblique ankle projection. How can this mispositioning be identified on an AP oblique ankle projection? _____

   _____

167. How is the patient positioned to demonstrate the calcaneus distal to the lateral mortise and fibula on an AP oblique ankle projection?

   _____

   _____

168. Accurate central ray centering on an AP oblique ankle projection is accomplished by centering a _____ (A) central ray to the ankle midline at the level of the _____ (B).

169. Which anatomic structures are included on an AP ankle projection with accurate positioning?

   _____

For the following descriptions of AP oblique ankle projections with poor positioning, state how the patient would have been mispositioned for such a projection to be obtained.

170. Mortise oblique: The lateral mortise is closed and the medial mortise is demonstrated as an open space. The tarsal sinus is not shown.

   _____

171. Mortise oblique: The lateral and medial mortises are closed and the tarsal sinus is demonstrated.

_____

172. 45-degree oblique: The lateral and medial mortises are closed, the fibula is demonstrated without tibial superimposition, and the tarsal sinus is demonstrated.

_____

173. Mortise oblique: The tibiotalar joint space is expanded, the anterior tibial margin is projected superior to the posterior margin, and the tibial articulating surface is demonstrated.

_____

174. 45-degree oblique: The calcaneus is obscuring the distal aspect of the lateral mortise and the distal fibula.

_____

For the following AP oblique ankle projections with poor positioning, state which anatomic structures are misaligned and how the patient should be repositioned for an optimal projection to be obtained.

Figure 6-32

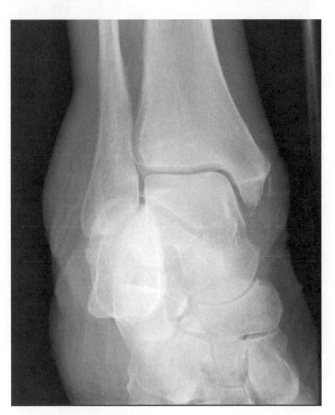

175. Figure 6-32 (mortise oblique): _____

_____

_____

_____

Figure 6-33

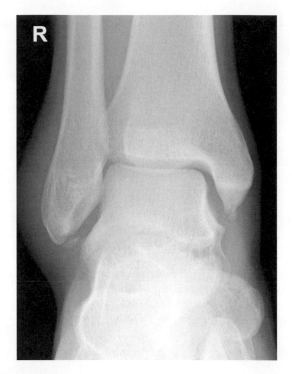

176. Figure 6-33 (mortise oblique): _____

_____

_____

_____

Figure 6-34

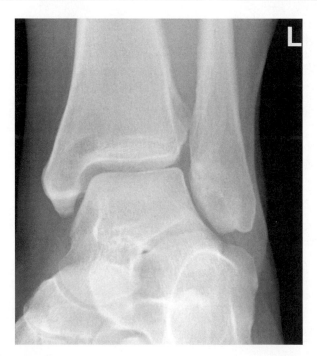

177. Figure 6-34 (45-degree oblique): _____

_____

_____

_____

Figure 6-35

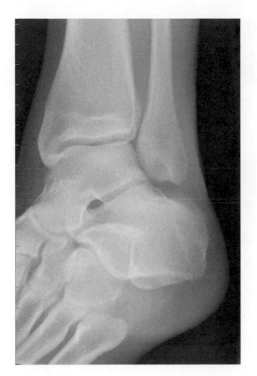

178. Figure 6-35 (45-degree oblique): _____

_____

_____

_____

Figure 6-36

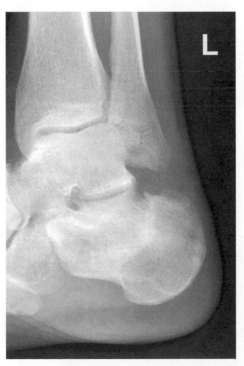

179. Figure 6-36 (45-degree oblique): _____

_____

_____

_____

Figure 6-37

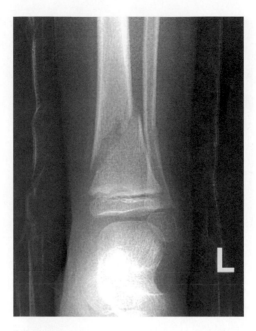

180. Figure 6-37 (trauma, 45-degree oblique): _____

_____

_____

_____

Ankle: Lateral Projection (Mediolateral)

181. Identify the labeled anatomy in Figure 6-38.

Figure 6-38

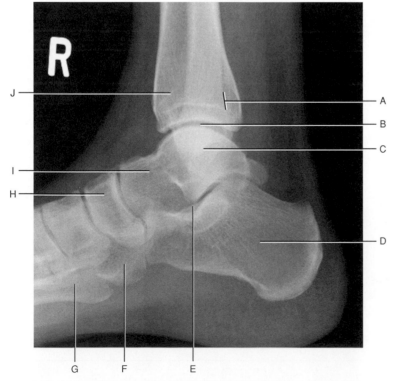

A. _____

B. _____

C. _____

D. _____

E. _____

F. _____

G. _____

H. _____

I. _____

J. _____

182. Complete the statements below referring to lateral ankle projection analysis criteria.

> **Lateral Ankle Projection Analysis Criteria**
>
> • Contrast and density are adequate to demonstrate the anterior pretalar and posterior pericapsular fat pads.
>
> • The talar domes are superimposed, the tibiotalar joint is _____ (A), and the distal fibula is superimposed by the posterior half of the _____ (B).
>
> • The long axis of the foot is positioned at a 90-degree angle with the _____ (C).
>
> • The _____ (D) is at the center of the exposure field.

183. Why is the visualization of the anterior pretalar and posterior pericapsular fat pads important on a lateral ankle projection? _____

_____

184. To obtain a lateral ankle projection with accurate positioning, the patient's leg is extended with the lower leg positioned _____ (A) to the imaging table and the foot dorsiflexed with its _____ (B) surface aligned parallel to the IR.

185. The height of the longitudinal arch can be determined on a lateral ankle projection with accurate positioning by measuring the amount of cuboid that appears _____ (A) to the _____ (B). The average ankle projection demonstrates approximately _____ (C) inch of the cuboid, whereas a high-arched patient demonstrates approximately _____ (D) inch and a low-arched patient demonstrates approximately _____ (E) inch.

186. Which anatomic structures form the structures referred to as the talar domes on a lateral foot projection?

_____

_____

187. Accurate lower leg positioning for a lateral ankle projection ensures accurate _____ alignment of the talar domes.

188. If the distal tibia is positioned farther from the imaging table than the proximal tibia for a lateral ankle projection, the _____ (A) dome is demonstrated _____ (B) to the _____ (C) talar dome and the longitudinal foot arch appears _____ (D) on the resulting projection.

189. If the proximal tibia is positioned farther from the imaging table than the distal tibia for a lateral ankle projection, the _____ (A) dome is demonstrated _____ (B) to the _____ (C) talar dome and the longitudinal foot arch appears _____ (D) on the resulting projection.

190. Accurate lateral foot surface positioning for a lateral ankle projection ensures proper _____ alignment of the talar domes.

191. If the calcaneus is positioned too close to the IR and the toes are raised off the IR for a lateral ankle projection, the _____ (A) talar dome is demonstrated _____ (B) to the _____ (C) talar dome and the fibula is demonstrated too far _____ (D) on the tibia.

192. If the toes are positioned too close to the IR and the calcaneus is raised off the IR for a lateral ankle projection, the _____ (A) talar domes are demonstrated _____ (B) to the _____ (C) talar dome and the fibula is demonstrated too far _____ (D) on the tibia.

193. Why is it important to dorsiflex the foot to a 90-degree angle with the lower leg?

   A. _____

   B. _____

   C. _____

194. Accurate central ray centering on a lateral ankle projection is accomplished by centering a _____ (A) central ray to the _____ (B).

195. Which anatomic structures are included on a lateral ankle projection with accurate positioning?

   _____

   _____

196. What is a Jones fracture? _____

197. Why should the transversely collimated field remain open to include 3 inches (7.5 cm) of the proximal forefoot?

   _____

   _____

For the following descriptions of lateral ankle projections with poor positioning, state how the patient would have been mispositioned for such a projection to be obtained.

198. The tibiotalar joint space is obscured, one talar dome is demonstrated proximal to the other dome, and the navicular bone is superimposed over most of the cuboid.

   _____

199. Average longitudinal arch: The tibiotalar joint space is obscured, one talar dome is demonstrated proximal to the other dome, and more than 0.5 inch (1.25 cm) of the cuboid appears posterior to the navicular bone.

   _____

200. The tibiotalar joint is obscured, one talar dome is demonstrated anterior to the other dome, and the fibula is demonstrated too posterior on the tibia.

   _____

201. The tibiotalar joint is obscured, one talar dome is demonstrated anterior to the other dome, and the fibula is demonstrated too anterior on the tibia.

   _____

Chapter **6** **Lower Extremity**

For the following lateral ankle projections with poor positioning, state which anatomic structures are misaligned and how the patient should be repositioned for an optimal projection to be obtained.

Figure 6-39

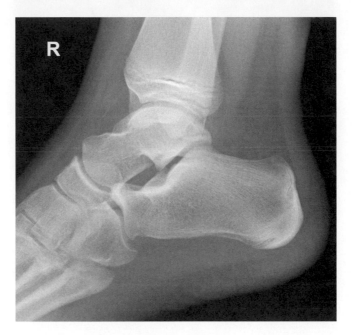

202. Figure 6-39: _____

_____

_____

_____

Figure 6-40

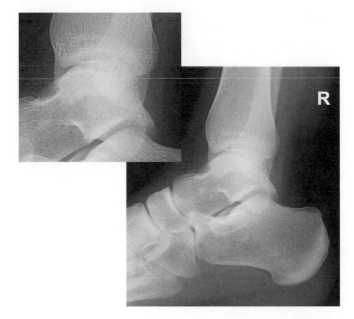

203. Figure 6-40: _____

_____

_____

_____

Figure 6-41

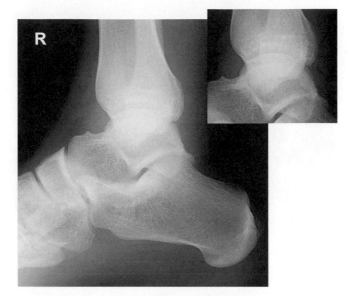

204. Figure 6-41: _____

_____

_____

_____

Figure 6-42

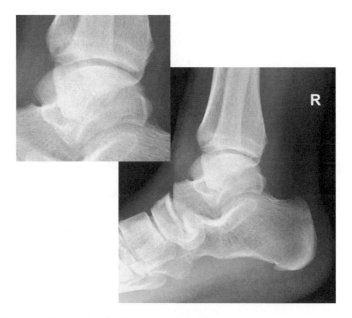

205. Figure 6-42 (trauma, lateromedial projection): _____

_____

_____

_____

Figure 6-43

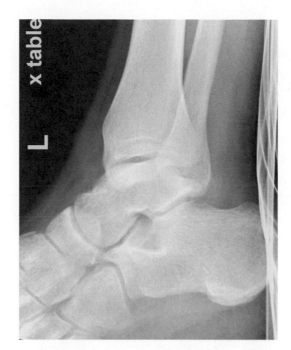

206. Figure 6-43 (trauma, lateromedial projection): _____

_____

_____

_____

Figure 6-44

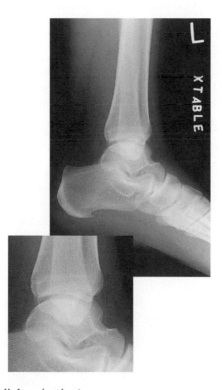

207. Figure 6-44 (trauma, lateromedial projection): _____

_____

_____

_____

Figure 6-45

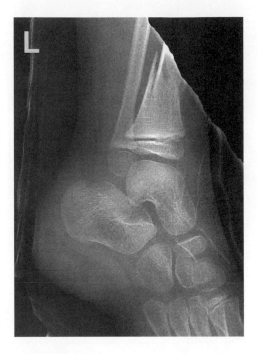

208. Figure 6-45 (trauma, lateromedial projection): _____
_____
_____
_____

Lower Leg: Anteroposterior Projection

209. Identify the labeled anatomy in Figure 6-46.

Figure 6-46

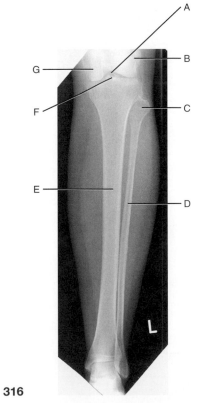

A. _____

B. _____

C. _____

D. _____

E. _____

F. _____

G. _____

210. Complete the statements below referring to AP lower leg projection analysis criteria.

> **Anteroposterior Lower Leg Projection Analysis Criteria**
>
> - Projection density is uniform across the lower leg.
> - The tibia demonstrates only minimal superimposition of the proximal and distal fibula, and the fibular midshaft is demonstrated free of _____ (A) superimposition.
> - The knee and tibiotalar joint spaces are _____ (B).
> - The _____ (C) is at the center of the exposure field.

211. How should the lower leg be positioned with respect to the x-ray tube to take advantage of the anode heel effect?

_____

_____

212. An AP projection of the lower leg is obtained by _____ (A) the patient's knee and _____ (B) rotating the leg until the medial and lateral _____ (C) are positioned at equal distances from the IR.

213. An AP projection of the distal lower leg is demonstrated when the _____ mortise is open.

214. Describe the relationship of the tibia and fibula at the knee, midshaft, and ankle on an AP lower leg projection with accurate positioning.

   A. Knee: _____

   B. Midshaft: _____

   C. Ankle: _____

215. Describe how the tibia and fibula on an AP lower leg projection are misaligned at the knee and ankle if the leg is internally rotated.

   A. Knee: _____

   B. Ankle: _____

216. A patient from the emergency room is unable to position the ankle and knee in an AP projection simultaneously for an AP lower leg projection. If the area of interest is closer to the knee joint, how should the leg be positioned for the projection?

_____

217. Are the femorotibial and tibiotalar joint spaces closed on an AP lower leg projection with accurate positioning?

   A. _____ (Yes/No)

   Explain how the divergence of the x-ray beam used to record these two joints affects their openness.

   B. _____

218. Why is it necessary for the IR to extend at least 1 inch (2.5 cm) beyond the ankle and knee joints when the lower leg is projectioned in an AP projection?

_____

219. The ankle joint is located at the level of the palpable _____ (A), and the knee joint is located 1 inch (2.5 cm) _____ (B) to the palpable _____ (C).

220. The _____ is centered to the collimated field on an AP lower leg projection with accurate positioning.

221. Which anatomic structures are included on an AP lower leg projection with accurate positioning?

_____

For the following descriptions of AP lower leg projections with poor positioning, state how the patient would have been mispositioned for such a projection to be obtained.

222. The medial mortise is closed, and the tibia and talus demonstrate excessive fibular superimposition.

_____

223. The distal fibula is free of talar superimposition, and the proximal fibula is free of tibial superimposition.

_____

For the following AP lower leg projection with poor positioning, state which anatomic structures are misaligned and how the patient should be repositioned for an optimal projection to be obtained.

Figure 6-47

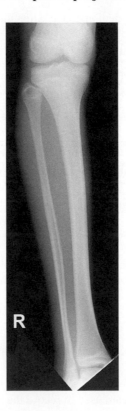

224. Figure 6-47: _____

_____

_____

_____

Lower Leg: Lateral Projection (Mediolateral)

225. Identify the labeled anatomy in Figure 6-48.

Figure 6-48

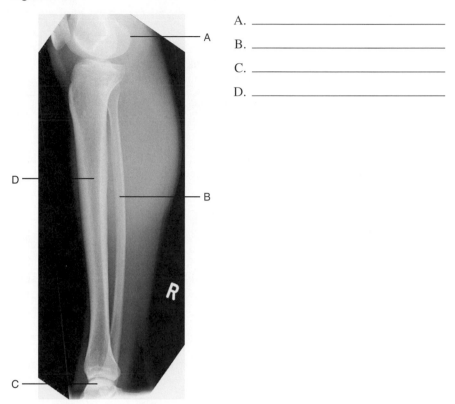

A. _____

B. _____

C. _____

D. _____

226. Complete the statements below referring to lateral lower leg projection analysis criteria.

Lateral Lower Leg Projection Analysis Criteria

• Projection density is uniform across the lower leg.

• The distal fibula is superimposed by the _____ (A) half of the distal tibia.

• The fibular _____ (B) is free of tibial superimposition.

• The tibia is partially superimposed over the fibular head and the medial femoral condyle is demonstrated posterior to the lateral condyle if the leg is _____ (C) or the condyles are superimposed if the knee is flexed to at least _____ (D) degrees.

• The _____ (E) is at the center of the exposure field.

227. State how the lower leg is positioned with respect to the x-ray tube to take advantage of the anode heel effect.

_____

_____

228. Which aspect of the patient's leg is positioned against the IR for a lateral lower leg projection with accurate positioning? _____ (medial/lateral)

229. Describe the anatomic relationship of the tibia and fibula at the knee, midshaft, and ankle on a lateral lower leg projection with accurate positioning.

A. Knee: _____

B. Midshaft: _____

C. Ankle: _____

230. How does the relationship between the tibia and fibula at the knee and ankle described in question 229 change if the patient's medial femoral epicondyle is rotated anterior to the lateral epicondyle for the projection?

A. Knee: _____

B. Ankle: _____

231. The degree of knee flexion determines how superimposed the femoral condyles will be on a lateral lower leg projection. Will the femoral condyles be superimposed if the projection is obtained with the knee extended?

A. _____ (Yes/No)

If the projection is obtained with the knee flexed 30 degrees?

B. _____ (Yes/No)

232. A patient from the emergency room is unable to projection the knee and ankle in a true lateral position simultaneously for a lateral lower leg projection. If the area of interest is closest to the ankle joint, how should the leg be positioned for this projection?

_____

233. To ensure that both joints are included on a lateral lower leg projection, how far should the IR and longitudinally collimated field extend beyond the knee and ankle joints?

_____

234. The _____ is centered to the collimated field on a lateral lower leg projection with accurate positioning.

235. Which anatomic structures are included on a lateral lower leg projection with accurate positioning?

_____

For the following descriptions of lateral lower leg projections with poor positioning, state how the patient would have been mispositioned for such a projection to be obtained.

236. The distal fibula is situated too far posterior on the tibia, the medial talar dome is anterior to the lateral dome, and the fibular head is free of tibial superimposition.

_____

237. The distal fibula is situated too far anterior on the tibia, the medial talar dome is posterior to the lateral dome, and the fibular head and midshaft are superimposed by the tibia.

_____

For the following lateral lower leg projections with poor positioning, state which anatomic structures are misaligned and how the patient should be repositioned for an optimal projection to be obtained.

Figure 6-49

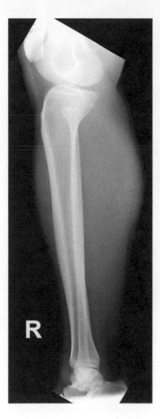

238. Figure 6-49: _____

_____

_____

_____

Figure 6-50

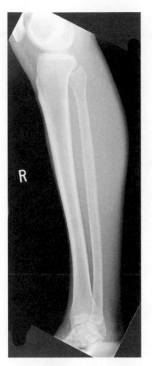

239. Figure 6-50: _____

_____

_____

_____

Knee: Anteroposterior Projection

240. Identify the labeled anatomy in Figure 6-51.

Figure 6-51

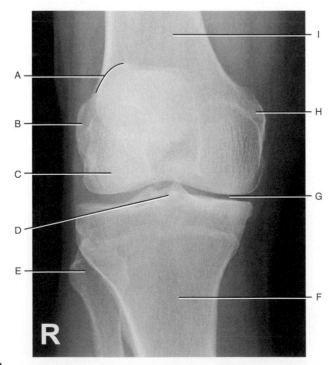

A. _____

B. _____

C. _____

D. _____

E. _____

F. _____

G. _____

H. _____

I. _____

241. Complete the statements below referring to AP knee projection analysis criteria.

Anteroposterior Knee Projection Analysis Criteria

- The medial and lateral femoral epicondyles are in _____ (A), the femoral condyles are symmetrical, the intercondylar eminence is centered within the intercondylar fossa, and the tibia is superimposed over _____ (B) inch of the fibular head.

- The knee joint space is open, the anterior and posterior condylar margins of the tibia are superimposed, and the fibular head is demonstrated approximately 0.5 inch (1.25 cm) distal to the _____ (C).

- The patella lies just _____ (D) to the patellar surface of the femur and is situated slightly _____ (E) to the knee midline. The intercondylar fossa is partially demonstrated.

- The _____ (F) is at the center of the exposure field.

242. A grid is used for a knee projection if the patient's knee measures more than _____ cm.

243. An AP knee projection is obtained by placing the patient supine with the knee _____ (A) and leg _____ (B) rotated until the femoral epicondyles are placed at _____ (C) from the IR.

244. Is the proximal tibia superimposed over the proximal fibula or is the proximal fibula superimposed over the proximal tibia when the knee is in an AP projection?

_____

245. If the knee is rotated from an AP projection, will the femoral condyle positioned closer to or farther away from the IR appear larger on the resulting projection? _____

246. If the patient's leg is not internally rotated to accurately position the femoral epicondyles, how will the appearances of the femoral condyles and the alignment of the tibia and fibula change? _____

_____

247. How does the central ray have to be aligned with the femorotibial joint space and tibial plateau to demonstrate them as open spaces on an AP knee projection? _____

248. Describe the slope of the tibial plateau. _____

_____

249. Why is it necessary to vary the degree of central ray angulation for AP knee projections in patients with different upper thigh and buttock thicknesses? _____

_____

250. Should the patient's abdominal thickness be included in the anterior superior iliac spine (ASIS)-to-imaging table measurement obtained for a patient undergoing AP knee imaging? _____ (Yes/No)

251. What central ray angulation is used when obtaining an AP knee projection in a patient with a large (more than 24 cm) ASIS-to-imaging table measurement?

A. _____

When imaging a patient with a small (less than 18 cm) ASIS-to-imaging table measurement?

B. _____

252. If the wrong central ray angle is used for an AP knee projection, the shape of the fibular head and its proximity to the tibial plateau change from that demonstrated on an AP knee projection in which an accurate central ray angle was used. For each situation that follows, state the change that occurs.

A. Central ray angled too cephalically: _____

_____

B. Central ray angled too caudally: _____

_____

253. Which knee compartment on an AP knee projection is narrower when a valgus deformity is present?

A. _____

When a varus deformity is present?

B. _____

254. Which deformity is demonstrated in Figure 6-52? _____

Figure 6-52

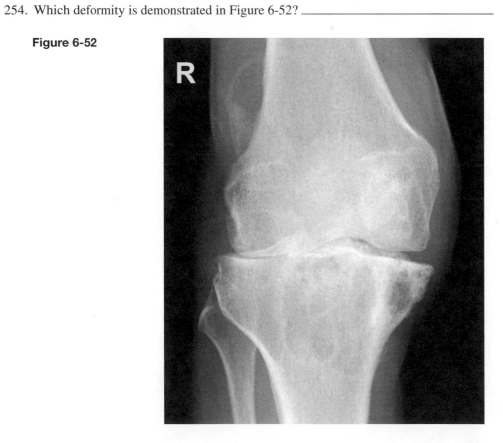

255. An AP knee projection is requested for a patient who is unable to fully extend the knee. The technologist angled the central ray until it was perpendicular to the anterior surface of the lower leg and obtained a 10-degree cephalic angle. How is this angle adjusted to align the central ray parallel with the tibial plateau and obtain an open femorotibial joint? _____

256. State the location of the patella on an AP knee projection with accurate positioning and without pathology.

257. When the knee is flexed, the patella shifts _____ (proximally/distally) (A) and _____ (medially/laterally) (B) onto the patellar surface of the femur and then _____ (medially/laterally) (C) onto the intercondylar fossa.

258. State the location of the patella for each of the following degrees of knee flexion.

A. 10 degrees: _____

B. 20 degrees: _____

C. 60 degrees: _____

259. Where is the patella demonstrated on an AP knee projection with accurate positioning in a patient with a subluxed patella?

A. _____

What type of knee rotation situates the patella in the same location?

B. _____

How can one distinguish patellar subluxation from knee rotation on an AP knee projection?

C. _____

260. Accurate central ray centering on an AP knee projection is accomplished by centering the central ray _____ (A) inch _____ (B) to the palpable _____ (C).

261. Which anatomic structures are included on an AP knee projection with accurate positioning? _____

For the following descriptions of AP knee projections with poor positioning, state how the patient or central ray would have been mispositioned for such a projection to be obtained.

262. The medial femoral condyle appears larger than the lateral condyle, and the head, neck, and shaft of the fibula are almost entirely superimposed by the tibia.

263. The lateral femoral condyle appears larger than the medial condyle, and the tibia demonstrates very little superimposition of the fibular head.

264. The femorotibial joint space is obscured, the tibial plateau is demonstrated, and the fibular head is foreshortened and demonstrated more than 0.5 inch (1.25 cm) distal to the tibial plateau.

_____

265. The medial femorotibial joint space is closed, and the fibular head is elongated and demonstrated less than 0.5 inch (1.25 cm) distal to the tibial plateau.

_____

For the following AP knee projections with poor positioning, state which anatomic structures are misaligned and how the patient should be repositioned for an optimal projection to be obtained.

Figure 6-53

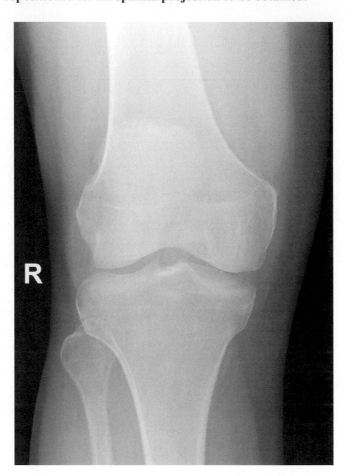

266. Figure 6-53: _____

_____

_____

_____

Figure 6-54

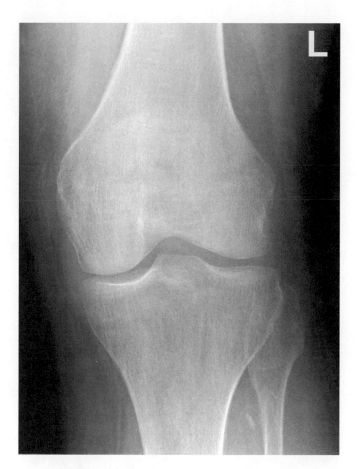

267. Figure 6-54: _____

_____

_____

_____

Figure 6-55

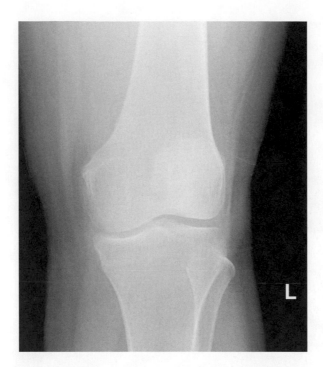

268. Figure 6-55: _____
_____
_____
_____

Figure 6-56

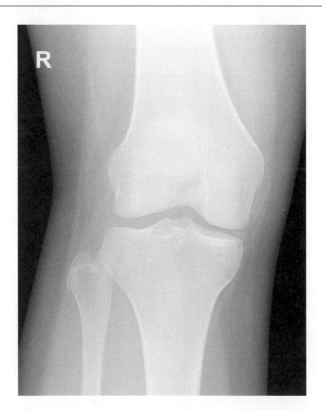

269. Figure 6-56: _____
_____
_____

Figure 6-57

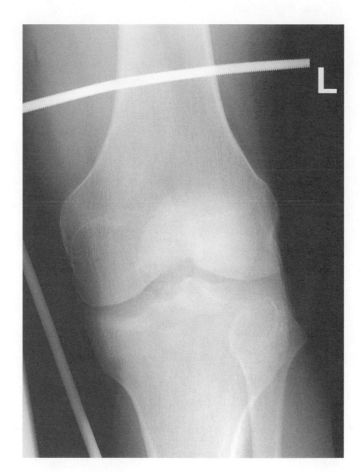

270. Figure 6-57 (trauma): _____

_____

_____

_____

Figure 6-58

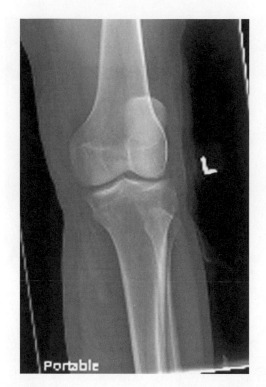

271. Figure 6-58 (trauma): _____

_____

_____

_____

Figure 6-59

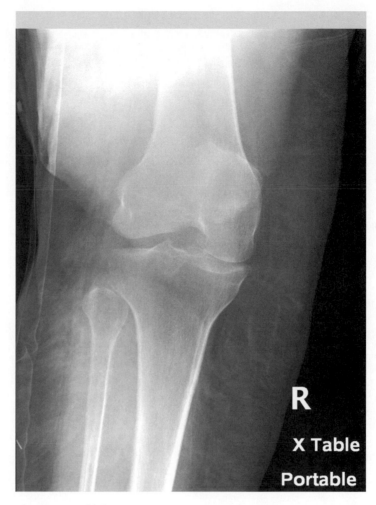

272. Figure 6-59 (trauma, taken cross-table): _____

_____

_____

_____

Knee: Anteroposterior Oblique Projection (Medial and Lateral Rotation)

273. Identify the labeled anatomy in Figure 6-60.

Figure 6-60

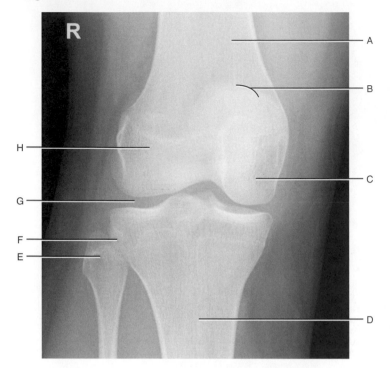

A. _____

B. _____

C. _____

D. _____

E. _____

F. _____

G. _____

H. _____

274. Identify the labeled anatomy in Figure 6-61.

Figure 6-61

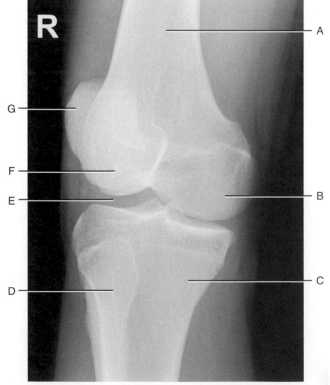

A. _____

B. _____

C. _____

D. _____

E. _____

F. _____

G. _____

275. Complete the statements below referring to AP oblique knee projection analysis criteria.

Anteroposterior Oblique Knee Projection Analysis Criteria
• The knee joint space is open, the anterior and posterior condylar margins of the tibia are superimposed, and the fibular head is approximately 0.5 inch (1.25 cm) _____ (A) to the _____ (B).
• Medial oblique: The fibular head is seen free of _____ (C) superimposition and the lateral femoral condyle is in profile without superimposing the medial condyle.
• Lateral oblique: The fibular head, neck, and shaft are aligned with the _____ (D) edge of the tibia and the medial femoral condyle is in profile without superimposing the lateral condyle.
• The _____ (E) is at the center of the exposure field.

276. For an internal or external oblique knee projection, an imaginary line drawn between the femoral epicondyles should form a _____-degree angle with the imaging table.

277. What is the relationship of the fibular head and tibia on an accurately rotated medial knee projection?

A. _____

_____

Which femoral condyle is demonstrated in profile?

B. _____

278. How can one determine from a knee projection with internal rotation that the patient was overrotated?

_____

_____

279. What is the relationship of the tibia and fibular head on a knee projection with accurate external rotation?

A. _____

_____

Which femoral condyle is demonstrated in profile?

B. _____

280. How can one determine from a knee projection with external rotation that the patient was overrotated?

_____

281. What degree of central ray angulation is used for a knee projection with lateral rotation in a patient whose ASIS-to-imaging table measurement is 12 cm?

A. _____

Why is it not uncommon to need a cephalic angle for the medially (internally) oblique knee projection?

B. _____

To need a caudal angle for the lateral (externally) oblique projection?

C. _____

282. The central ray is centered to the _____ (A) at the level of the _____ (B) for AP oblique knee projections.

333

283. Which anatomic structures are included on an oblique knee projection with accurate positioning?

_____

For the following descriptions of AP oblique knee projections with poor positioning, state how the patient or central ray would have been mispositioned for such a projection to be obtained.

284. On an internally rotated knee projection, the tibia is partially superimposed over the fibular head.

_____

285. On an externally rotated knee projection, the lateral femoral condyle is superimposed over the medial condyle, and the fibula is located in the center of the tibia.

_____

286. On an externally rotated knee projection, the fibula is not entirely superimposed by the tibia.

_____

287. On an internally rotated knee projection, the femorotibial joint space is obscured, and the fibular head is foreshortened and demonstrated more than 0.5 inch (1.25 cm) distal to the tibial plateau.

_____

For the following AP oblique knee projections with poor positioning, state which anatomic structures are misaligned and how the patient should be repositioned for an optimal projection to be obtained.

Figure 6-62

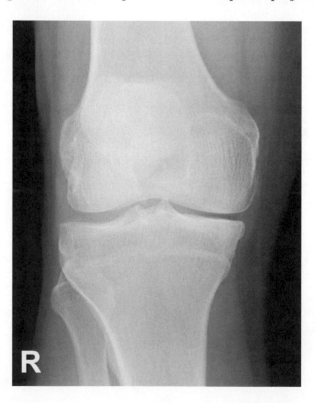

288. Figure 6-62 (internal oblique): _____

_____

_____

_____

Figure 6-63

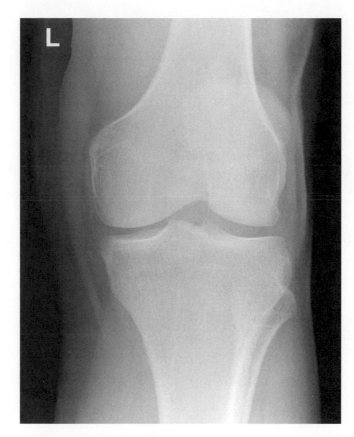

289. Figure 6-63 (external oblique): _____

_____

_____

_____

Figure 6-64

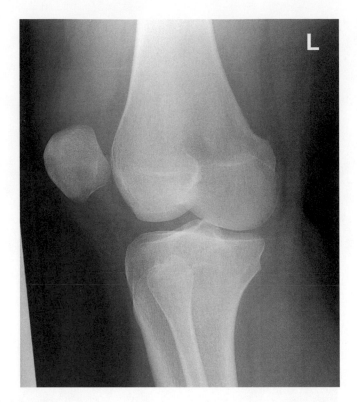

290. Figure 6-64 (external oblique): _____

_____

_____

_____

Knee: Lateral Projection (Mediolateral)

291. Identify the labeled anatomy in Figure 6-65.

Figure 6-65

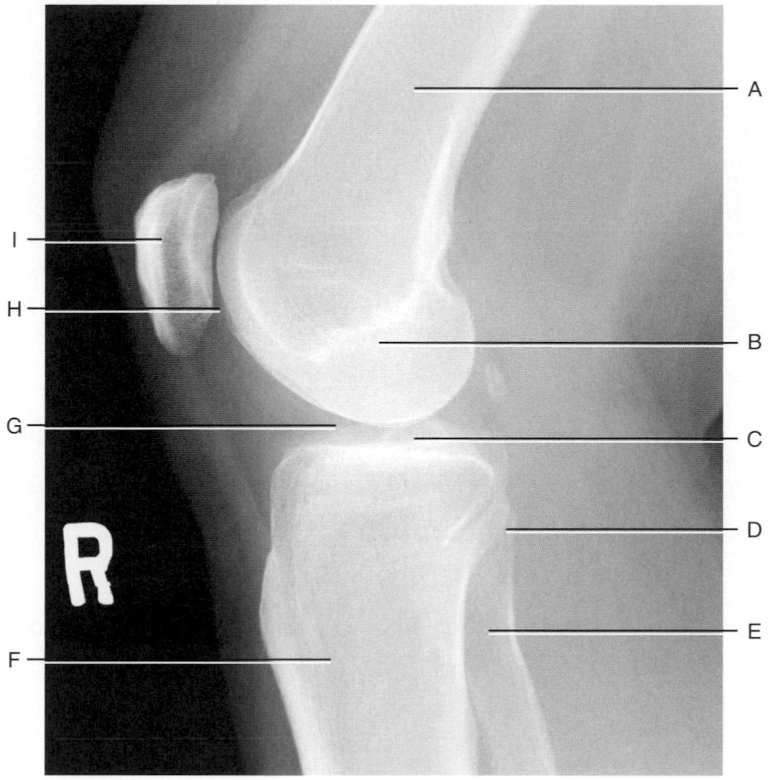

A. _____

B. _____

C. _____

D. _____

E. _____

F. _____

G. _____

H. _____

I. _____

292. Complete the statements below referring to lateral knee projection analysis criteria.

Lateral Knee Projection Analysis Criteria
• Contrast and density are adequate to demonstrate the _____ (A) fat pad.
• The patella is situated _____ (B) to the patellar surface of the femur and the patellofemoral joint is open.
• The distal articulating surfaces of the medial and lateral _____ (C) are superimposed, and the knee joint space is open.
• The anterior and posterior surfaces of the medial and lateral femoral condyles are superimposed, and the tibia is partially superimposed over the _____ (D).
• The _____ (E) is at the center of the exposure field.

293. List the two soft tissue structures on a lateral knee projection that can be used to diagnose joint effusion.

A. _____

B. _____

294. Why can a joint effusion diagnosis be made when evaluating a lateral knee projection if the knee is flexed less than 20 degrees but becomes difficult to make when the knee is flexed more than 20 degrees?

_____

_____

295. When a patient is erect, the distal femoral condylar surfaces are aligned _____ (A) to the floor and the femoral shaft inclines _____ (B) approximately _____ (C) degrees. A patient that demonstrates the greatest femoral inclination will have a _____ (wide/narrow) (D) pelvis and _____ (long/short) (E) femoral shaft length.

296. When the average patient is placed in a recumbent position for a lateral knee projection, the femoral shaft inclination displayed in the erect position is reduced, causing the _____ (A) condyle to be projected _____ (B) to the _____ (C) condyle.

297. To obtain superimposed distal femoral condylar surfaces when imaging the average patient for a lateral knee projection, a _____-degree (A) cephalic central ray angulation is used to shift the _____ (B) condyle anteriorly and proximally. The central ray angulation is _____ (increased/reduced) (C) when imaging a patient with a narrow pelvis and long femora.

298. State two methods of distinguishing the medial femoral condyle from the lateral femoral condyle on a lateral knee projection with poor positioning.

    A. _____

    B. _____

299. When is it necessary to use a cephalic central ray angulation for a lateral knee projection in a patient in a supine position?

_____

_____

300. What is the relationship between the tibia and the fibular head on a lateral knee projection with accurate positioning if superimposed condyles were obtained by aligning the femoral epicondyles perpendicular to the IR and directing the central ray across the femur to project the medial condyle anteriorly and proximally?

    A. _____

How will this relationship change if superimposed condyles are obtained by rolling the patient's patella approximately 0.25 inch (0.6 cm) closer to the IR and directing the central ray toward the femur so it only moves the medial condyle proximally?

    B. _____

301. Why is the medial condyle shifted more than the lateral condyle when the degree of central ray angulation is adjusted?

_____

302. If the distal surfaces of the femoral condyles are demonstrated without superimposition, how does one determine the degree of central ray adjustment that would be required to superimpose them?

_____

_____

303. The abductor tubercle is located _____ (anteriorly/posteriorly) (A) on the _____ (B) condyle.

304. Is the proximal fibula superimposed over the tibia or is the tibia superimposed over the proximal fibula on a mediolateral knee projection with accurate positioning?

_____

305. If the medial condyle is demonstrated anterior to the lateral condyle on a lateral knee projection with poor positioning, what will the tibia and fibular relationship be?

_____

306. If the lateral condyle is demonstrated anterior to the medial condyle on a lateral knee projection with poor positioning, what will the tibia and fibular relationship be?

_____

307. Accurate central ray centering on a lateral knee projection is accomplished by centering the central ray to the midline of the knee at a level _____ inch (A) _____ (B) to the palpable _____ (C).

308. Which anatomic structures are included on a lateral knee projection with accurate positioning?

_____

For the following descriptions of lateral knee projections with poor positioning, state how the patient or central ray would have been mispositioned for such a projection to be obtained.

309. The patient's patella is in contact with the patellar surface of the femur, and the suprapatellar fat pads are obscured.

_____

310. The distal articulating surfaces of the femoral condyles are demonstrated without superimposition. The condyle that has the adductor tubercle attached to it is demonstrated approximately 0.25 inch (0.6 cm) distal to the other condyle.

_____

311. The distal articulating surfaces of the femoral condyles are demonstrated without superimposition. The condyle that has the flattest distal surface is demonstrated approximately 0.5 inch (1.25 cm) distal to the other condyle.

_____

312. The anterior and posterior aspects of the femoral condyles are demonstrated without superimposition. The medial condyle is demonstrated posteriorly.

_____

313. The anterior and posterior aspects of the femoral condyles are demonstrated without superimposition. The medial condyle is demonstrated anteriorly.

_____

For the following lateral knee projections with poor positioning, state which anatomic structures are misaligned and how the patient should be repositioned for an optimal projection to be obtained.

Figure 6-66

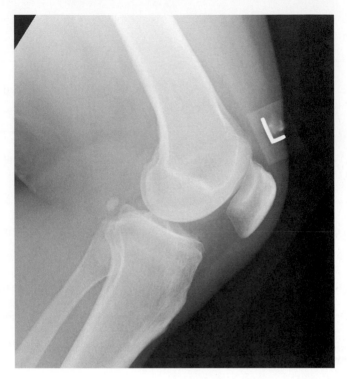

314. Figure 6-66: _____

_____

_____

_____

Figure 6-67

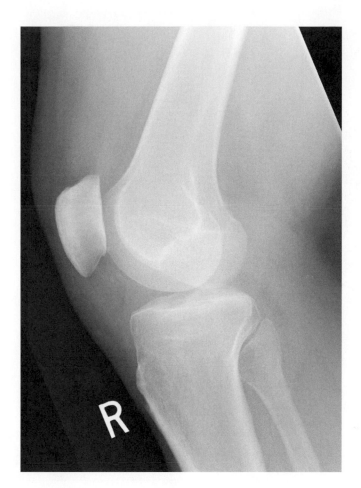

315. Figure 6-67: _____

_____

_____

_____

Figure 6-68

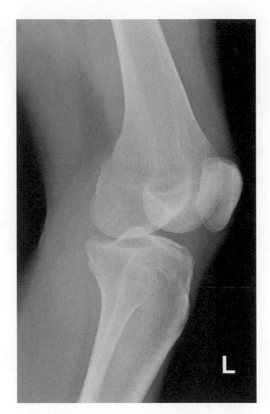

316. Figure 6-68: _____

_____

_____

_____

Figure 6-69

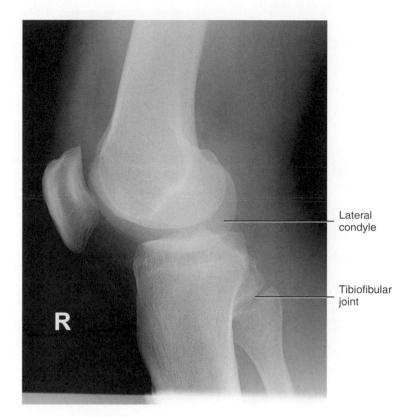

Lateral
condyle

Tibiofibular
joint

R

317. Figure 6-69: _____

_____

_____

_____

Figure 6-70

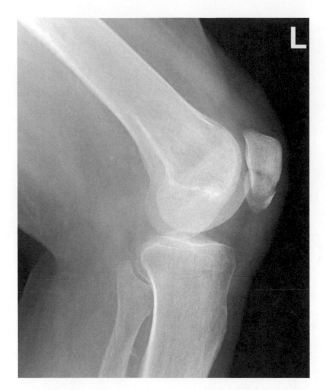

318. Figure 6-70 (trauma, mediolateral projection): _____

_____

_____

_____

Figure 6-71

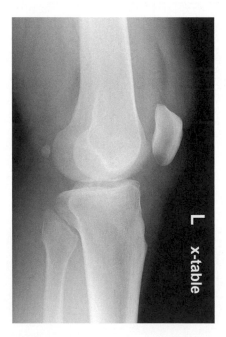

319. Figure 6-71(trauma, lateromedial projection): _____

_____

_____

_____

Figure 6-72

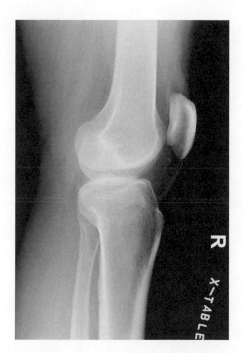

320. Figure 6-72 (trauma, lateromedial projection): _____
_____
_____
_____

Figure 6-73

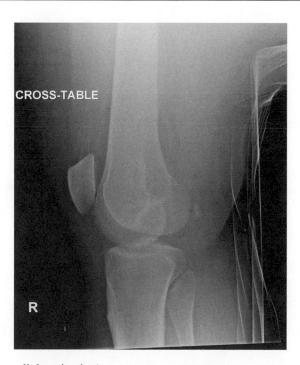

321. Figure 6-73 (trauma, lateromedial projection): _____
_____
_____
_____

Intercondylar Fossa: Posteroanterior Axial Projection (Holmblad Method)

322. Identify the labeled anatomy in Figure 6-74.

Figure 6-74

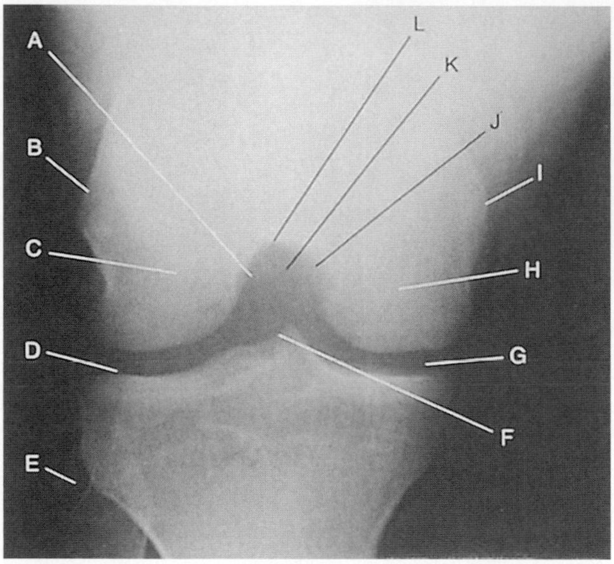

A. _____

B. _____

C. _____

D. _____

E. _____

F. _____

G. _____

H. _____

I. _____

J. _____

K. _____

L. _____

323. Complete the statements below referring to PA axial (Holmblad method) knee projection analysis criteria.

Posteroanterior Axial (Holmblad Method) Knee Projection Analysis Criteria
• The medial and lateral surfaces of the intercondylar fossa and the femoral epicondyles are in profile and the _____ (A) is partially superimposed over the proximal tibia.
• The proximal surfaces of the intercondylar fossa are _____ (B), and the patellar apex is demonstrated _____ (C) to the intercondylar fossa.
• The knee joint space is _____ (D) and the tibial plateau and intercondylar eminence and the tubercles are in profile. The fibular head is demonstrated approximately 0.5 inch (1.25 cm) _____ (E) to the tibial plateau.
• The _____ (F) is at the center of the exposure field.

324. How are the femur and foot positioned to demonstrate superimposed medial and lateral intercondylar fossa surfaces on a PA axial knee projection?

A. Femur: _____

B. Foot: _____

325. Which direction does the patella move when the patient is positioned for a PA axial knee projection and the heel is rotated as indicated below?

A. Medially: _____

B. Laterally: _____

326. To superimpose the proximal surfaces of the intercondylar fossa in the PA axial knee projection, position the patient's femur at _____ degrees (A) from vertical or _____ (B) degrees from the imaging table.

327. What direction does the patella move when the knee is flexed? _____ (proximally/distally)

328. If the knee is flexed more than needed to superimpose the proximal surfaces of the intercondylar fossa, is the patella demonstrated proximally or distally to where it is demonstrated on a PA axial knee projection with accurate positioning?

_____

329. What is the relationship of the tibial plateau margins when the foot is plantar-flexed on a PA axial knee?

A. _____

How is the patient positioned for the anterior and posterior condylar margins of the tibia to be superimposed on a PA axial knee projection?

B. _____

This positioning also demonstrates an open _____ (C) joint space and the _____ (D) and _____ (E) without foreshortening.

330. Accurate central ray centering on a PA axial knee projection is accomplished by centering a _____ (A) central ray to the midline of the knee at a level _____ inch (B) distal to the palpable _____ (C).

331. Which anatomic structures are included on a PA axial knee projection with accurate positioning?

_____

For the following descriptions of PA axial (Holmblad method) knee projections with poor positioning, state how the patient would have been mispositioned for such a projection to be obtained.

332. The medial and lateral aspects of the intercondylar fossa are demonstrated without superimposition, and the patella is situated laterally.

_____

333. The medial and lateral aspects of the intercondylar fossa are demonstrated without superimposition, the patella is situated medially, and the tibia is demonstrated without fibular head superimposition.

_____

334. The proximal surfaces of the intercondylar fossa are demonstrated without superimposition, and the patella is positioned within the intercondylar fossa.

_____

335. The proximal surfaces of the intercondylar fossa are demonstrated without superimposition, and the patella is positioned too far proximal to the intercondylar fossa.

_____

336. The femorotibial joint is obscured, and the tibial plateau is demonstrated.

_____

For the following PA axial (Holmblad method) knee projections with poor positioning, state which anatomic structures are misaligned and how the patient should be repositioned for an optimal projection to be obtained.

Figure 6-75

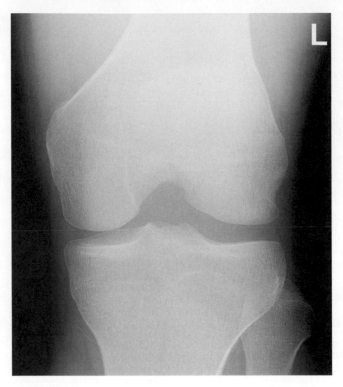

337. Figure 6-75: _____

_____

_____

_____

Figure 6-76

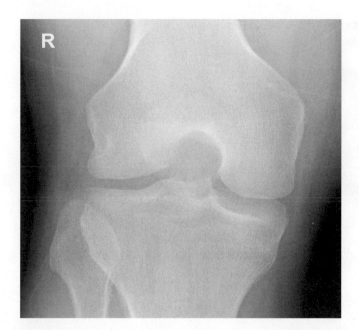

338. Figure 6-76: _____

_____

_____

_____

Figure 6-77

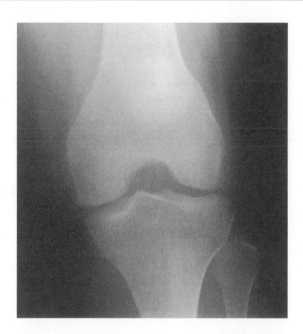

339. Figure 6-77: _____

_____

_____

_____

Intercondylar Fossa: Anteroposterior Axial Projection (Béclère Method)

340. Identify the labeled anatomy in Figure 6-78.

Figure 6-78

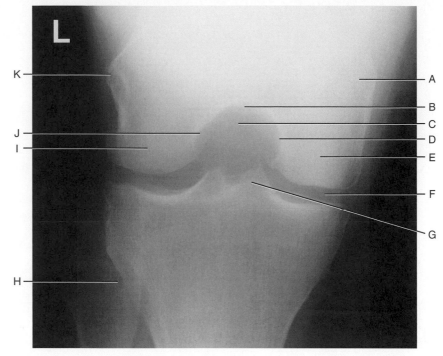

A. _____

B. _____

C. _____

D. _____

E. _____

F. _____

G. _____

H. _____

I. _____

J. _____

K. _____

341. Complete the statements below referring to AP axial (Béclère method) intercondylar fossa projection analysis criteria.

Anteroposterior Axial (Béclère Method) Intercondylar Fossa Projection Analysis Criteria
• The intercondylar fossa is shown in its entirety, the medial and lateral surfaces of the intercondylar fossa, the _____ (A) are in profile, and the tibia is partially superimposed over the _____ (B). • The proximal surface of the intercondylar fossa is in profile and the patellar apex is demonstrated _____ (C) to the fossa. • The knee joint space is open, the anterior and posterior condylar margins of the tibia are _____ (D), the intercondylar eminence and tubercles are in profile, and the fibular head is demonstrated approximately _____ (E) distal to the tibial plateau. • The _____ (F) is at the center of the exposure field.

342. How is the knee positioned to superimpose the medial and lateral surfaces on the PA axial projection?

_____

_____

343. How are the central ray and the patient positioned to obtain a projection that demonstrates the proximal surfaces of the intercondylar fossa in profile?

A. Central ray: _____

B. Patient: _____

344. As the knee is flexed, the patella shifts _____ (A) onto the patellar surface of the femur and then into the _____ (B) with increased flexion.

345. For an open knee joint space and demonstration of the intercondylar eminence and tubercles in profile, the _____ (A) and _____ (B) must be aligned parallel with each other.

346. Accurate central ray centering on an AP axial projection is accomplished by first positioning the central ray _____ (A) with the anterior lower leg surface, and then _____ (B) the obtained angulation by 5 degrees and centering the central ray 1 inch (2.5 cm) distal to the _____ (C).

347. Which anatomic structures are included on an AP axial knee projection with accurate positioning?

_____

For the following descriptions of AP axial (Béclère method) knee projections with poor positioning, state how the patient would have been mispositioned for such a projection to be obtained.

348. The medial and lateral aspects of the intercondylar fossa are not superimposed, the lateral femoral condyle is wider than the lateral condyle, and the fibular head demonstrates decreased tibial superimposition.

_____

349. The medial and lateral aspects of the intercondylar fossa are not superimposed, the medial femoral condyle is wider than the medial condyle, and the fibular head demonstrates increased tibial superimposition.

_____

350. The proximal surfaces of the intercondylar fossa are not superimposed, and the patellar apex is demonstrated within the intercondylar fossa.

_____

351. The proximal surfaces of the intercondylar fossa are not superimposed, and the patellar apex is demonstrated proximal to the intercondylar fossa.

_____

352. The knee joint space is closed, and the fibular head is shown less than 0.5 inch (1.25 cm) distal to the tibial plateau.

_____

353. The knee joint space is closed, and the fibular head is shown more than 0.5 inch (1.25 cm) distal to the tibial plateau.

_____

For the following AP axial (Béclère method) knee projections with poor positioning, state which anatomic structures are misaligned and how the patient should be repositioned for an optimal projection to be obtained.

Figure 6-79

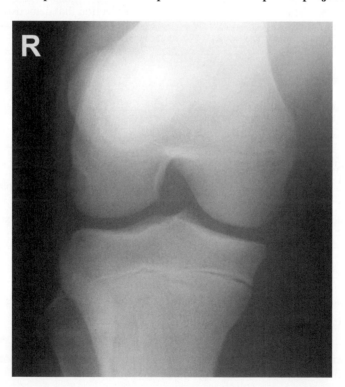

354. Figure 6-79: _____

_____

_____

_____

Figure 6-80

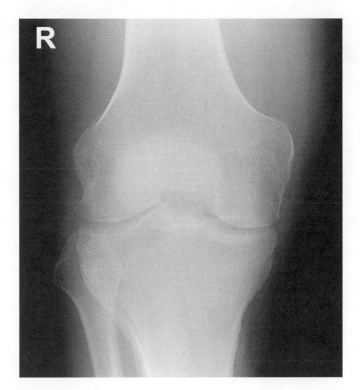

355. Figure 6-80: _____

_____

_____

_____

Patella and Patellofemoral Joint: Tangential Projection (Merchant Method)

356. Identify the labeled anatomy in Figure 6-81.

Figure 6-81

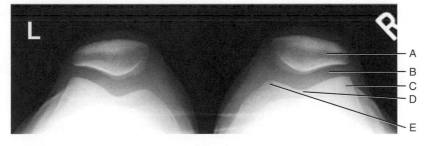

A. _____

B. _____

C. _____

D. _____

E. _____

357. Complete the statements below referring to tangential (Merchant method) patella projection analysis criteria.

Tangential (Merchant Method) Patella and Patellofemoral Joint Projection Analysis Criteria

- The patellae, anterior femoral condyles, and intercondylar sulci are seen superiorly, and the _____
  (A) femoral condyle demonstrates slightly more height than the _____ (B) condyle.

- The patellofemoral joint spaces are _____ (C), with no superimposition of the upper anterior thigh
  soft tissue, patellae, or tibial tuberosities.

- A point midway between the _____ (D) is at the center of the exposure field.

---

358. Why is a grid not required for a tangential projection knee projection? _____

359. What open joint spaces are demonstrated on a tangential projection knee projection?

_____

360. How are the patient's legs positioned to prevent rotation on a tangential projection knee projection?

_____

361. How do the positions of the patellae and femoral condyles change when the knees are in external rotation for a
tangential projection knee projection?

A. Patellae: _____

B. Femoral condyles: _____

362. The tangential projection knee projection is most often obtained to demonstrate which patient condition?

A. _____

How is this condition demonstrated on a tangential projection knee projection with accurate positioning?

B. _____

How can one distinguish this condition from rotation on a tangential projection knee projection?

C. _____

363. Why is it important for the patient to relax the quadriceps femoris muscles for the tangential projection knee projection?

_____

364. How are the long axes of the patient's femurs positioned to obtain a tangential projection knee projection with
accurate positioning?

_____

365. Where are the long axes of the patient's posterior knee curves positioned with respect to the axial viewer for a
tangential projection knee projection with accurate positioning?

_____

366. How is the positioning setup for a tangential projection knee projection adjusted when imaging a patient with large
posterior calves?

A. _____

_____

If this positioning setup is not changed, which anatomic misalignment appears on the resulting projection?

B. _____

_____

367. What are the standard direction and degree of central ray angulation used for the tangential projection?

_____

368. What is the sum of the central ray angle and the angle of the axial viewer for all tangential projections?

_____

369. Why is a 72-inch (183-cm) SID used for the tangential projection?

_____

370. On a tangential projection knee projection with accurate positioning, the _____ are centered along the longitudinal axis of the collimated field.

371. Which anatomic structures are included on a tangential projection knee projection with accurate positioning?

_____

For the following descriptions of tangential projection knee projections with poor positioning, state how the patient would have been mispositioned for such a projection to be obtained.

372. The patellae are demonstrated directly above the intercondylar sulci and rotated laterally. The medial femoral condyles demonstrate more height than the lateral condyles.

_____

373. Soft tissue from the patient's anterior thighs has been projected onto the patellae and patellofemoral joint spaces.

_____

374. The patellae are resting against the intercondylar sulci, obscuring the patellofemoral joint spaces.

_____

375. The tibial tuberosities are demonstrated within the patellofemoral joint spaces. The patient's calves were not large.

_____

For the following tangential (axial) projection knee projections with poor positioning, state which anatomic structures are misaligned and how the patient should be repositioned for an optimal projection to be obtained.

Figure 6-82

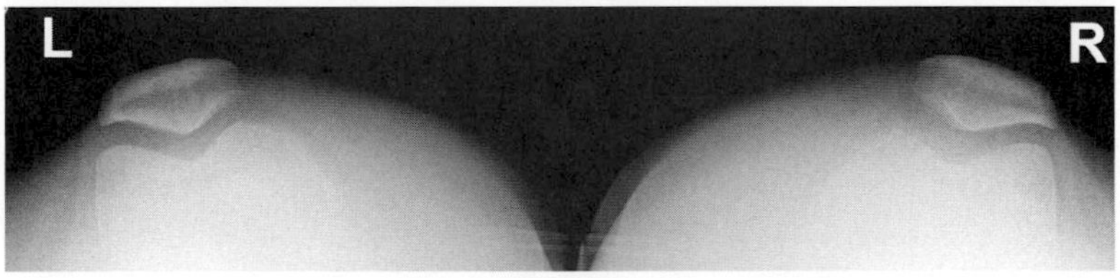

376. Figure 6-82: _____

_____

_____

_____

Figure 6-83

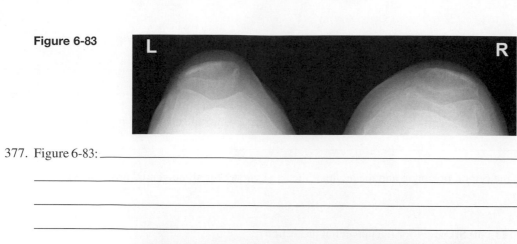

377. Figure 6-83: _____

_____

_____

_____

Figure 6-84

378. Figure 6-84: _____

_____

_____

_____

Figure 6-85

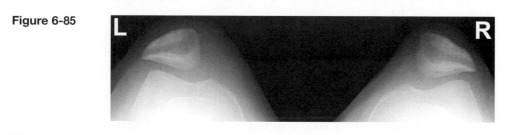

379. Figure 6-85: _____

_____

_____

_____

Femur: Anteroposterior Projection

380. Identify the labeled anatomy in Figure 6-86.

Figure 6-86

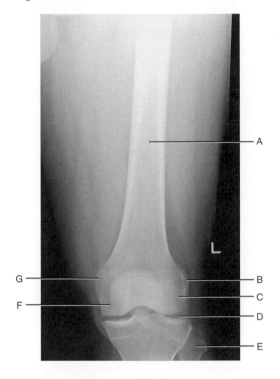

A. _____

B. _____

C. _____

D. _____

E. _____

F. _____

G. _____

381. Identify the labeled anatomy in Figure 6-87.

Figure 6-87

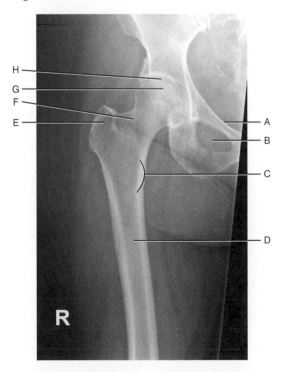

A. _____

B. _____

C. _____

D. _____

E. _____

F. _____

G. _____

H. _____

382. Complete the statements below referring to AP distal femur projection analysis criteria

---

Anteroposterior Distal Femur Projection Analysis Criteria

- Projection density is uniform across the femur.
- The medial and lateral epicondyles are in _____ (A), the femoral condyles are symmetrical in shape, and the tibia is superimposed over 0.25 inch (0.6 cm) of the _____ (B).
- The knee joint space is open but narrowed, and the anterior and posterior margins of the proximal tibia are superimposed.
- The _____ (C) is at the center of the exposure field.

---

383. Complete the statements below referring to AP proximal femur projection analysis criteria.

Anteroposterior Proximal Femur Projection Analysis Criteria

- Projection density is uniform across the femur.
- The ischial spine is aligned with the _____ (A) and the obturator foramen is open.
- The femoral neck is demonstrated without foreshortening, the _____ (B) trochanter is in profile laterally, and the _____ (C) trochanter is completely superimposed by the proximal femur.
- The _____ (D) is at the center of the exposure field.

---

384. How is the femur positioned with respect to the x-ray tube for an AP femoral projection to take advantage of the anode heel effect? _____

_____

385. Why is it necessary to include all the femoral soft tissue when imaging the femur?

_____

386. An AP distal femur is obtained by placing the patient in a _____ (A) position with the knee _____ (B) and leg _____ (C) rotated until the femoral epicondyles are at equal distances from the IR.

387. Should the technologist rotate a patient with a suspected fractured femur in an attempt to position the leg in an AP projection?

A. _____ (Yes/No)

Justify your answer.

B. _____

388. Why is the femorotibial joint space narrowed on an AP femoral projection?

_____

389. Accurate central ray centering on a distal femoral projection is accomplished by positioning the lower IR edge approximately _____ inches (A) below the _____ (B) joint.

390. Which anatomic structures are included on an AP distal femur projection with accurate positioning?

_____

391. How can the patient be positioned to prevent pelvic rotation on an AP proximal femur projection?

_____

392. How are the femoral epicondyles positioned for an AP proximal femur projection?

A. _____

How will this positioning demonstrate the femoral neck and greater trochanter on the resulting projection?

B. _____

393. On an AP proximal femur projection with accurate positioning, the _____ (A) is centered within the collimated field. This is accomplished by placing the upper IR edge at the level of the _____ (B).

394. Why should the surrounding soft tissue be included on femoral projections?

_____

395. Which anatomic structures are included on an AP proximal femur projection with accurate positioning?

_____

For the following descriptions of AP femoral projections with poor positioning, state how the patient would have been mispositioned for such a projection to be obtained.

396. The medial femoral condyle appears larger than the lateral condyle, and the intercondylar eminence is not centered within the intercondylar fossa.

_____

397. The lateral femoral condyle appears larger than the medial condyle, and the intercondylar eminence is not centered within the intercondylar fossa.

_____

398. The affected side's obturator foramen is narrowed, and the iliac spine is demonstrated without pelvic brim superimposition.

_____

399. The affected side's obturator foramen is open, and the ischial spine is not aligned with the pelvic brim but is demonstrated closer to the acetabulum.

_____

400. The femoral neck is partially foreshortened, and the lesser trochanter is demonstrated in profile.

_____

For the following AP femoral projections with poor positioning, state which anatomic structures are misaligned and how the patient should be repositioned for an optimal projection to be obtained.

Figure 6-88

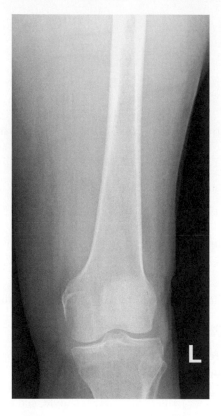

401. Figure 6-88 (distal femur): _____

_____

_____

_____

Figure 6-89

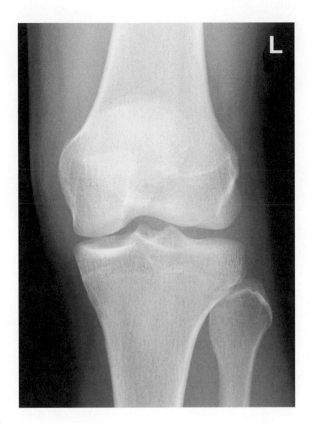

402. Figure 6-89 (distal femur): _____

_____

_____

_____

Figure 6-90

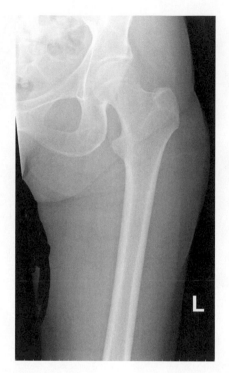

403. Figure 6-90 (proximal femur): _____

_____

_____

_____

Femur: Lateral Projection (Mediolateral)

404. Identify the labeled anatomy in Figure 6-91.

Figure 6-91

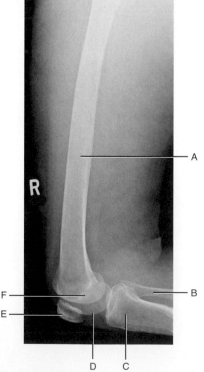

A. _____

B. _____

C. _____

D. _____

E. _____

F. _____

405. Identify the labeled anatomy in Figure 6-92.

Figure 6-92

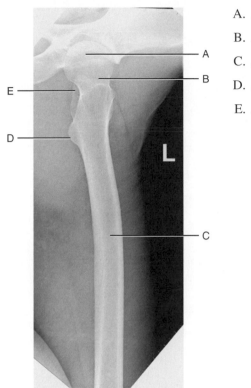

A. _____

B. _____

C. _____

D. _____

E. _____

406. Identify the labeled anatomy in Figure 6-93.

Figure 6-93

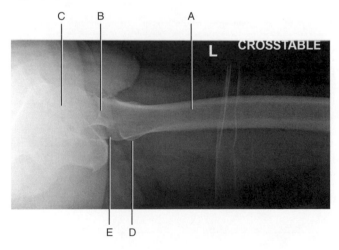

A. _____

B. _____

C. _____

D. _____

E. _____

407. Complete the statements below referring to lateral distal femur projection analysis criteria.

Lateral Distal Femur Projection Analysis Criteria

- Projection density is uniform across the femur.
- The anterior and posterior margins of the medial and lateral _____ (A) condyles are aligned and the tibia is partially superimposed by the _____ (B).
- The _____ (C) femoral condyle is projected distal to the _____ (D) femoral condyle, closing the knee joint space.
- The _____ (E) is at the center of the exposure field.

408. Complete the statements below referring to lateral proximal femur projection analysis criteria.

Lateral Proximal Distal Femur Projection Analysis Criteria

- Projection density is uniform across the femur.
- The lesser trochanter is in profile _____ (A) and the femoral neck and head are superimposed over the _____ (B).
- The femoral shaft is seen without foreshortening, the femoral neck is demonstrated on end, and the _____ (C) trochanter is demonstrated at the same transverse level as the femoral head.
- The long axis of the femoral shaft is aligned with the long axis of the collimated field.
- The _____ (D) is at the center of the exposure field.

409. To take advantage of the anode heel effect, how is the femur positioned with respect to the x-ray tube for a lateral femur projection?

_____

_____

410. A lateral distal femur projection is obtained by rotating the patient onto the _____ (medial/lateral) (A) aspect of the affected femur until an imaginary line connecting the femoral epicondyles is aligned _____ (B) to the IR.

411. Which of the femoral condyles is positioned distally on a lateral distal femur projection with accurate positioning?

A. _____

What causes this distal positioning?

B. _____

C. _____

412. How is a lateral distal femur projection obtained in a patient with a known or suspected femur fracture?

_____

_____

413. What advantage is gained by aligning the long axis of the femoral shaft with the long axis of the collimated field?

_____

414. Accurate central ray centering on a lateral distal femur projection is accomplished by placing the lower IR edge approximately _____ inches (A) below the _____ (B).

415. Which anatomic structures are included on a lateral distal femur projection with accurate positioning?

_____

_____

416. How is the patient positioned to place the lesser trochanter in profile and the greater trochanter beneath the femoral neck on a lateral proximal femur projection? _____

_____

417. How is the patient positioned for a lateral proximal femur projection to demonstrate the femoral shaft without fore-shortening and the femoral neck on end? _____

_____

418. Which position is performed to demonstrate a lateral proximal femur when a fracture is suspected or known to be present? _____

_____

419. On a lateral proximal femoral projection with accurate positioning, the _____ (A) is centered within the collimated field. This is accomplished by positioning the upper IR edge at the level of the

_____ (B).

420. Which anatomic structures are included on a lateral proximal femoral projection with accurate positioning?

_____

For the following descriptions of lateral femoral projections with poor positioning, state how the patient would have been mispositioned for such a projection to be obtained.

421. The anterior and posterior surfaces of the medial and lateral femoral condyles are demonstrated without alignment. The medial condyle is posterior to the lateral condyle.

_____

422. The anterior and posterior surfaces of the medial and lateral femoral condyles are demonstrated without alignment. The medial condyle is anterior to the lateral condyle.

_____

423. The greater trochanter is demonstrated medially (next to the ischial tuberosity), and the lesser trochanter is obscured.

_____

424. The greater trochanter is demonstrated laterally, and the lesser trochanter is obscured.

_____

For the following lateral femoral projections with poor positioning, state which anatomic structures are misaligned and how the patient should be repositioned for an optimal projection to be obtained.

Figure 6-94

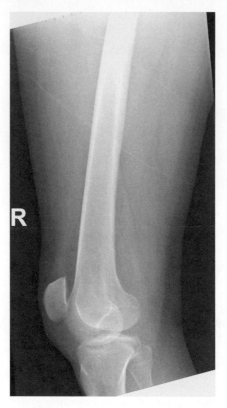

425. Figure 6-94 (distal femur): _____

_____

_____

_____

Figure 6-95

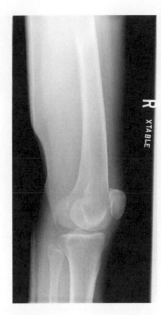

426. Figure 6-95 (trauma, lateromedial distal femur): _____

_____

_____

_____

Figure 6-96

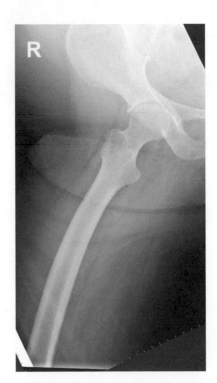

427. Figure 6-96 (proximal femur): _____

_____

_____

_____

Figure 6-97

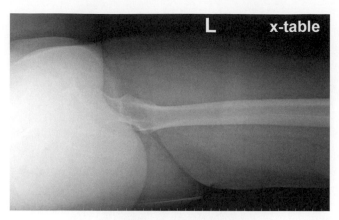

428. Figure 6-97 (proximal femur): _____

_____

_____

_____

Figure 6-98

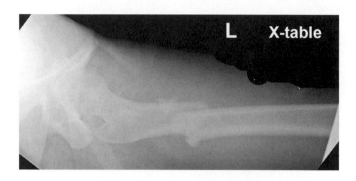

429. Figure 6-98 (trauma, proximal femur): _____

_____

_____

_____

7 Hip and Pelvis

STUDY QUESTIONS

1. Describe how the following hip and pelvic projections should be displayed on a view box or digital monitor.

   A. Left axiolateral hip: _____

   _____

   B. AP pelvis: _____

   _____

   C. Left AP oblique sacroiliac joints: _____

   _____

2. Which anatomic artifact is common on AP hip and pelvic projections?

   _____

3. List the four soft tissue structures that are demonstrated on accurately exposed AP hip and pelvis projections, and describe their locations.

   A. _____

   B. _____

   C. _____

   D. _____

   Why is it important that these soft tissue structures be visualized?

   E. _____

4. Complete Exercise 7-1.

EXERCISE 7-1 Hip and Pelvis Technical Data				
Projection	kVp	Grid	AEC Chamber(s)	SID
AP, hip				
PA oblique, hip				
Axiolateral, hip				
AP, pelvis				
AP oblique, pelvis				
AP axial, sacroiliac joints				
AP oblique, sacroiliac joints				

AEC, Automatic exposure control; *kVp*, kilovoltage peak; *SID*, source–image receptor distance.

Hip: Anteroposterior Projection

5. Identify the labeled anatomy in Figure 7-1.

Figure 7-1

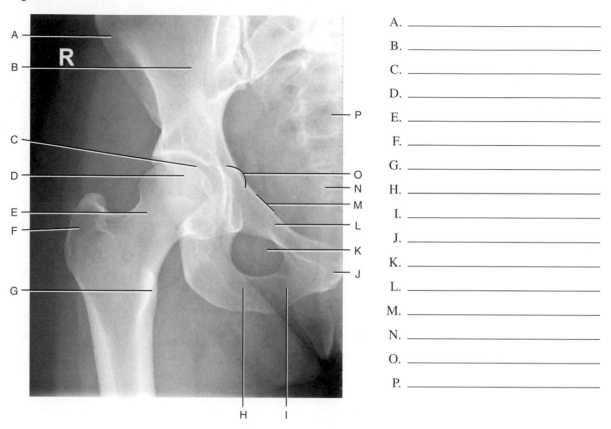

A. _____

B. _____

C. _____

D. _____

E. _____

F. _____

G. _____

H. _____

I. _____

J. _____

K. _____

L. _____

M. _____

N. _____

O. _____

P. _____

6. Complete the statements below referring to AP hip projection analysis criteria.

Anteroposterior Hip Projection Analysis Criteria
• The ischial spine is aligned with the _____ (A), the sacrum and coccyx are aligned with the _____ (B), and the obturator foramen is open.
• The femoral neck is demonstrated without foreshortening, the greater trochanter is in profile _____ (C), and the lesser trochanter is superimposed by the _____ (D).

7. How can patient positioning be evaluated to ensure that pelvic rotation is not present on an AP hip projection?

_____

8. Describe the relationship that would result between the following anatomic structures on an AP hip projection if the affected side were rotated away from the IR.

A. Sacrum and symphysis pubis: _____

B. Iliac spine and pelvic brim: _____

9. If the affected hip is rotated toward the IR for an AP hip projection, how will the obturator foramen appear in comparison with a nonrotated AP hip projection? _____

10. The demonstration of the femoral neck and lesser trochanter on an AP hip projection depends on the position of the femoral epicondyles. For each epicondyle position in the following list, describe how the femoral neck and lesser trochanter are demonstrated on an AP hip projection.

   A. Leg is externally rotated, with the foot at a 45-degree angle and an imaginary line connecting the femoral epicondyles at a 60- to 65-degree angle with the imaging table:

   _____

   B. Leg is internally rotated, with the foot vertical and an imaginary line connecting the femoral epicondyles at a 15- to 20-degree angle with imaging table:

   _____

   C. Leg is internally rotated, with the foot 15 to 20 degrees from vertical and an imaginary line connecting the femoral epicondyles aligned parallel with imaging table:

   _____

11. How are the patient's foot and femoral epicondyles positioned to obtain an AP hip projection with accurate positioning? _____

   _____

12. Should the technologist attempt to rotate the leg of a patient with a suspected fracture or dislocated hip?

   A. _____ (Yes/No)

   Defend your answer.

   B. _____

13. Accurate central ray centering on an AP hip projection is accomplished by centering a _____ (A) central ray 1.5 inches (4 cm) _____ (B) to the midpoint of a line connecting the anterior superior iliac spine (ASIS) and superior _____ (C).

14. Which anatomic structures are included on an AP hip projection with accurate positioning?

   _____

15. How may the positioning procedure require adjusting if the patient has a prosthesis? _____

   _____

16. State whether gonadal shielding should be used for an AP hip projection for the following:

   A. Male: _____

   B. Female: _____

For the following descriptions of AP hip projections with poor positioning, state how the patient would have been mispositioned for such a projection to be obtained.

17. The ischial spine is demonstrated without pelvic brim superimposition, the sacrum and coccyx are not aligned with the symphysis pubis but are rotated away from the affected hip, and the obturator foramen is narrowed.

   _____

18. The ischial spine is not aligned with the pelvic brim but is demonstrated closer to the acetabulum, the sacrum and coccyx are not aligned with the symphysis pubis but are rotated toward the affected hip, and the obturator foramen is clearly demonstrated.

_____

19. The femoral neck is completely foreshortened, and the lesser trochanter is demonstrated in profile.

_____

For the following AP hip projections with poor positioning, state which anatomic structures are misaligned and how the patient should be repositioned for an optimal projection to be obtained.

Figure 7-2

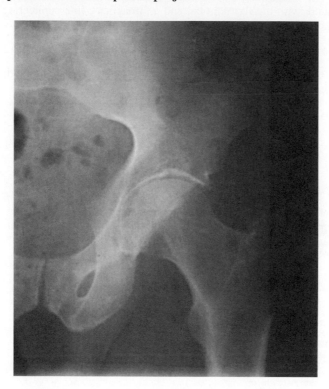

20. Figure 7-2: _____

_____

_____

_____

_____

_____

Figure 7-3

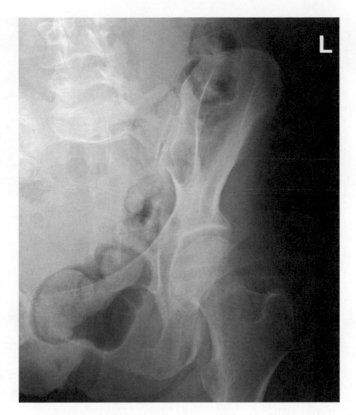

21. Figure 7-3: _____

_____

_____

_____

_____

_____

Figure 7-4

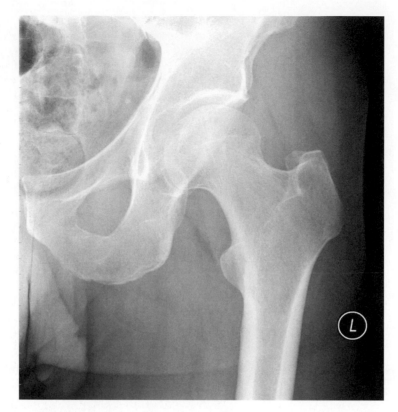

22. Figure 7-4: _____

_____

_____

_____

_____

_____

Figure 7-5

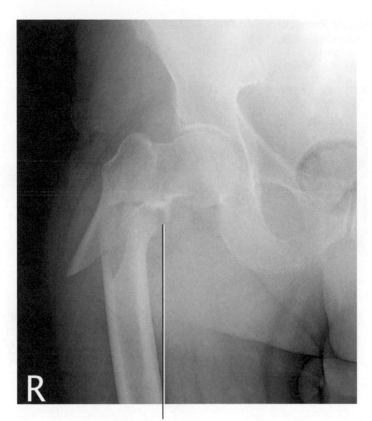

Lesser trochanter

23. Figure 7-5 (fracture): _____

_____

_____

_____

_____

_____

_____

Hip: Anteroposterior Oblique Projection (Modified Cleaves Method)

24. Identify the labeled anatomy in Figure 7-6.

Figure 7-6

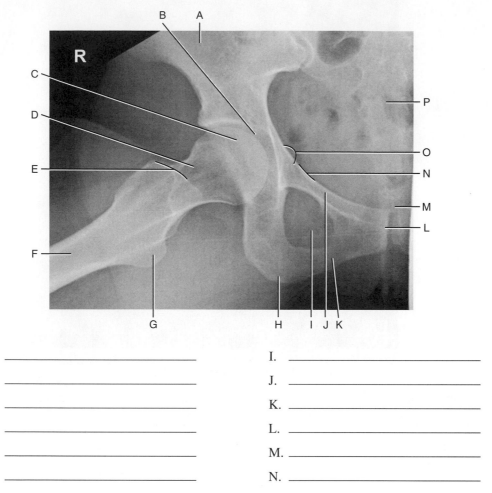

A. _____

B. _____

C. _____

D. _____

E. _____

F. _____

G. _____

H. _____

I. _____

J. _____

K. _____

L. _____

M. _____

N. _____

O. _____

P. _____

25. Complete the statements below referring to an AP oblique hip projection analysis criteria.

Anteroposterior Oblique Hip Projection (Modified Cleaves Method) Analysis Criteria
• The _____ (A) is aligned with the pelvic brim, the sacrum and coccyx are aligned with the symphysis pubis, and the obturator foramen is open.
• The _____ (B) is in profile medially and the _____ (C) is superimposed over the greater trochanter.
• The _____ (D) is partially foreshortened and the proximal _____ (E) is demonstrated at a transverse level halfway between the femoral head and the lesser trochanter.

26. How can rotation of the pelvis be avoided when positioning a patient for an AP oblique hip projection?

_____

27. For the Lauenstein and Hickey lateral hip methods, the patient's pelvis is rotated _____ (toward/away from) (A) the affected hip until the femur is placed _____ (B).

28. The degree of patient knee and hip flexion determines whether the greater and lesser trochanter will be in

_____.

29. At what degree with the imaging table is the femur placed to accurately demonstrate the lesser trochanter on an AP oblique hip projection in profile? _____

30. The degree of femoral abduction for an AP oblique hip projection will determine which two proximal femur anatomic relationships?

A. _____

B. _____

31. Describe the position of the greater trochanter and degree of femoral neck foreshortening demonstrated on an AP oblique hip projection if the femur is abducted as stated for each of the following:

A. Femur is abducted until it is placed next to the imaging table:

_____

B. Femur is abducted to a 45-degree angle with the imaging table:

_____

C. Femur is abducted 20 to 30 degrees from vertical:

_____

32. Accurate central ray centering on an AP oblique hip projection is accomplished by centering a _____ (A) central ray _____ (B) inches distal to the midpoint of a line connecting the _____ (C) and superior symphysis pubis.

33. Which anatomic structures are included on an AP oblique hip projection with accurate positioning?

_____

_____

For the following descriptions of AP oblique hip projections with poor positioning, state how the patient would have been mispositioned for such a projection to be obtained.

34. The ischial spine is demonstrated without pelvic brim superimposition, the sacrum and coccyx are not aligned with the symphysis pubis but are rotated away from the affected hip, and the obturator foramen is narrowed.

_____

35. The greater trochanter is positioned medially, and the lesser trochanter is obscured.

_____

36. The greater trochanter is positioned laterally.

_____

37. The femoral neck is demonstrated on end, and the greater trochanter is demonstrated on the same transverse level as the femoral head.

_____

For the following AP oblique hip projections with poor positioning, state which anatomic structures are misaligned and how the patient should be repositioned for an optimal projection to be obtained.

Figure 7-7

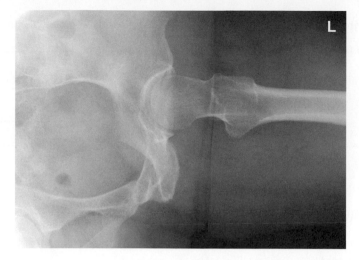

38. Figure 7-7: _____

_____

_____

_____

Figure 7-8

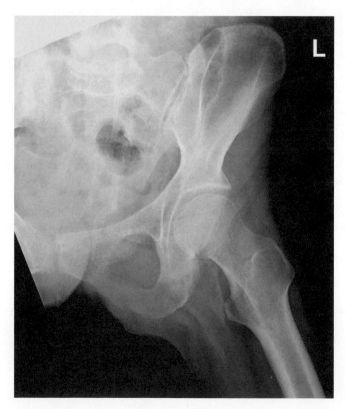

39. Figure 7-8: _____

_____

_____

Figure 7-9

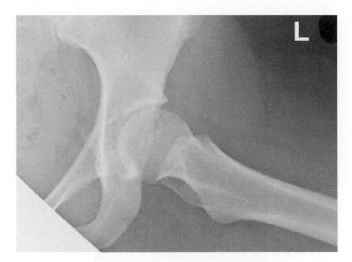

40. Figure 7-9: _____

_____

_____

_____

Figure 7-10

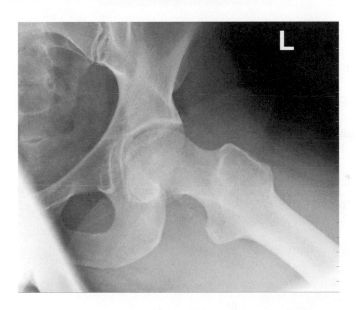

41. Figure 7-10: _____

_____

_____

_____

Figure 7-11

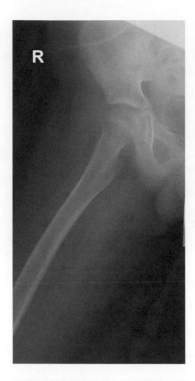

42. Figure 7-11: _____

_____

_____

_____

Hip: Axiolateral (Inferosuperior) Projection (Danelius-Miller Method)

43. Identify the labeled anatomy in Figure 7-12.

Figure 7-12

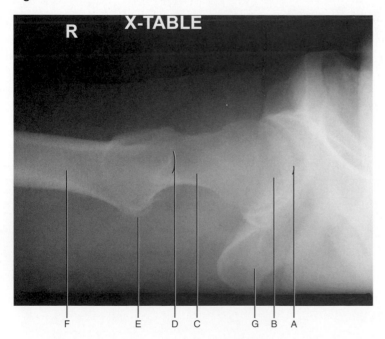

A. _____

B. _____

C. _____

D. _____

E. _____

F. _____

G. _____

44. Complete the statements below referring to axiolateral hip projection analysis criteria.

> **Axiolateral Hip Projection Analysis Criteria**
>
> - The proximal femur demonstrates uniform density across it.
> - The femoral neck is demonstrated without foreshortening, and the _____ (A) and lesser trochanters are demonstrated at approximately the same level.
> - The lesser trochanter is in profile _____ (B) and the greater trochanter is superimposed by the _____ (C).

45. State three ways that scatter radiation can be reduced on an axiolateral hip projection.

    A. _____

    B. _____

    C. _____

46. Describe how a wedge compensating filter is positioned if used for an axiolateral hip projection.

    _____

47. How is the unaffected leg positioned for an axiolateral hip projection to prevent its soft tissue from superimposing the affected hip?

    _____

    _____

48. Where is the IR placed for an axiolateral hip projection?

    A. _____

    How is it aligned with the femoral neck?

    B. _____

    How is the position of the IR changed if the patient has a large amount of lateral soft tissue thickness?

    C. _____

    How should the central ray be positioned with respect to the IR and femoral neck?

    D. _____

49. Describe how to localize the femoral neck when positioning for an axiolateral hip projection.

    _____

    _____

50. Describe the appearance of the femoral neck and greater trochanter if the central ray is not accurately aligned with the femoral neck for an axiolateral hip projection.

    A. Femoral neck: _____

    B. Greater trochanter: _____

51. Forced internal rotation of a dislocated hip or fractured proximal femur may cause _____

    _____

52. How is the patient's leg positioned to accurately position the lesser trochanter on an axiolateral hip projection?

_____

_____

53. On an axiolateral hip projection with accurate positioning, the _____ is centered within the collimated field.

54. Which anatomic structures are included on an axiolateral hip projection with accurate positioning?

_____

For the following descriptions of axiolateral hip projections with poor positioning, state how the patient or central ray would have been mispositioned for such a projection to be obtained.

55. The soft tissue from the unaffected thigh is superimposed over the acetabulum and femoral head of the affected hip.

_____

56. The greater trochanter is demonstrated at a transverse level that is proximal to the lesser trochanter, and the femoral neck is partially foreshortened.

_____

57. The greater trochanter is demonstrated posteriorly, and the lesser trochanter is superimposed over the femoral shaft.

_____

For the following axiolateral hip projections with poor positioning, state which anatomic structures are misaligned and how the patient or central ray should be repositioned for an optimal projection to be obtained.

Figure 7-13

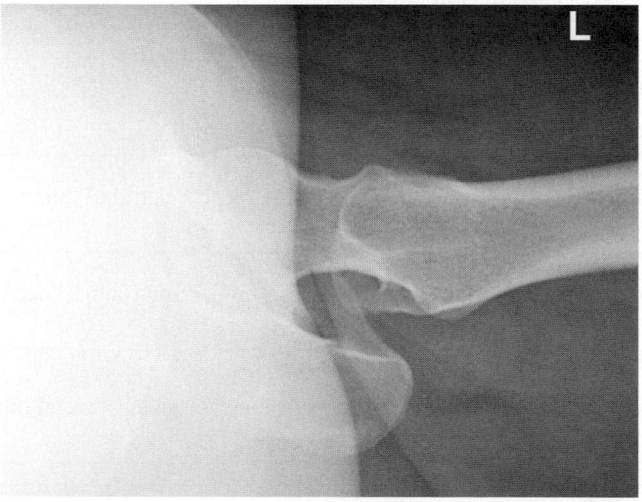

58. Figure 7-13: _____

_____

_____

_____

Figure 7-14

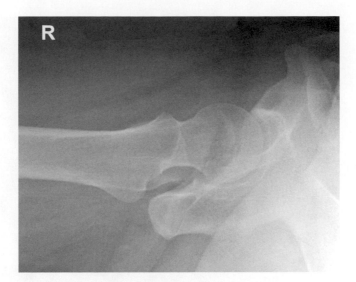

59. Figure 7-14: _____

_____

_____

_____

Figure 7-15

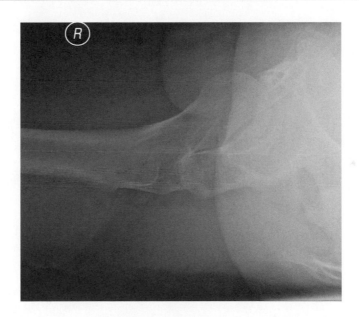

60. Figure 7-15: _____

_____

_____

_____

Figure 7-16

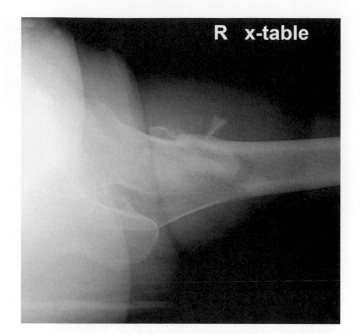

R   x-table

61. Figure 7-16 (fracture): _____

_____

_____

_____

Pelvis: Anteroposterior Projection

62. Identify the labeled anatomy in Figure 7-17.

Figure 7-17

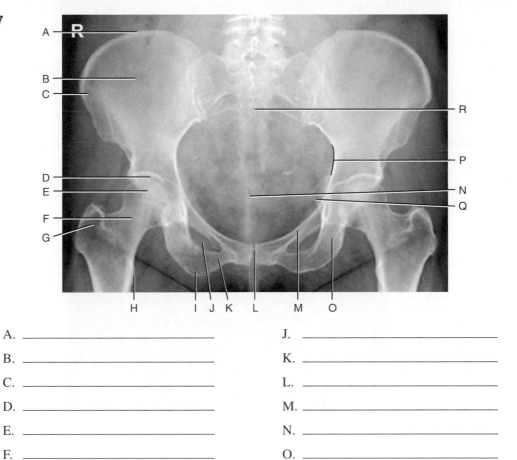

A. _____   J. _____

B. _____   K. _____

C. _____   L. _____

D. _____   M. _____

E. _____   N. _____

F. _____   O. _____

G. _____   P. _____

H. _____   Q. _____

I. _____   R. _____

63. Complete Exercise 7-2.

EXERCISE 7-2 Male and Female Pelvic Differences		
Parameter	**Male**	**Female**
Overall shape		
Ala		
Pubic arch angle		
Inlet shape		
Obturator foramen		

64. Complete the statements below referring to AP pelvis projection analysis criteria.

Anteroposterior Pelvis Projection Analysis Criteria

- The ischial spines are aligned with the _____ (A), the sacrum and coccyx are aligned with the symphysis pubis, and the obturator foramina are open and uniform in size and shape.

- The femoral necks are demonstrated without foreshortening, the _____ (B) trochanters are in

   profile laterally, and the _____ (C) trochanters are superimposed by the femoral necks.

65. State whether the following pelvis projections are from a female or male patient:

Figure 7-18

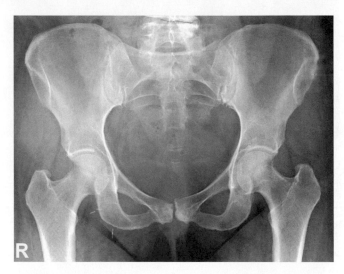

A. Figure 7-18: _____

Figure 7-19

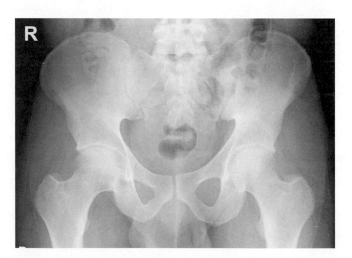

B. Figure 7-19: _____

66. How can patient positioning be evaluated to ensure that pelvic rotation is not present on an AP pelvic projection?

_____

67. Describe the relationship of the sacrum and coccyx to the symphysis pubis and that of the iliac spine to the pelvic brim on an AP pelvic projection in which the patient's left side was rotated away from the IR.

_____

_____

68. Following are descriptions of the femoral neck appearance on different AP pelvic projections. For each description, state the position of the patient's feet and humeral epicondyles that would result in the described projection.

A. Femoral necks without foreshortening: _____

_____

B. Femoral necks on end: _____

_____

C. Femoral necks partially foreshortened: _____

_____

69. How are the patient's feet and femoral epicondyles positioned for an AP pelvic projection with accurate positioning to be obtained?

_____

_____

70. Accurate central ray centering on an AP pelvic projection is accomplished by centering a _____

(A) central ray to the midsagittal plane at a level halfway between the _____ (B) and an imaginary line connecting the _____ (C).

71. Which anatomic structures are included on an AP pelvic projection with accurate positioning?

_____

_____

For the following descriptions of AP pelvic projections with poor positioning, state how the patient would have been mispositioned for such a projection to be obtained.

72. The right obturator foramen is narrowed, the right ischial spine is demonstrated without pelvic brim superimposition, and the sacrum and coccyx are rotated toward the left hip.

_____

73. The femoral necks are foreshortened, and the lesser trochanters are demonstrated in profile.

_____

For the following AP pelvic projections with poor positioning, state which anatomic structures are misaligned and how the patient should be repositioned for an optimal projection to be obtained.

Figure 7-20

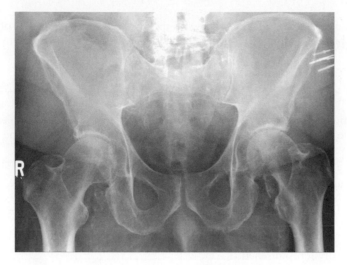

74. Figure 7-20: _____

_____

_____

_____

_____

Figure 7-21

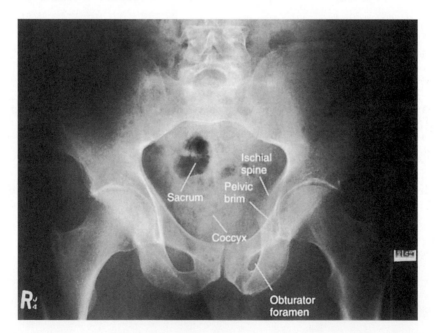

75. Figure 7-21: _____

_____

_____

_____

Figure 7-22

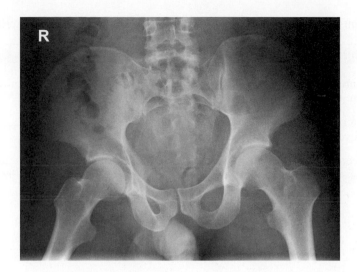

76. Figure 7-22: _____

_____

_____

_____

Pelvis: Anteroposterior Oblique Projection (Modified Cleaves Method)

77. Identify the labeled anatomy in Figure 7-23.

Figure 7-23

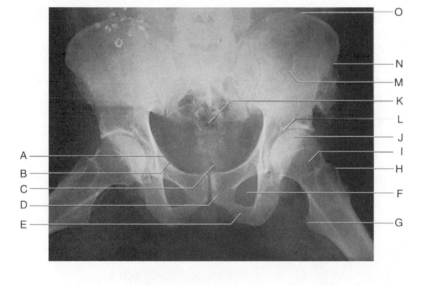

A. _____

B. _____

C. _____

D. _____

E. _____

F. _____

G. _____

H. _____

I. _____

J. _____

K. _____

L. _____

M. _____

N. _____

O. _____

78. Complete the statements below referring to AP oblique pelvis projection analysis criteria.

Anteroposterior Oblique Pelvis Projection (Modified Cleaves Method) Analysis Criteria
• The ischial spines are aligned with the pelvic brim, the sacrum and coccyx are aligned with the symphysis pubis, and the obturator foramina are open and uniform in size and shape.
• The lesser trochanters are in profile _____ (A) and the _____ (B) are superimposed over the adjacent greater trochanters.
• The femoral necks are partially foreshortened and the _____ (C) are demonstrated at the same transverse level halfway between the femoral heads and lesser trochanters.

79. How can the rotation of the pelvis be avoided when positioning a patient for an AP oblique pelvic projection?

_____

80. Describe the relationship of the sacrum and coccyx to the symphysis pubis and that of the iliac spine to the pelvic brim that result on an AP pelvic projection if the patient's right side is rotated away from the IR.

_____

_____

_____

81. The degree of patient knee and hip flexion determines whether the greater and lesser trochanters will be in

_____.

82. At what degree with the imaging table are the femurs placed to position the greater and lesser trochanters on an AP oblique pelvic projection accurately?

_____

83. The patient's knees and hips were flexed 20 degrees with the imaging table for an AP oblique pelvic projection. How can this misposition be identified on the resulting projection?

_____

84. The degree of femoral abduction for an AP oblique pelvic projection determines which two anatomic relationships?

A. _____

B. _____

85. Describe the position of the greater trochanters and the degree of femoral neck foreshortening demonstrated on an AP oblique pelvic projection if the femurs are abducted as follows:

A. Femurs are abducted until placed against the imaging table:

_____

B. Femurs are abducted to a 45-degree angle with the imaging table:

_____

C. Femurs are abducted only 20 to 30 degrees from vertical:

_____

86. Accurate central ray centering on an AP oblique pelvic projection is accomplished by centering a _____ (A) central ray to the _____ (B) plane at a level _____ (C) superior to the _____ (D).

87. Which anatomic structures are included on an AP oblique pelvic projection with accurate positioning?

_____

_____

For the following descriptions of AP oblique pelvic projections with poor positioning, state how the patient would have been mispositioned for such a projection to be obtained.

88. The left obturator foramen is narrowed, the left ischial spine is demonstrated without pelvic brim superimposition, and the sacrum and coccyx are rotated toward the right hip.

_____

89. The femoral necks are demonstrated on end and the greater trochanters are demonstrated on the same transverse level as the femoral heads.

_____

For the following AP oblique pelvic projections with poor positioning, state which anatomic structures are misaligned and how the patient should be repositioned for an optimal projection to be obtained.

Figure 7-24

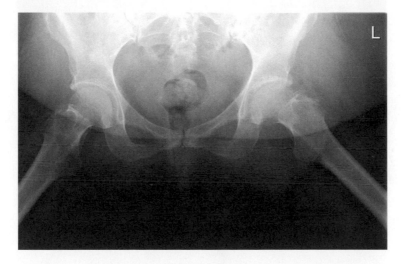

90. Figure 7-24: _____

_____

_____

_____

Figure 7-25

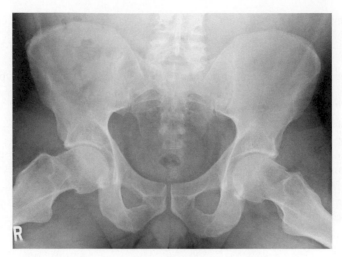

91. Figure 7-25: _____

_____

_____

_____

Figure 7-26

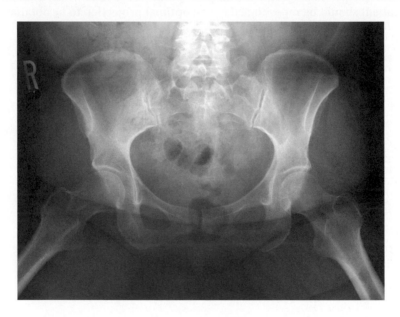

92. Figure 7-26: _____

_____

_____

_____

Figure 7-27

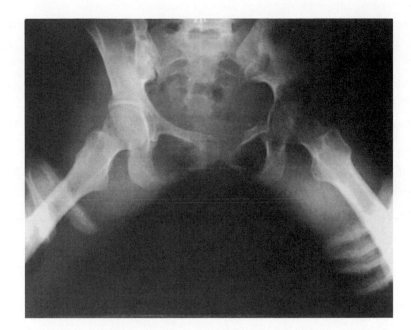

93. Figure 7-27: _____

_____

_____

_____

Sacroiliac Joints: Anteroposterior Axial Projection

94. Identify the labeled anatomy in Figure 7-28.

Figure 7-28

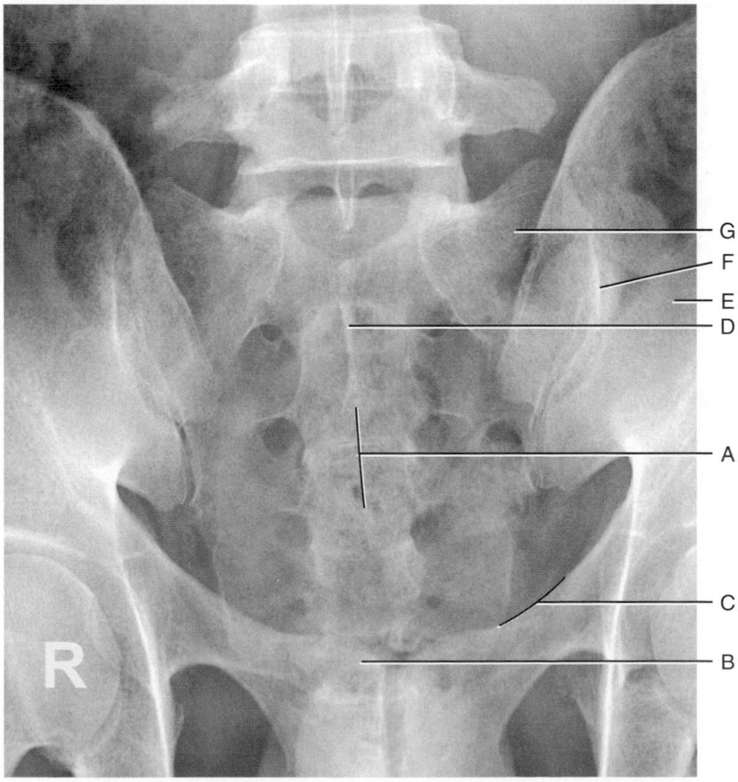

A. _____

B. _____

C. _____

D. _____

E. _____

F. _____

G. _____

95. Complete the statements below referring to AP axial sacroiliac joint projection analysis criteria.

> **Anteroposterior Axial Sacroiliac Joints Projection Analysis Criteria**
>
> • The median sacral crest is aligned with the _____ (A) and the sacrum is at equal distance from the lateral wall of the pelvic brim on both sides.
>
> • The sacroiliac joints are demonstrated without foreshortening and the sacrum is elongated, with the
>
> _____ (B) superimposed over the inferior sacral segments.
>
> • The long axis of the median sacral crest is aligned with the long axis of the collimated field.

96. How can patient positioning be evaluated to ensure that pelvic rotation is not present on an AP sacroiliac joint projection?

_____

97. When a patient is rotated for an AP sacroiliac joint projection, the sacrum rotates in the _____ (same/ opposite) (A) direction as the symphysis pubis and is positioned next to the lateral wall of the pelvic brim situated

_____ (closer/farther) (B) to/from the IR.

98. How are the patient and central ray positioned to demonstrate the sacroiliac joints without foreshortening?

A. For a male patient: _____

B. For a female patient: _____

C. For a patient with greater than average lumbosacral curvature:

_____

_____

D. For a patient with less than average lumbosacral curvature:

_____

_____

99. Why is the median sacral crest aligned with the long axis of the collimated field for an AP sacroiliac joint projection?

A. _____

B. _____

100. Accurate central ray centering on an AP sacroiliac joint projection is obtained by positioning the central ray to

the patient's _____ (A) plane at a level halfway between an imaginary line connecting the

_____ (B) and _____ (C).

101. Which anatomic structures are included on an AP sacroiliac joint projection with accurate positioning? _____

_____

For the following descriptions of AP sacroiliac joint projections with poor positioning, state how the patient or central ray would have been mispositioned for such a projection to be obtained.

102. The sacrum is situated closer to the right pelvic brim than to the left.

_____

103. The sacroiliac joints are foreshortened, and the inferior sacrum is demonstrated without symphysis pubis superimposition.

_____

For the following AP sacroiliac joint projections with poor positioning, state which anatomic structures are misaligned and how the patient should be repositioned for an optimal projection to be obtained.

Figure 7-29

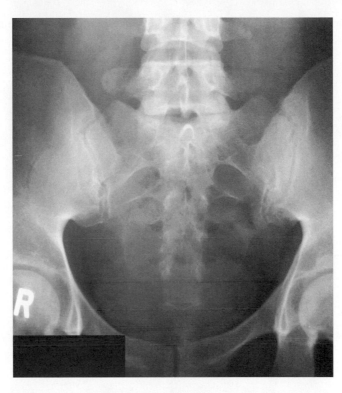

104. Figure 7-29: _____

_____

_____

_____

_____

Figure 7-30

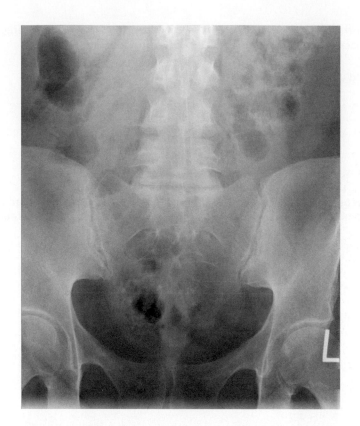

105. Figure 7-30: _____

_____

_____

Figure 7-31

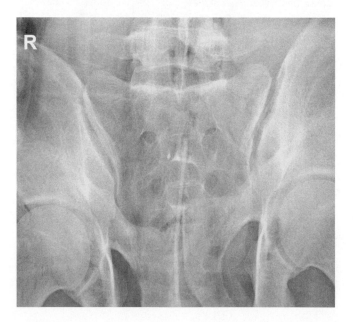

106. Figure 7-31: _____

_____

_____

_____

Sacroiliac Joints: Anteroposterior Oblique Projection (Left and Right Posterior Oblique Positions)

107. Identify the labeled anatomy in Figure 7-32.

Figure 7-32

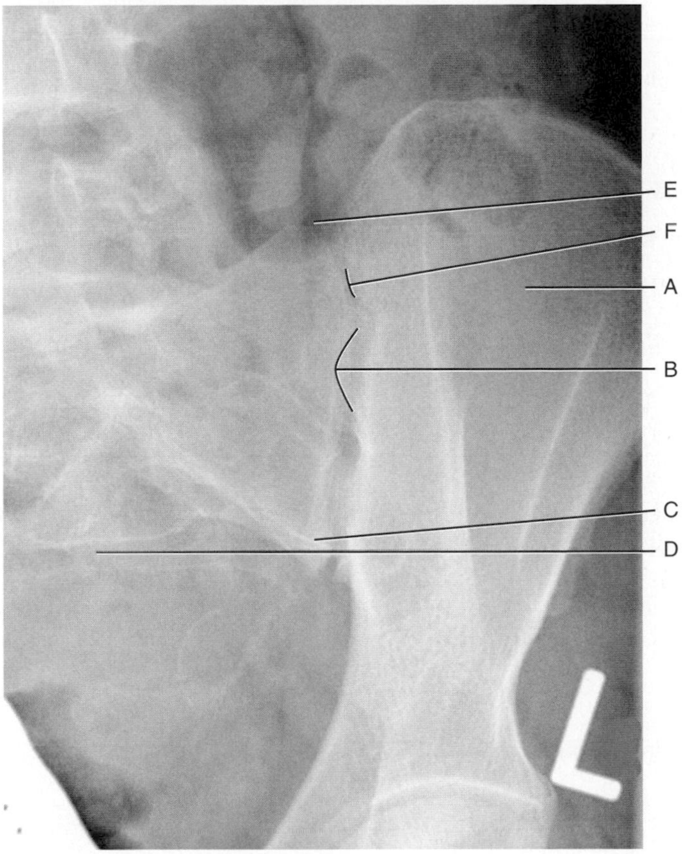

A. _____

B. _____

C. _____

D. _____

E. _____

F. _____

108. Complete the statements below referring to AP oblique sacroiliac joint projection analysis criteria.

Anteroposterior Oblique Sacroiliac Joint Projection Analysis Criteria
• A right or left marker identifying the sacroiliac joint positioned farther from the IR is present on the projection and is not superimposed over the anatomy of interest.
• The ilium and _____ (A) are demonstrated without superimposition, and the sacroiliac joint is open.
• The long axis of the sacroiliac joint is aligned with the _____ (B) of the collimated field.

IR, Image receptor.

109. Which two bony structures articulate to form the sacroiliac joints?

A. _____

B. _____

110. An open sacroiliac joint is obtained when the _____ (A) and _____ (B) are demonstrated without superimposition.

111. For an open sacroiliac joint to be obtained on an AP oblique sacroiliac joint projection, the patient is rotated until the _____ (A) plane is at a _____-degree (B) angle with the imaging table and IR.

112. Which sacroiliac joint is open when the patient is placed in a left posterior oblique (LPO) position?

A. _____

Which sacroiliac joint is open if the patient is placed in a right anterior oblique (RAO) position?

B. _____

113. The affected sacroiliac joint is centered within the collimated field on an AP oblique sacroiliac joint projection with accurate positioning. This centering is obtained by placing the central ray 1 to 1.5 inches _____ (medial/lateral) (A) to the elevated _____ (B).

114. Which anatomic structures are included on an AP oblique sacroiliac joint projection with accurate positioning?

_____

_____

For the following descriptions of AP oblique sacroiliac joint projections with poor positioning, state how the patient would have been mispositioned for such a projection to be obtained.

115. The sacroiliac joint is closed, the superior and inferior sacral ala are demonstrated without iliac superimposition, and the lateral sacral ala is superimposed over the iliac tuberosity.

_____

116. The sacroiliac joint is closed, and the ilium is superimposed over the lateral sacral ala and inferior sacrum.

_____

For the following AP oblique sacroiliac joint projections with poor positioning, state which anatomic structures are misaligned and how the patient should be repositioned for an optimal projection to be obtained.

Figure 7-33

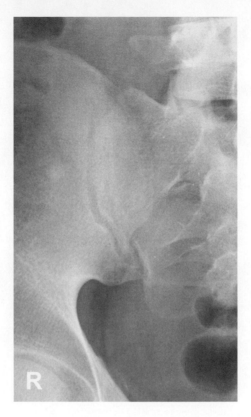

117. Figure 7-33: _____

_____

_____

_____

Figure 7-34

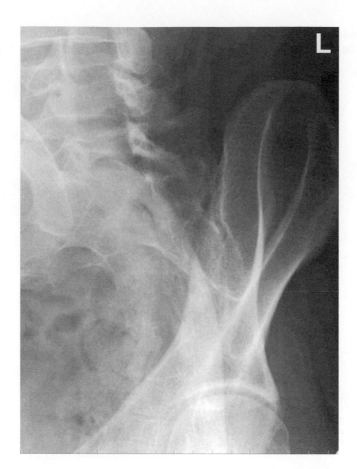

118. Figure 7-34: _____

_____

_____

_____

8 Cervical and Thoracic Vertebrae

1. Describe how the following vertebral projections should be displayed on a view box or digital monitor.

   A. AP cervical vertebrae: _____

   _____

   B. PA oblique cervical vertebrae (right anterior oblique [RAO] position): _____

   _____

   C. Lateral cervicothoracic (Twining method): _____

   _____

   D. Lateral thoracic vertebrae: _____

   _____

2. Complete Exercise 8-1.

EXERCISE 8-1 Cervical and Thoracic Vertebrae Technical Data				
Projection	kVp	Grid	AEC Chamber(s)	SID
AP axial, cervical vertebrae				
AP, open-mouth, C1 and C2				
Lateral, cervical vertebrae				
AP axial oblique, cervical vertebrae				
Lateral (Twining method), cervicothoracic vertebrae				
AP, thoracic vertebrae				
Lateral, thoracic vertebrae				

AEC, Automatic exposure control; *kVp,* kilovoltage peak ; *SID,* source–image receptor distance.

3. Define the following:

   A. Acanthiomeatal line: _____

   _____

   B. Costal breathing: _____

   _____

   C. EAM: _____

   _____

D. IOML: _____

_____

E. Occlusal plane: _____

_____

Cervical Vertebrae: Anteroposterior Axial Projection

4. Identify the labeled anatomy in Figure 8-1.

Figure 8-1

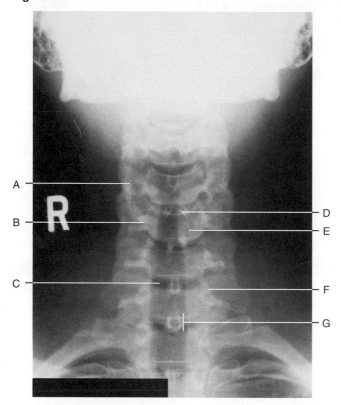

A. _____

B. _____

C. _____

D. _____

E. _____

F. _____

G. _____

5. Complete the statements below referring to AP axial cervical vertebrae projection analysis criteria.

Anteroposterior Axial Cervical Vertebrae Projection Analysis Criteria

• The _____ (A) are aligned with the midline of the cervical bodies, the mandibular angles and mastoid tips are at equal distances from the cervical vertebrae, the articular pillars

and pedicles are symmetrically visualized _____ (B) and to the cervical bodies, and the distance from the vertebral column to the medial clavicular ends is equal.

• The intervertebral disk spaces are open, the vertebral bodies are demonstrated without distortion, and each

vertebra's spinous process is visualized at the level of its _____ (C) intervertebral disk space.

• The third cervical vertebra is demonstrated in its entirety and the posterior occiput and mandibular mentum

are _____ (D).

• The long axis of the cervical column is aligned with the long axis of the exposure field.

---

6. If the transversely collimated field is coned to a 6-inch (15-cm) field size, where is the marker placed to ensure that it will be within the collimated field? _____

7. How is the patient positioned for an AP axial cervical projection to prevent rotation of the upper and lower cervical vertebrae?

A. Upper: _____

_____

B. Lower: _____

_____

8. When the patient and cervical vertebrae are rotated away from the AP axial projection, the vertebral bodies will move toward the side positioned _____ (closer to/farther from) (A) the IR, and the spinous processes will move toward the side positioned _____ (closer to/farther from) (B) the IR.

9. Will rotation on an AP axial cervical projection with poor positioning always be demonstrated throughout the entire cervical column?

A. _____ (Yes/No)

Defend your answer.

B. _____

_____

10. A patient wearing a collar and on a backboard is taken to the x-ray department for a cervical vertebrae series. Should the collar be removed before the x-rays are taken?

A. _____ (Yes/No)

The patient's head is rotated. Should it be adjusted?

B. _____ (Yes/No)

Defend your answers to parts A and B.

C. _____

_____

11. What is the curvature of the cervical vertebral column?

_____

12. How do the intervertebral disk spaces slant on the cervical vertebrae?

A. _____

Is the degree of slant higher when the patient is upright or supine?

B. _____

What central ray angulation is used for an AP axial cervical projection in a supine patient?

C. _____

In an upright patient?

D. _____

What causes this difference?

E. _____

13. If the central ray angulation is not adequately angled for an AP axial cervical projection, the intervertebral disk spaces are _____ (A) and each vertebra's spinous process is demonstrated within _____ (B).

14. Where is each vertebra's spinous process demonstrated if the central ray angulation is too cephalad?

_____

15. Does too much or too little cephalad angulation cause elongation of the uncinate processes on an AP axial cervical projection? _____

16. The third cervical vertebra is demonstrated in its entirety on an AP axial cervical projection with accurate positioning. How was the patient positioned to accomplish this demonstration? _____

_____

_____

17. Accurate central ray centering on an AP axial cervical projection is obtained by placing the central ray at the patient's _____ (A) plane at a level halfway between the _____ (B) and _____ (C).

18. Which anatomic structures are demonstrated on an AP axial cervical projection with accurate positioning?

_____

_____

For the following descriptions of AP axial cervical projections with poor positioning, state how the patient or central ray would have been mispositioned for such a projection to be obtained.

19. The spinous processes are not aligned with the midline of the cervical bodies and the pedicles and articular pillars are not symmetrically demonstrated lateral to the vertebral bodies. The right mandibular angle is visible, the left mandibular angle is superimposed over the cervical vertebrae, and the medial end of the right clavicle is demonstrated without vertebral column superimposition.

_____

20. The anteroinferior aspects of the cervical bodies are obscuring the intervertebral disk spaces, and each vertebra's spinous process is demonstrated within the vertebral body.

_____

21. The posteroinferior aspects of the cervical bodies are obscuring the intervertebral disk spaces, the uncinate processes are elongated, and each vertebra's spinous process is demonstrated within the inferior adjoining vertebral body.

_____

22. A portion of the third cervical vertebra is superimposed over the posterior occipital bone.

_____

_____

23. The mandible is superimposed over a portion of the third cervical vertebra.

_____

24. The upper cervical vertebra is tilted toward the left side.

_____

For the following AP axial cervical projections with poor positioning, state which anatomic structures are misaligned and how the patient should be repositioned for an optimal projection to be obtained.

Figure 8-2

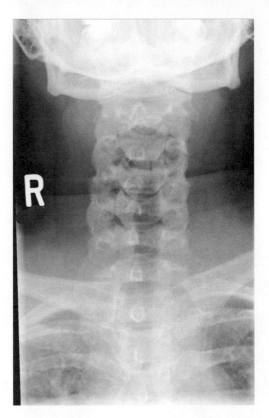

25. Figure 8-2: _____

_____

_____

_____

Figure 8-3

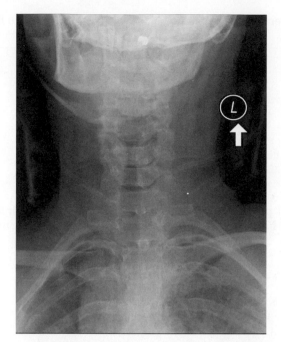

26. Figure 8-3: _____

_____

_____

_____

Figure 8-4

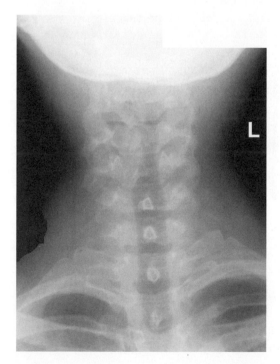

27. Figure 8-4: _____

_____

_____

_____

Figure 8-5

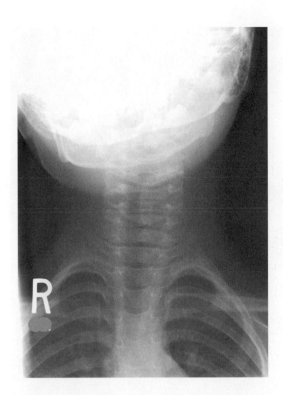

28. Figure 8-5: _____

_____

_____

_____

Figure 8-6

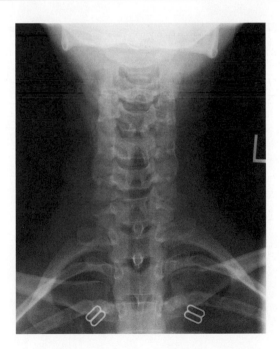

29. Figure 8-6: _____

_____

_____

_____

Figure 8-7

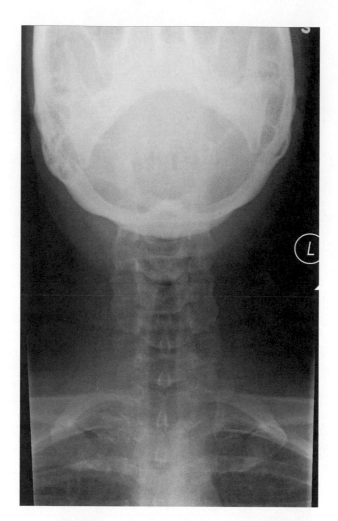

30. Figure 8-7: _____

_____

_____

_____

Figure 8-8

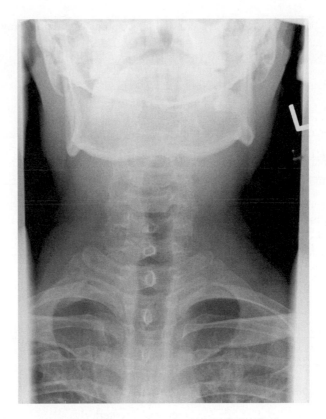

31. Figure 8-8: _____

_____

_____

_____

Cervical Atlas and Axis: Anteroposterior Projection (Open-Mouth)

32. Identify the labeled anatomy in Figure 8-9.

Figure 8-9

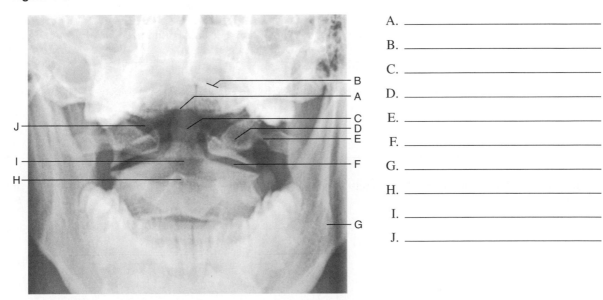

A. _____

B. _____

C. _____

D. _____

E. _____

F. _____

G. _____

H. _____

I. _____

J. _____

33. Complete the statements below referring to AP cervical atlas and axis vertebrae projection analysis criteria.

Anteroposterior Cervical Atlas and Axis Projection Analysis Criteria

- The atlas is symmetrically seated on the _____ (A), with the atlas's lateral masses at equal distances from the (B) _____ (B).

- The spinous processes of the axis is aligned with the midline of the _____ (C) body, and the mandibular rami are visualized at equal distances from the _____ (D).

- The upper incisors and base of the skull are seen _____ (E) to the dens and the atlantoaxial joint.

- The atlantoaxial joint is open and the axis's spinous process is demonstrated in the _____ (F) and slightly inferior to the dens.

---

34. How is the patient positioned to obtain an AP projection of the atlas and axis without rotation?

_____

_____

35. On head rotation, the atlas pivots around the dens. This results in the lateral mass located on the side toward which the face is turned being displaced _____ (anteriorly/posteriorly) (A) and the side away from which the face is turned being displaced _____ (anteriorly/posteriorly) (B).

36. How is the patient positioned for an AP projection of the atlas and axis to demonstrate the upper incisor and posterior occiput superior to the dens and atlantoaxial joint?

A. _____

_____

How is a patient without upper teeth positioned?

B. _____

_____

37. Why is it necessary to use a 5-degree cephalic central ray angulation on an AP atlas and axis projection? _____

_____

38. Describe how to determine the central ray angulation to use for an AP atlas and axis projection on a trauma patient in a collar.

_____

_____

39. How can one determine from an AP atlas or axis projection that the patient's neck was in flexion for the projection?

A. _____

_____

That it was in extension for the projection?

B. _____

_____

40. Accurate central ray centering on an AP atlas and axis projection is accomplished by centering the central ray through the open mouth to the _____.

41. Which anatomic structures are included on an AP atlas and axis projection with accurate positioning?

_____

_____

For the following descriptions of AP atlas and axis cervical projections with poor positioning, state how the patient or central ray would have been mispositioned for such a projection to be obtained.

42. The distances from the atlas's lateral masses to the dens and from the mandibular rami to the dens are narrower on the right side of the patient than on the left side, and the axis's spinous process is shifted from the midline.

_____

43. The upper incisors are demonstrated approximately 1 inch (2.5 cm) inferior to the posterior occiput's inferior edge, obscuring the dens and atlantoaxial joint, and the posterior occiput's inferior edge is demonstrated directly superior to the dens. The acanthiomeatal line was aligned perpendicular to the imaging table.

_____

44. The upper incisors are superimposed over the dens, and the posterior occiput's inferior edge is demonstrated superior to the dens and upper incisors. A 5-degree cephalic angulation was used to obtain this projection.

A. Patient: _____

_____

B. Central ray: _____

45. The dens is superimposed over the posterior occiput and the upper incisors are demonstrated approximately 2 inches (5 cm) superior to the posterior occiput's inferior edge.

A. Patient: _____

_____

B. Central ray: _____

For the following AP atlas and axis cervical projections with poor positioning, state which anatomic structures are misaligned and how the patient should be repositioned for an optimal projection to be obtained.

Figure 8-10

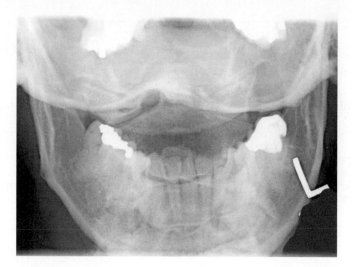

46. Figure 8-10: _____

_____

_____

_____

Figure 8-11

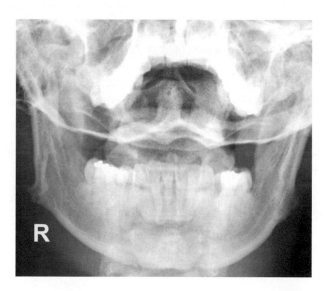

47. Figure 8-11: _____

_____

_____

_____

Figure 8-12

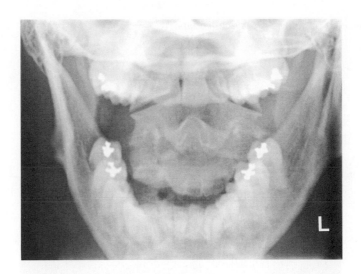

48. Figure 8-12: _____

_____

_____

_____

Figure 8-13

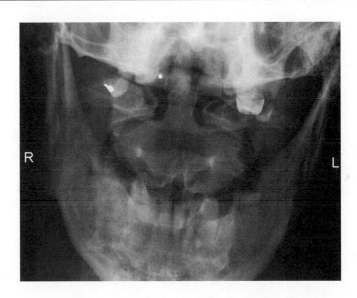

49. Figure 8-13: _____

_____

_____

_____

50. Figure 8-14 (taken with the patient in a cervical collar):

Figure 8-14

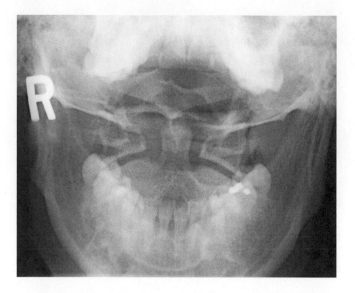

_____

_____

_____

_____

Cervical Vertebrae: Lateral Projection

51. Identify the labeled anatomy in Figure 8-15.

Figure 8-15

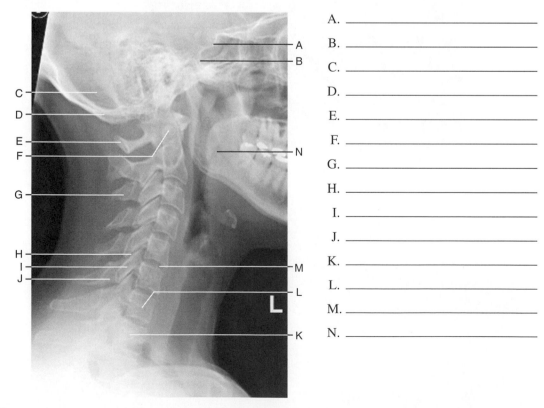

A. _____

B. _____

C. _____

D. _____

E. _____

F. _____

G. _____

H. _____

I. _____

J. _____

K. _____

L. _____

M. _____

N. _____

52. Complete the statements below referring to lateral cervical vertebrae projection analysis criteria.

Lateral Cervical Vertebrae Projection Analysis Criteria
• Contrast and density are adequate to visualize the _____ (A) fat stripe.
• The anterior and posterior aspects of the right and left articular pillars and right and left zygapophyseal joints of each cervical vertebra are _____ (B) and the spinous processes are in _____ (C).
• The posterior arch of C1 and spinous process of C2 are in profile without _____ (D) superimposition, their bodies are seen without mandibular superimposition, the cranial cortices and the mandibular rami are _____ (E), the superior and inferior aspects of the right and left articular pillars and the _____ (F) of each cervical vertebra are superimposed, and the intervertebral disk spaces are open.
• The long axis of the cervical vertebral column is aligned with the long axis of the exposure field.

53. Which soft tissue structure found on a lateral cervical projection can be used to detect and localize cervical fractures or masses?

_____

54. Why is a long source–image receptor distance (SID) used for the lateral cervical vertebrae projection?

_____

55. Which body plane is positioned perpendicular to the IR for a lateral cervical projection? _____

56. Which anatomic structures are aligned with the IR to prevent rotation when positioning the patient for a lateral cervical projection?

_____

57. How can rotation be identified on a lateral cervical projection with poor positioning?

_____

_____

58. How must the patient's head be positioned for a lateral cervical projection to demonstrate the posterior arch of C1 and the spinous process of C2 in profile without posterior occiput superimposition and the bodies of C1 and C2 without mandibular rami superimposition?

_____

_____

59. How must the patient's head be positioned for a lateral cervical projection to demonstrate superimposed inferior cranial and mandibular cortices and to obtain open superior intervertebral disk spaces?

_____

_____

60. What are two advantages of aligning the long axis of the cervical vertebral column with the long axis of the collimated field for a lateral cervical projection?

A. _____

B. _____

61. Why are lateral flexion and extension projections of the cervical vertebrae obtained?

_____

62. How is patient positioning adjusted from a neutral lateral cervical projection to achieve a flexed lateral projection?

_____

_____

63. How is patient positioning adjusted from a neutral lateral cervical projection to achieve an extended lateral projection?

_____

_____

64. Accurate central ray centering on a lateral cervical projection is accomplished by centering the central ray to the

_____ (A) plane at a level halfway between the _____ (B) and _____ (C).

65. Which anatomic structures are included on a lateral cervical projection with accurate positioning?

_____

_____

66. Why should the clivus be included on all lateral cervical projections?

_____

_____

67. It is often difficult to demonstrate C7 on a routine lateral cervical projection because of shoulder thickness. How should the patient be positioned to increase shoulder depression and improve C7 demonstration?

A. _____

B. _____

C. _____

68. Which special view can be taken to demonstrate C7 when the procedure referred to in question 67 fails?

_____

For the following descriptions of lateral cervical projections with poor positioning, state how the patient would have been mispositioned for such a projection to be obtained.

69. The articular pillars and zygapophyseal joints of one side of the patient are situated anterior to the opposite side's pillars and zygapophyseal joints.

_____

70. Neither the posterior nor the anterior cortices of the cranium nor the mandible are superimposed.

_____

71. The inferior cortices of the cranium and mandible are demonstrated without superimposition, and the vertebral foramen of C1 is demonstrated.

_____

For the following lateral cervical projections with poor positioning, state which anatomic structures are misaligned and how the patient should be repositioned for an optimal projection to be obtained.

Figure 8-16

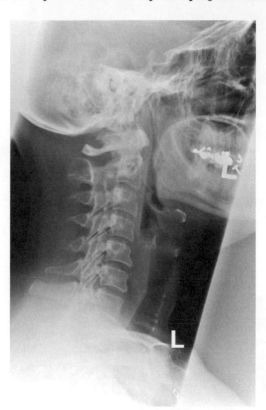

72. Figure 8-16: _____

_____

_____

_____

Figure 8-17

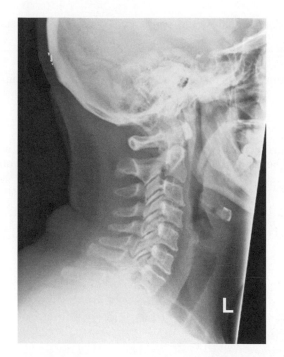

73. Figure 8-17: _____

_____

_____

_____

Figure 8-18

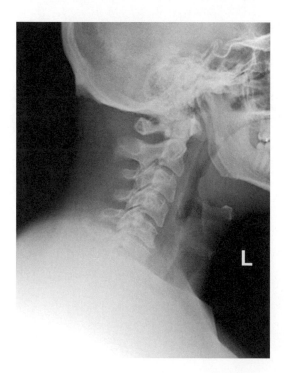

74. Figure 8-18: _____

_____

_____

_____

Figure 8-19

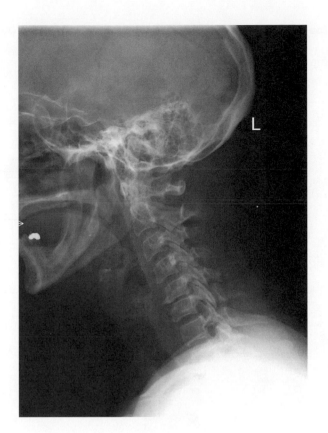

L

75. Figure 8-19: _____

_____

_____

_____

Cervical Vertebrae: Posteroanterior-Anteroposterior Axial Oblique Projection (Anterior and Posterior Oblique Positions)

76. Identify the labeled anatomy in Figure 8-20.

Figure 8-20

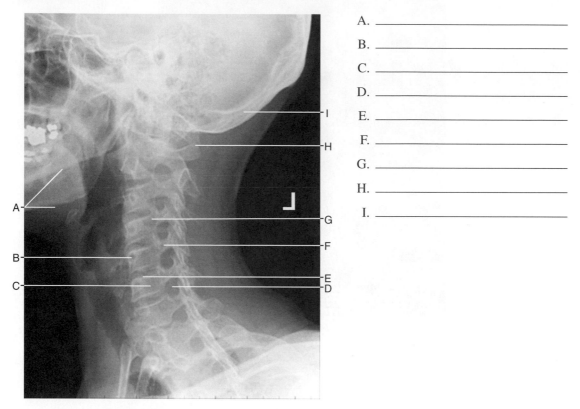

A. _____

B. _____

C. _____

D. _____

E. _____

F. _____

G. _____

H. _____

I. _____

77. Complete the statements below referring to PA-AP axial oblique cervical vertebrae projection analysis criteria.

Posteroanterior-Anteroposterior Axial Oblique Cervical Vertebrae Projection Analysis Criteria
• The second through _____ (A) intervertebral foramina are open, demonstrating uniform size and shape, the pedicles of interest are shown in _____ (B), and the opposite pedicles are aligned with the _____ (C) vertebral bodies.
• The intervertebral disk spaces are open, the cervical bodies are seen as individual structures and are uniform in shape, and the posterior arch of the atlas is seen without foreshortening, demonstrating the _____ (D).
• The inferior outline of the outer cranial cortices and the mandibular rami are seen without superimposition.
• Oblique cranium: The upper cervical vertebrae are seen with posterior occipital and mandibular superimposition.
• Lateral cranium: The upper cervical vertebrae are seen without occipital or mandibular superimposition, and the right and left posterior cortices of the cranium and the mandible are aligned.

78. Why is a long SID used for AP axial oblique cervical projections?

_____

79. Why is it not necessary to use a grid, even though a high kilovoltage peak (kVp) level is used for AP axial oblique cervical projections?

_____

_____

80. For the following AP-PA axial oblique cervical vertebrae projections, state whether the right or left intervertebral foramina will be demonstrated.

A. Right PA axial oblique (RAO position): _____

B. Left AP axial oblique (left posterior oblique [LPO] position): _____

C. Left PA axial oblique (left anterior oblique [LAO] position): _____

D. Right AP axial oblique (right posterior oblique [RPO] position): _____

81. Which degree of body rotation is used for AP-PA axial oblique cervical projections? _____

82. Which body plane is used to set up the degree of obliquity? _____

83. Describe how to position the image receptor (IR) beneath a trauma patient to demonstrate the right intervertebral foramina for an AP axial oblique cervical projection.

A. _____

_____

How is the central ray angled and positioned?

B. _____

_____

84. What degree and direction of central ray angulation are used for PA axial oblique cervical projections?

A. _____

For AP axial oblique cervical projections?

B. _____

Why is it necessary to use an angled central ray for AP-PA axial oblique cervical projections?

C. _____

_____

85. How should the patient be positioned to demonstrate the alignment of the right and left posterior cranium and mandible cortices and to demonstrate the upper cervical vertebrae without occipital or mandibular superimposition for an AP-PA axial oblique cervical projection?

_____

_____

86. How should the central ray be adjusted from the routinely used angle for a PA axial oblique cervical vertebrae projection in a patient who has severe kyphosis to demonstrate the lower cervical vertebrae better?

_____

87. Which cranial and mandibular cortices will be demonstrated inferiorly on a right PA axial oblique cervical projection?

A. _____

On a left AP axial oblique cervical projection?

B. _____

Which aspect of the positioning setup causes these cortices to be projected one superior to the other?

C. _____

_____

88. Accurate central ray centering on a PA axial oblique cervical projection is accomplished by centering the central ray

to the _____ (A) plane at a level halfway between the _____ (B)

and _____ (C).

89. Which anatomic structures are included on oblique cervical projections with accurate positioning?

_____

_____

For the following descriptions of PA-AP axial oblique cervical projections with poor positioning, state how the patient or central ray would have been mispositioned for such a projection to be obtained.

90. A left PA axial oblique cervical projection (LAO position), obtained with the patient's head in an oblique position, demonstrates obscured pedicles and intervertebral foramina, and the vertebral column is superimposed over a portion of the left sternoclavicular joint and medial clavicular end.

_____

91. A right PA axial oblique cervical projection (RAO position), obtained with the patient's head in a lateral position, demonstrates the intervertebral foramina, the right pedicles (although they are not in true profile), the left pedicles in the midline of the vertebral bodies, and the right zygapophyseal joints.

_____

92. On a left PA axial oblique cervical projection (LAO position), the intervertebral disk spaces are closed, the vertebral bodies are distorted, the posterior tubercles are demonstrated within the vertebral foramina, the C1 vertebral foramen is not demonstrated, and the inferior mandibular rami and the cranial cortices are demonstrated with superimposition.

_____

93. The upper cervical vertebrae are obscured by the patient's cranium and mandible.

_____

94. The atlas and its posterior arch are obscured. The inferior cranial cortices demonstrate more than 0.25 inch (0.6 cm) of distance between them, and the inferior cortices of the mandibular rami demonstrate more than 0.5 inch (1.25 cm) of distance between them.

_____

For the following PA-AP axial oblique cervical projections with poor positioning, state which anatomic structures are misaligned and how the patient should be repositioned for such a projection to be obtained.

Figure 8-21

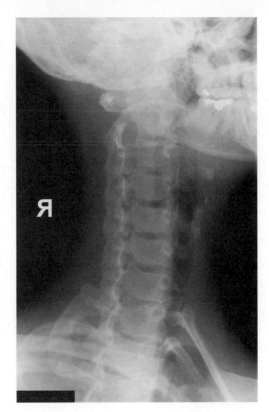

95. Figure 8-21: _____

_____

_____

_____

Figure 8-22

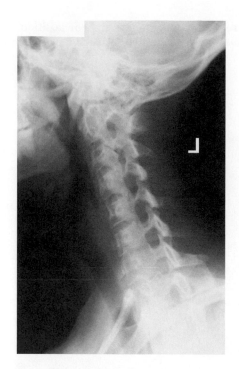

96. Figure 8-22: _____

_____

_____

_____

Figure 8-23

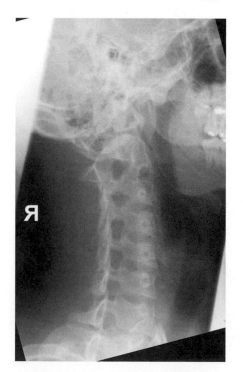

97. Figure 8-23: _____

_____

_____

Figure 8-24

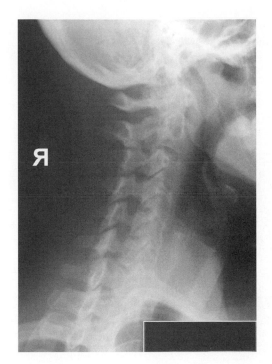

98. Figure 8-24: _____

_____

_____

_____

Figure 8-25

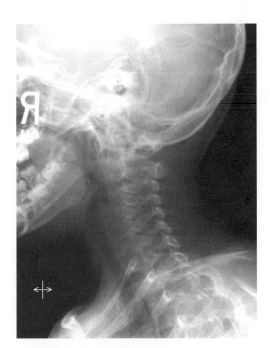

99. Figure 8-25: _____

_____

_____

_____

Cervicothoracic Vertebrae: Lateral Projection (Twining Method; Swimmer's Technique)

100. Identify the labeled anatomy in Figure 8-26.

Figure 8-26

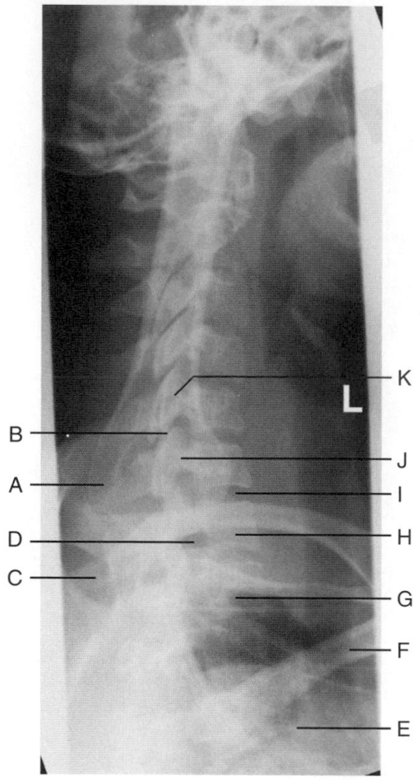

A. _____

B. _____

C. _____

D. _____

E. _____

F. _____

G. _____

H. _____

I. _____

J. _____

K. _____

101. Complete the statements below referring to lateral cervicothoracic vertebrae projection (Twining method) analysis criteria.

Lateral Cervicothoracic Vertebrae Projection Analysis Criteria
• The humerus elevated above the patient's head is aligned with the _____ (A), and the right and left cervical zygapophyseal joints, articular pillars, and posterior ribs are _____ (B).
• The intervertebral disk spaces are open, and the vertebral bodies are demonstrated without distortion.

102. List two situations in which a cervicothoracic lateral projection would be indicated.

A. _____

B. _____

_____

103. List three ways to reduce the amount of scatter radiation that reaches the IR when using the cervicothoracic lateral projection.

A. _____

B. _____

C. _____

104. What respiration is used for the cervicothoracic lateral projection? _____

105. To obtain a cervicothoracic lateral projection, how is the arm adjacent to the imaging table positioned?

A. _____

How is the arm situated farther from the imaging table positioned?

B. _____

106. How is the patient positioned to prevent rotation on a lateral cervicothoracic projection?

A. Cervical rotation: _____

_____

B. Thoracic rotation: _____

_____

107. How can rotation be identified on a lateral cervicothoracic projection?

_____

_____

108. How is the patient positioned for a lateral cervicothoracic projection to demonstrate open intervertebral disk spaces and undistorted vertebral bodies?

_____

_____

109. Accurate central ray centering on a lateral cervicothoracic projection is accomplished by centering a perpendicular central ray to the _____ (A) plane at a level 1 inch (2.5 cm) superior to the _____ (B) or at the level of the _____ (C).

110. When should a 5-degree caudal central ray angulation be used with the cervicothoracic lateral projection?

_____

_____

111. Which anatomic structures are included on a lateral cervicothoracic projection with accurate positioning?

_____

_____

For the following descriptions of lateral cervicothoracic projections with poor positioning, state how the patient would have been mispositioned for such a projection to be obtained.

112. The right and left articular pillars, zygapophyseal joints, and posterior ribs are demonstrated without superimposition. The humerus that was raised and situated closer to the IR is demonstrated posterior to the vertebral column.

_____

113. The right and left articular pillars, zygapophyseal joints, and posterior ribs are demonstrated without superimposition. The humerus demonstrating the lesser amount of magnification is situated anterior to the vertebral column.

_____

114. The intervertebral disk spaces are closed and the vertebral bodies are distorted.

_____

For the following lateral cervicothoracic projections with poor positioning, state which anatomic structures are misaligned and how the patient should be repositioned for an optimal projection to be obtained.

Figure 8-27

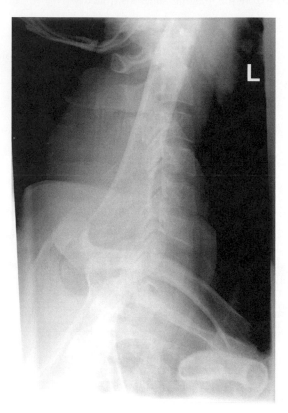

115. Figure 8-27: _____

_____

_____

_____

Figure 8-28

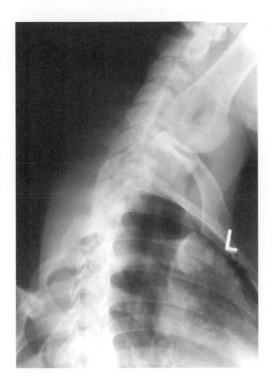

116. Figure 8-28: _____

_____

_____

_____

Thoracic Vertebrae: Anteroposterior Projection

117. Identify the labeled anatomy in Figure 8-29.

Figure 8-29

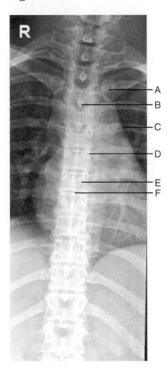

A. _____

B. _____

C. _____

D. _____

E. _____

F. _____

118. Complete the statements below referring to AP thoracic vertebrae projection analysis criteria.

Anteroposterior Thoracic Vertebrae Projection Analysis Criteria
• There is uniform density across the thoracic vertebrae.   • The spinous processes are aligned with the midline of the _____ (A) and the distances from the vertebral column to the sternoclavicular ends and from the pedicles to the _____ (B) are equal on the two sides.   • The intervertebral disk spaces are _____ (C) and the vertebral bodies are seen without foreshortening.

119. How tightly can one transversely collimate on an AP projection of the thoracic vertebrae?

_____

120. List two methods of achieving uniform projection density of the thoracic vertebrae on an AP projection.

A. _____

B. _____

121. Describe how to position the compensating filter for an AP thoracic projection accurately.

_____

_____

122. How can the patient be positioned with respect to the x-ray tube for an AP thoracic projection to take advantage of the anode heel effect?

_____

_____

123. What patient respiration is used for an AP thoracic projection to demonstrate the vertebrae and posterior ribs?

_____

_____

124. How is the patient positioned to ensure that rotation will not be demonstrated on an AP thoracic projection?

_____

_____

125. When rotation is present on an AP thoracic projection, the side demonstrating the greater distance between the spinous processes and pedicles will be _____ (closer to/farther from) the IR.

126. Which patient condition can simulate rotation on an AP thoracic projection?

A. _____

Describe how this condition can be distinguished from rotation.

B. _____

_____

127. What type of curvature does the thoracic vertebral column demonstrate?

A. _____

How can the patient be positioned to reduce this curvature and better align the x-ray beams with the intervertebral disk spaces?

B. _____

_____

128. Accurate central ray centering on an AP thoracic projection is accomplished by centering the central ray to the _____ (A) plane at a level halfway between the _____ (B) and xiphoid.

129. Which anatomic structures are included on an AP thoracic projection with accurate positioning?

_____

_____

For the following descriptions of AP thoracic projections with poor positioning, state how the patient would have been mispositioned for such a projection to be obtained.

130. The lower thoracic intervertebral disk spaces are obscured and the vertebral bodies are distorted.

_____

131. The distance from the left pedicles to the spinous processes is greater than the distance from the right pedicles to the spinous processes.

_____

132. The upper thoracic vertebrae are overexposed and the lower thoracic vertebrae demonstrate adequate density.

_____

For the following AP thoracic projections with poor positioning, state which anatomic structures are misaligned and how the patient should be repositioned for an optimal projection to be obtained.

Figure 8-30

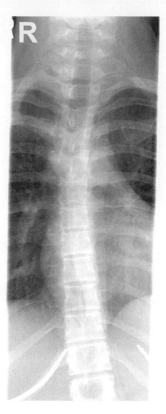

133. Figure 8-30: _____

_____

_____

_____

Figure 8-31

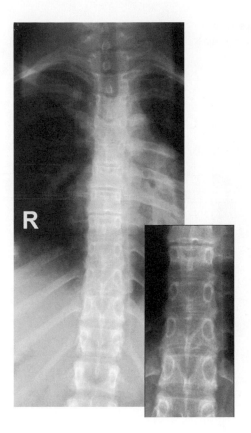

134. Figure 8-31: _____

_____

_____

_____

Thoracic Vertebrae: Lateral Projection

135. Identify the labeled anatomy in Figure 8-32.

Figure 8-32

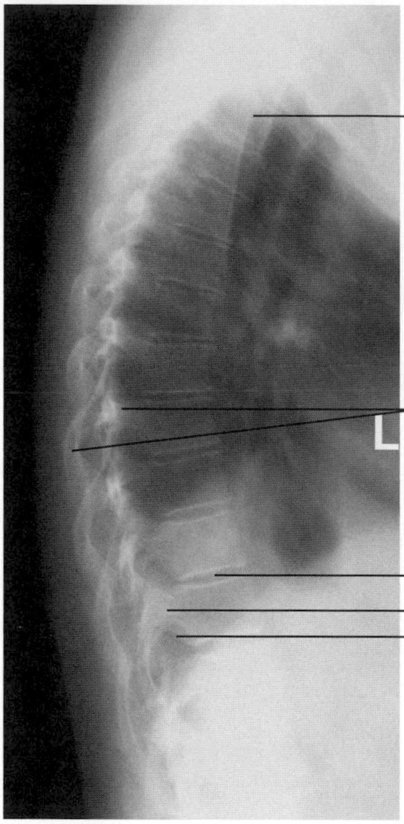

A. _____

B. _____

C. _____

D. _____

E. _____

136. Complete the statements below referring to lateral thoracic vertebrae projection analysis criteria.

Lateral Thoracic Vertebrae Projection Analysis Criteria

- The thoracic vertebrae are seen through overlying lung and rib structures.

- The intervertebral foramina are clearly demonstrated, the pedicles are in _____ (A), the posterior surfaces of each vertebral body are superimposed, and no more than _____ inch (B) of space is demonstrated between the posterior ribs.

- The intervertebral disk spaces are _____ (C) and the vertebral bodies are demonstrated without distortion.

---

137. What advantage does using a breathing technique over a nonbreathing technique have when imaging the thoracic vertebrae in the lateral projection? _____

_____

138. If patient motion cannot be avoided on a lateral thoracic projection when using a breathing technique, what respiration should be used?

_____

139. List two reasons why the patient's arms should be positioned at a 90-degree angle with the body for a lateral thoracic projection.

A. _____

_____

B. _____

_____

140. How is the patient positioned to prevent rotation on a lateral thoracic projection?

_____

_____

141. How can rotation be identified on a lateral thoracic projection?

_____

_____

142. How can scoliosis be distinguished from rotation on a lateral thoracic projection? _____

_____

143. When the thoracic vertebrae are in a lateral projection, the posterior ribs are positioned on top of each other. Why does the resulting projection demonstrate the posterior ribs without superimposition?

_____

_____

144. How is the patient positioned to obtain open intervertebral disk spaces on a lateral thoracic projection?

_____

145. Describe the patient body form that demonstrates the greatest thoracic vertebral sagging when the patient is placed in a lateral projection.

A. _____

_____

State where the radiolucent sponge is positioned to offset this sagging.

B. _____

_____

State how the central ray can be adjusted to offset this sagging.

C. _____

146. Accurate central ray centering on a lateral thoracic vertebral projection is accomplished by centering the central ray

to the _____ when the patient's arm is positioned at a 90-degree angle with the body.

147. Which anatomic structures are included on a lateral thoracic projection with accurate positioning?

_____

148. List two methods of confirming which is the twelfth thoracic vertebra on a lateral thoracic projection.

A. _____

B. _____

_____

149. List two methods of confirming which is the first thoracic vertebra on a lateral thoracic projection.

A. _____

B. _____

150. If the first, second, or third thoracic vertebra is not included on a routine lateral thoracic projection, which supplementary position is used to demonstrate these vertebrae?

_____

For the following descriptions of lateral thoracic projections with poor positioning, state how the patient would have been mispositioned for such a projection to be obtained.

151. The posterior surfaces of the vertebral bodies are demonstrated without superimposition and more than 0.5 inch (1.25 cm) of space is demonstrated between the posterior ribs.

_____

152. The posterior surfaces of the vertebral bodies are demonstrated without superimposition and the posterior ribs are superimposed.

_____

153. The eighth through twelfth thoracic intervertebral disk spaces are obscured and the vertebral bodies are distorted.

_____

For the following lateral thoracic projections with poor positioning, state which anatomic structures are misaligned and how the patient should be repositioned for an optimal projection to be obtained.

Figure 8-33

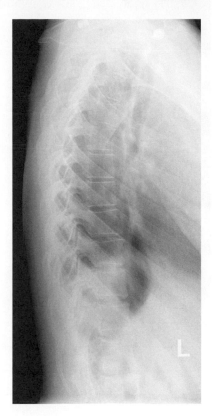

154. Figure 8-33: _____

_____

_____

_____

Figure 8-34

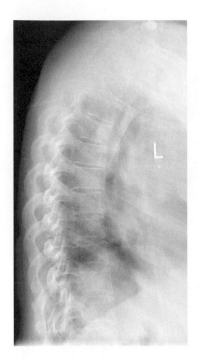

155. Figure 8-34: _____

_____

_____

_____

Figure 8-35

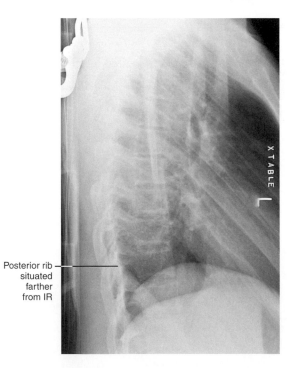

Posterior rib
situated
farther
from IR

156. Figure 8-35 (cross-table trauma projection): _____

_____

_____

_____

9 Lumbar Vertebrae, Sacrum, and Coccyx

STUDY QUESTIONS

1. Describe how the following lumbar projections should be displayed on a view box or digital monitor.

   A. AP lumbar vertebrae: _____

   B. AP oblique lumbar vertebrae (right postior oblique [RPO] position): _____

   _____

   C. Lateral coccyx: _____

2. Complete Exercise 9-1.

TABLE 9-1 Lumbar Vertebrae, Sacrum, and Coccyx Technical Data				
Projection	kVp	Grid	AEC Chamber(s)	SID
AP, lumbar vertebrae				
AP oblique, lumbar vertebrae				
Lateral, lumbar vertebrae				
Lateral, L5-S1 lumbosacral junction				
AP axial, sacrum				
Lateral, sacrum				
AP axial, coccyx				
Lateral, coccyx				

AEC, Automatic exposure control; *kVp,* kilovoltage peak ; *SID,* source–image receptor distance.

Lumbar Vertebrae: Anteroposterior Projection

3. Identify the labeled anatomy in Figure 9-1.

Figure 9-1

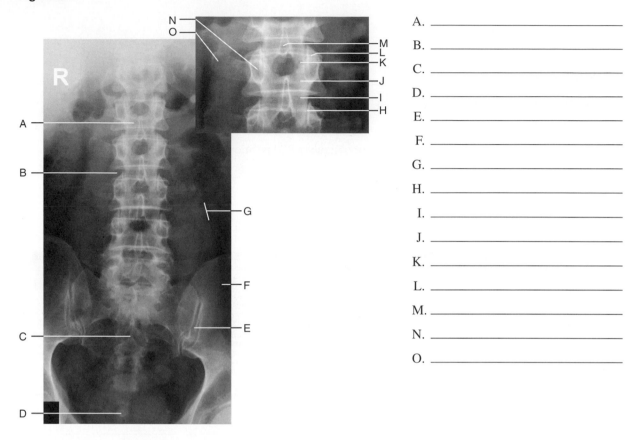

A. _____

B. _____

C. _____

D. _____

E. _____

F. _____

G. _____

H. _____

I. _____

J. _____

K. _____

L. _____

M. _____

N. _____

O. _____

4. Complete the statements below referring to AP lumbar vertebrae projection analysis criteria.

Anteroposterior Lumbar Vertebrae Projection Analysis Criteria

- The _____ (A) muscles are demonstrated and the distances from the pedicles

  to the _____ (B) and from the sacroiliac joints to the spinous processes are

  _____ (C) on both sides. The sacrum and coccyx should be centered within the inlet
  pelvis and aligned with the symphysis pubis.

- The intervertebral disk spaces are _____ (D), and the vertebral bodies are seen without
  distortion.

- The _____ (E) are aligned with the midline of the vertebral bodies.

- The long axis of the lumbar column is aligned with the long axis of the exposure field.

---

5. Which soft tissue structures are included on an AP lumbar projection when proper contrast and density exist?

   A. _____

   Where are these structures located?

   B. _____

6. How is the patient positioned to prevent rotation on an AP lumbar projection? _____

_____

7. How is rotation identified on an AP lumbar projection?

_____

_____

8. How can a rotated AP lumbar projection be distinguished from an AP lumbar projection in a patient with subtle scoliosis?

_____

_____

_____

9. How is the patient positioned to ensure that open intervertebral disk spaces and undistorted vertebral bodies are obtained?

_____

_____

10. What is the curvature of the lumbar vertebral column?

_____

11. What is the relationship of the iliac spine to the pelvic brim on an AP lumbar projection that was taken with the patient's legs extended?

_____

_____

12. Which anatomic structures can be used to ensure that the long axis of the lumbar vertebral column is aligned with the collimated field when positioning for an AP lumbar vertebral projection?

   A. _____

   _____

   Why is the patient's navel not a reliable structure to use when locating the lumbar vertebral column?

   B. _____

   _____

13. An AP lumbar projection demonstrates the vertebral column deviating laterally at the level of the second through fourth lumbar vertebrae, the sacrum is centered within the pelvic inlet, and the distances from the pedicles to the spinous processes of the eleventh thoracic vertebra and the fifth lumbar vertebra are almost equal. What has caused the appearance of this projection?

_____

14. Accurate central ray centering on an AP lumbar projection taken on an 11- × 14-inch (28- × 35-cm) lengthwise image receptor (IR) is accomplished by centering the central ray to the _____ (A) plane at a level 1.5 inches (4 cm) _____ (B) to the _____ (C).

15. Which anatomic structures are included on an AP lumbar projection with accurate positioning taken on an 11- × 14-inch (28- × 35-cm) lengthwise IR?

_____

16. Accurate central ray centering on an AP lumbar projection taken on a 14- × 17-inch (35- × 43-cm) lengthwise IR is accomplished by centering the central ray to the _____ (A) plane at the level of the _____ (B).

17. Which anatomic structures are included on an AP lumbar projection with accurate positioning taken on a 14- × 17-inch (35- × 43-cm) lengthwise IR?

_____

18. How tightly can the transversely collimated field be coned and still include all the required anatomic structures?

_____

19. When is gonadal shielding not used for an AP lumbar projection of a female patient?

_____

For the following descriptions of AP lumbar projections with poor positioning, state how the patient would have been mispositioned for such a projection to be obtained.

20. The distance from the right pedicles to the spinous processes is less than the distance from the left pedicles to the spinous processes, and the sacrum and coccyx are rotated toward the right lateral inlet pelvis.

_____

21. The first through third lumbar vertebrae are demonstrated without rotation, the fourth and fifth vertebrae are rotated, and the sacrum and coccyx are rotated toward the patient's left side.

_____

22. The intervertebral disk spaces between the twelfth thoracic vertebra and third lumbar vertebra are closed, and these lumbar bodies are distorted. The iliac spines are demonstrated without pelvic brim superimposition.

_____

For the following AP lumbar projections with poor positioning, state which anatomic structures are misaligned and how the patient should be repositioned for an optimal projection to be obtained.

Figure 9-2

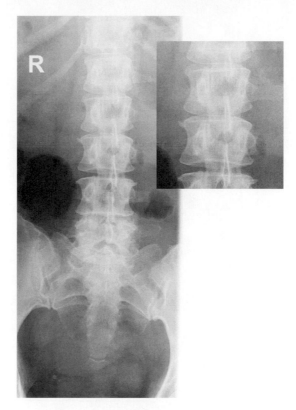

23. Figure 9-2: _____

_____

_____

_____

Figure 9-3

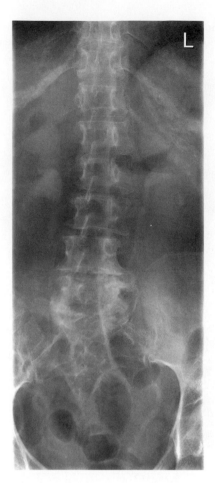

L

24. Figure 9-3: _____

_____

_____

_____

Figure 9-4

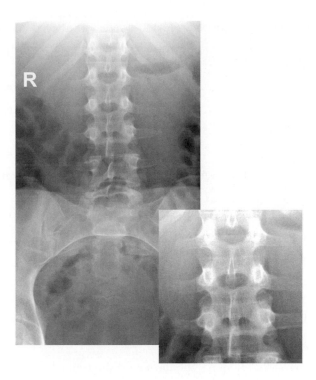

25. Figure 9-4: _____

_____

_____

_____

Lumbar Vertebrae: Anteroposterior Oblique Projection (RPO and LPO Positions)

26. Identify the labeled anatomy in Figure 9-5.

Figure 9-5

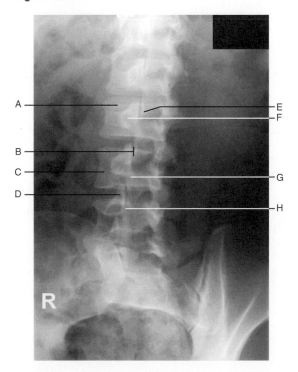

A. _____

B. _____

C. _____

D. _____

E. _____

F. _____

G. _____

H. _____

27. Complete the statements below referring to AP oblique lumbar vertebrae projection analysis criteria.

Anteroposterior Oblique Lumbar Vertebrae Projection Analysis Criteria
• The superior and inferior _____ (A) are in profile, the _____ (B) joints are demonstrated, and the _____ (C) are seen halfway between the midpoint of the vertebral bodies and the lateral border of the vertebral bodies.

28. For the following positions, state whether the right or left zygapophyseal joints are demonstrated on an AP oblique lumbar projection.

    A. RAO: _____

    B. Left posterior oblique (LPO): _____

    C. Right posterior oblique (RPO): _____

    D. Left anterior oblique (LAO): _____

29. Which body plane is used to determine patient obliquity for an AP oblique lumbar projection?

    A. _____

    How much is the patient's torso rotated for an AP oblique lumbar projection?

    B. _____

30. Name the anatomic structures of the lumbar vertebrae that correspond with the parts of the "Scottie dog" listed below.

    A. Ear: _____

    B. Nose: _____

    C. Body: _____

    D. Eye: _____

    E. Front leg: _____

31. Accurate central ray centering on an AP oblique lumbar projection is accomplished by centering the central ray 2 inches (5 cm) _____ (A) to the elevated _____ (B) at a level 1.5 inches (4 cm) superior to the _____ (C).

32. Which anatomic structures are included on an AP oblique lumbar projection with accurate positioning?

    _____

    _____

For the following descriptions of AP oblique lumbar projections with poor positioning, state how the patient would have been mispositioned for such a projection to be obtained.

33. The vertebrae's superior and inferior articular processes are not demonstrated in profile, their corresponding zygapophyseal joint spaces are closed, and their pedicles are demonstrated adjacent to the vertebrae's lateral vertebral body borders.

    _____

34. The vertebrae's superior and inferior articular processes are not demonstrated in profile, their corresponding zyga-pophyseal joint spaces are closed, their laminae are obscured, and their pedicles are shown at the midpoint of the vertebral bodies.

For the following oblique lumbar projections with poor positioning, state which anatomic structures are mis-aligned and how the patient should be repositioned for an optimal projection to be obtained.

Figure 9-6

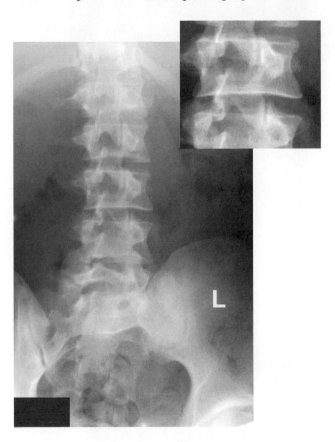

35. Figure 9-6: _____

_____

_____

_____

Figure 9-7

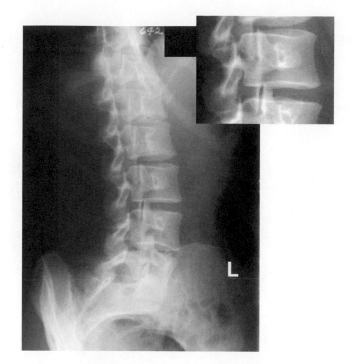

36. Figure 9-7: _____

_____

_____

_____

Figure 9-8

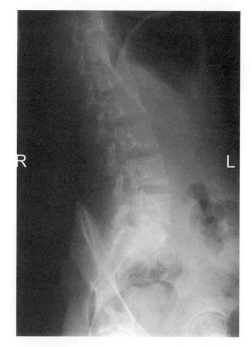

37. Figure 9-8: _____

_____

_____

_____

Lumbar Vertebrae: Lateral Projection

38. Identify the labeled anatomy in Figure 9-9.

Figure 9-9

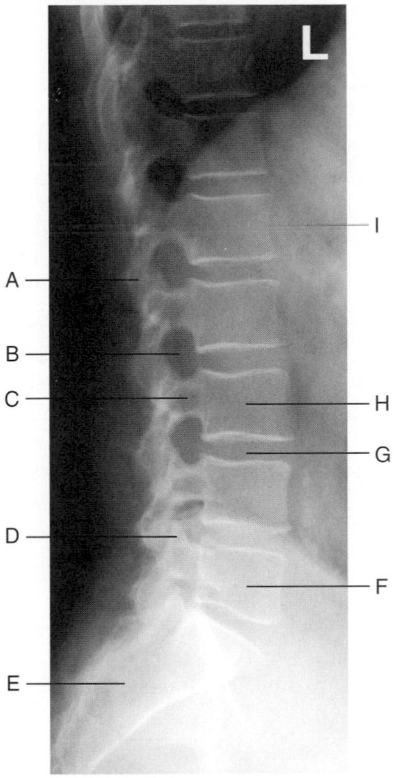

A. _____

B. _____

C. _____

D. _____

E. _____

F. _____

G. _____

H. _____

I. _____

39. Complete the statements below referring to lateral lumbar vertebrae projection analysis criteria.

Lateral Lumbar Vertebrae Projection Analysis Criteria
• The intervertebral foramina are demonstrated and the _____ (A) are in profile.
The right and left pedicles and the posterior surfaces of each vertebral body are _____ (B).
• The intervertebral disk spaces are open and the vertebral bodies are seen without distortion.
• The lumbar vertebral column is in a _____ (C) position, without anteroposterior flexion or extension.
• The long axis of the lumbar vertebral column is aligned with the long axis of the exposure field.

40. List three methods of controlling the amount of scatter radiation that reaches the IR when a lateral lumbar projection is produced.

A. _____

B. _____

C. _____

41. Controlling the amount of scatter radiation that reaches the IR will provide a _____ (higher/lower) (A) contrast projection and will _____ (increase/decrease) (B) the visibility of recorded details.

42. How is the patient positioned to prevent rotation on a lateral lumbar projection?

_____

_____

43. For a lateral lumbar projection, the patient may be placed on the imaging table in a left or right recumbent position unless the patient has which spinal condition?

A. _____

For this condition, how are the central ray and vertebral column positioned?

B. _____

44. What is accomplished by placing a pillow or sponge between the patient's legs for a lateral lumbar projection?

_____

_____

45. How can rotation be detected on a rotated lateral lumbar projection?

_____

_____

46. Will the upper and lower vertebrae on a lateral lumbar projection always demonstrate simultaneous rotation?

A. _____ (Yes/No)

Defend your answer.

B. _____

_____

47. Why is it difficult to determine which side of the body has been rotated anteriorly or posteriorly when a lateral lumbar projection demonstrates rotation?

_____

48. How is the patient positioned to ensure open intervertebral disk spaces and undistorted vertebral bodies on a lateral lumbar projection?

_____

49. Describe the body shape that requires a radiolucent sponge to be used to position the lumbar vertebral column parallel with the imaging table.

A. _____

Where is the sponge placed for such a patient?

B. _____

_____

If a sponge cannot be used with such a patient, what alternative method can be used?

C. _____

450

50. Why are flexion and extension lateral lumbar projections requested?

_____

51. Describe how patient positioning is adjusted from a neutral lateral projection to place the patient in maximum flexion for a lateral lumbar projection.

A. _____

Describe how patient positioning is adjusted from a neutral lateral position to place the patient in maximum extension for a lateral lumbar projection?

B. _____

_____

52. The lordotic curvature on a lumbar projection is _____ (increased/decreased) (A) when the patient is positioned in maximum flexion and is _____ (increased/decreased) (B) when the patient is positioned in maximum extension.

53. Describe how one can find the location of the lumbar vertebral column for an AP projection.

_____

_____

54. Accurate central ray centering on a lateral lumbar projection when an 11- × 14-inch (28- × 35-cm) lengthwise IR is used is accomplished by centering the central ray to the _____ (A) plane located halfway between the elevated _____ (B) and _____ (C) at a level 1.5 inches (4 cm) superior to the _____ (D).

55. Which anatomic structures are included on a lateral lumbar projection with accurate positioning taken on an 11- × 14-inch (28- × 35-cm) lengthwise IR?

_____

56. Accurate central ray centering on a lateral lumbar projection when a 14- × 17-inch (35- × 43-cm) lengthwise IR is used is accomplished by centering the central ray to the _____ (A) plane located halfway between the elevated _____ (B) and _____ (C) at the level of the _____ (D).

57. Which anatomic structures are included on a lateral lumbar projection with accurate positioning taken on a 14- × 17-inch (35- × 43-cm) lengthwise IR?

_____

58. Describe two situations in which a tightly collimated lateral view of the L5-S1 lumbar region is indicated after the lateral lumbar projection has been reviewed.

A. _____

B. _____

59. Explain how the shield is positioned for a lateral lumbar projection to protect the patient's gonads.

_____

_____

For the following descriptions of lateral lumbar projections with poor positioning, state how the patient would have been mispositioned for such a projection to be obtained.

60. The posterior surfaces of the first through fourth vertebral bodies and the posterior ribs are demonstrated without superimposition. The most magnified ribs are demonstrated anteriorly.

_____

61. The L4-5 and L5-S1 intervertebral disk spaces are closed, and the third through fifth vertebral bodies are distorted.

_____

62. Explain why the intervertebral joint spaces are closed on the lateral lumbar projection in Figure 9-10, even though the iliac crests and alae are perfectly superimposed.

Figure 9-10

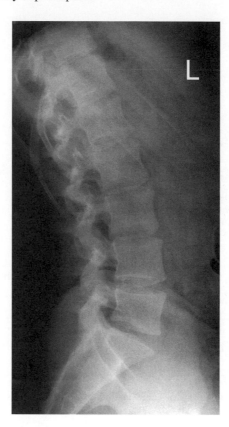

_____
_____
_____
_____

For the following lateral lumbar projections with poor positioning, state which anatomic structures are misaligned and how the patient should be repositioned for an optimal projection to be obtained.

Figure 9-11

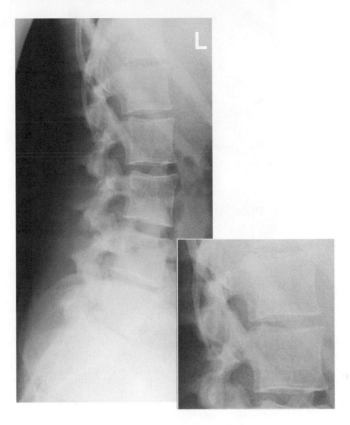

63. Figure 9-11: _____

_____

_____

_____

Figure 9-12

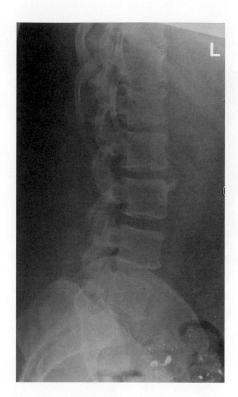

64. Figure 9-12: _____

_____

_____

_____

Figure 9-13

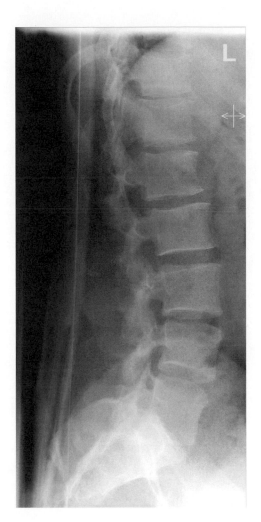

65. Figure 9-13: _____

_____

_____

_____

Figure 9-14

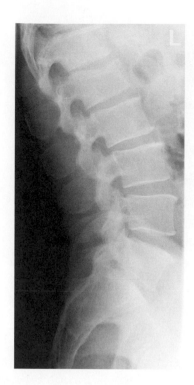

66. Figure 9-14: _____

_____

_____

_____

L5-S1 Lumbosacral Junction: Lateral Projection

67. Identify the labeled anatomy in Figure 9-15.

Figure 9-15

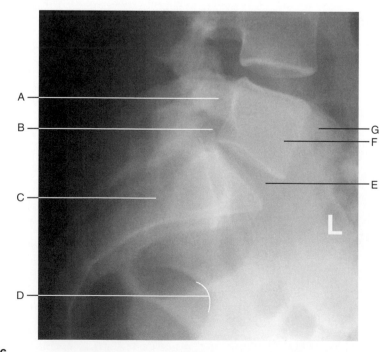

A. _____

B. _____

C. _____

D. _____

E. _____

F. _____

G. _____

68. Complete the statements below referring to lateral L5-S1 lumbosacral junction projection analysis criteria.

Lateral L5-S1 Lumbosacral Junction Projection Analysis Criteria
• The intervertebral foramina are demonstrated, the right and left _____ (A) are superimposed and in profile, and the greater sciatic notches and _____ (B) are almost superimposed. • The L5-S1 intervertebral disk space is _____ (C), the pelvic alae are superimposed, and the sacrum is seen without foreshortening.

69. How tightly can the transverse field be collimated and still include the needed anatomic information on a lateral L5-S1 projection?

_____

70. List three methods of controlling the amount of scatter radiation that reaches the IR when a lateral L5-S1 projection is produced.

A. _____

B. _____

C. _____

71. How is the patient positioned to prevent rotation on a lateral L5-S1 projection?

_____

_____

72. What is accomplished by placing a pillow or sponge between the patient's legs for a lateral L5-S1 projection?

_____

_____

73. How can rotation be detected on a rotated lateral L5-S1 projection?

_____

_____

74. How is the patient positioned to obtain open intervertebral disk spaces and undistorted vertebral bodies on a lateral L5-S1 projection?

_____

75. Which patient body shape requires that a radiolucent sponge be used to position the lumbar vertebral column parallel with the imaging table?

A. _____

_____

Where is the sponge placed on such a patient?

B. _____

If a sponge cannot be used on such a patient, what alternative method can be used?

C. _____

76. How should the central ray be adjusted to obtain an open L5-S1 joint space in a patient whose vertebral column curves upwardly?

_____

77. Accurate central ray centering on a lateral L5-S1 projection is accomplished by centering the central ray to a point

2 inches (5 cm) _____ (A) to the elevated _____ (B) and 1.5 inches (4 cm)

_____ (C) to the _____ (D).

78. Which anatomic structures are included on a lateral L5-S1 projection with accurate positioning?

_____

79. Describe how the gonads of male and female patients can be protected when a lateral L5-S1 projection is taken.

_____

_____

For the following descriptions of lateral L5-S1 lumbar projections with poor positioning, state how the patient would have been mispositioned for such a projection to be obtained.

80. The L5-S1 intervertebral foramen is obscured, and the greater sciatic notches and femoral heads are not superimposed.

_____

81. The L5-S1 intervertebral disk space is closed, and the pelvic alae are not superimposed.

_____

For the following lateral L5-S1 lumbar projections with poor positioning, state which anatomic structures are misaligned and how the patient should be repositioned for an optimal projection to be obtained.

Figure 9-16

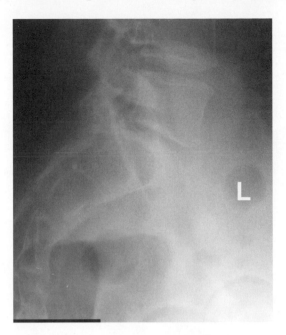

82. Figure 9-16: _____

_____

_____

_____

Figure 9-17

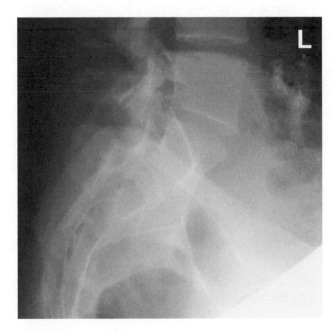

83. Figure 9-17: _____

_____

_____

_____

Sacrum: Anteroposterior Axial Projection

84. Identify the labeled anatomy in Figure 9-18.

Figure 9-18

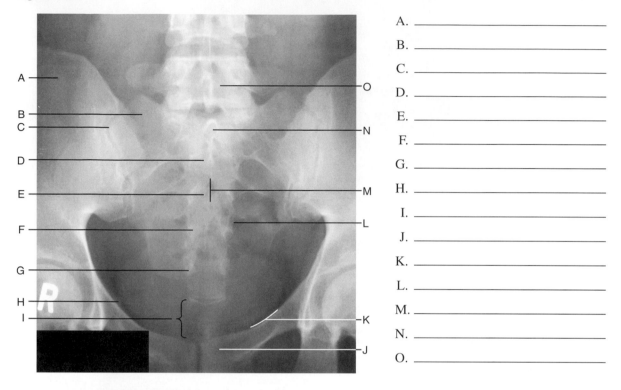

A. _____

B. _____

C. _____

D. _____

E. _____

F. _____

G. _____

H. _____

I. _____

J. _____

K. _____

L. _____

M. _____

N. _____

O. _____

85. Complete the statements below referring to AP axial sacrum projection analysis criteria.

Anteroposterior Axial Sacrum Projection Analysis Criteria
• There is no evidence of urine, gas, or fecal material superimposing the sacrum. • The ischial spines are equally demonstrated and are aligned with the _____ (A); the median sacral crest and the _____ (B) are aligned with the symphysis pubis. • The first through _____ (C) sacral segments are seen without foreshortening, the sacral foramina demonstrate equal spacing, and the _____ (D) is not superimposed over any portion of the sacrum.

86. Why is the patient instructed to empty the bladder and colon before an AP sacral projection is taken? _____

_____

87. How can patient positioning be evaluated to ensure that pelvic rotation will not be present on an AP sacral projection?

_____

88. When a patient is rotated for an AP sacral projection, the sacrum rotates in the _____ (opposite/same)

(A) direction as the symphysis pubis and is positioned next to the lateral pelvic brim situated _____ (closer/farther) (B) to/from the IR.

89. What is the curvature of the sacrum? _____

90. How must the patient and central ray be positioned to demonstrate the sacrum without foreshortening?

_____

_____

91. Why is the median sacral crest aligned with the long axis of the collimated field for an AP sacral projection?

_____

_____

92. Accurate central ray centering on an AP sacral projection is accomplished by positioning the central ray to the

_____ (A) plane at a level halfway between _____ (B) and the _____ (C).

93. Which anatomic structures are included on an AP sacral projection with accurate positioning? _____

_____

94. Is gonadal protection shielding used on all AP sacral projections?

A. _____ (Yes/No)

Defend your answer.

B. _____

_____

For the following descriptions of AP sacral projections with poor positioning, state how the patient or central ray would have been mispositioned for such a projection to be obtained.

95. The left ischial spine is demonstrated without pelvic brim superimposition, and the median sacral crest and coccyx are rotated toward the right hip.

_____

96. The first, second, and third sacral segments are foreshortened.

_____

97. The sacrum is elongated, and the symphysis pubis is superimposed over the fifth sacral segment.

_____

For the following AP sacral projections with poor positioning, state which anatomic structures are misaligned and how the patient should be repositioned for an optimal projection to be obtained.

Figure 9-19

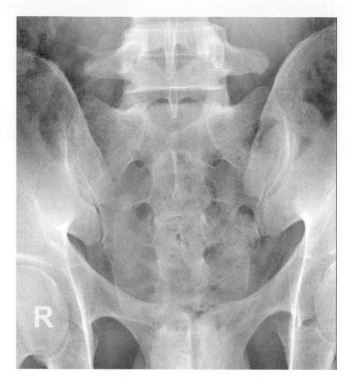

98. Figure 9-19: _____

_____

_____

_____

Figure 9-20

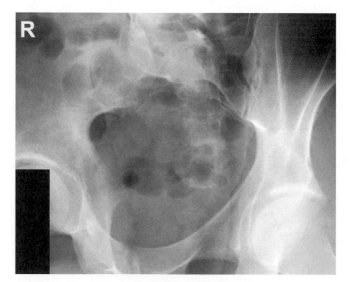

99. Figure 9-20: _____

_____

_____

_____

Figure 9-21

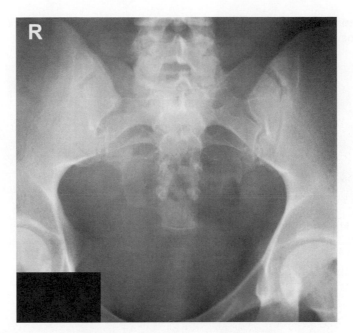

100. Figure 9-21: _____

_____

_____

_____

Figure 9-22

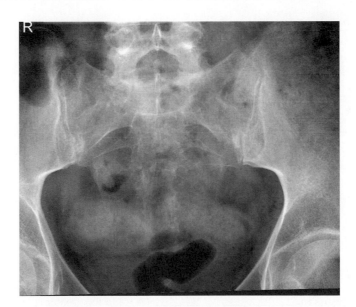

101. Figure 9-22: _____

_____

_____

_____

Sacrum: Lateral Projection

102. Identify the labeled anatomy in Figure 9-23.

Figure 9-23

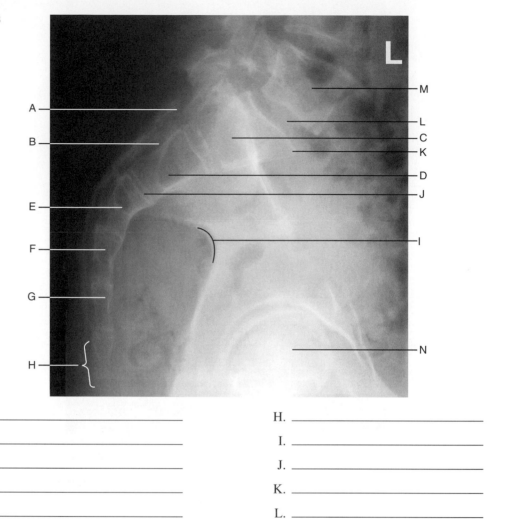

A. _____   H. _____

B. _____   I. _____

C. _____   J. _____

D. _____   K. _____

E. _____   L. _____

F. _____   M. _____

G. _____   N. _____

103. Complete the statements below referring to lateral sacrum projection analysis criteria.

Lateral Sacrum Projection Analysis Criteria

• The median sacral crest is in _____ (A), and the greater sciatic notches and

_____ (B) are almost superimposed.

• The L5-S1 disk space is open, the greater sciatic notches are _____ (C), and the sacrum is seen without foreshortening.

104. How is the patient positioned to prevent rotation on a lateral sacrum projection?

_____

_____

105. What is accomplished by placing a pillow or sponge between the patient's legs for a lateral sacrum projection?

_____

_____

106. How can rotation be detected on a rotated lateral sacrum projection?

_____

_____

107. When a lateral sacrum projection demonstrates rotation and the femoral heads are demonstrated on the projection, the hip that is projected inferiorly is situated _____ (closer to/farther away from) the IR.

108. How is the patient positioned to obtain an open L5-S1 disk space and an undistorted fifth lumbar body on a lateral sacrum projection?

_____

_____

109. Which patient body shape requires that a radiolucent sponge be used to position the lumbar vertebral column parallel with the imaging table for a lateral sacrum projection?

A. _____

Where is the sponge placed on such a patient?

B. _____

_____

If a sponge cannot be used on such a patient, what alternative method can be used?

C. _____

_____

110. How should the central ray be adjusted to obtain an open L5-S1 intervertebral joint space in a patient whose vertebral column curves upwardly?

_____

111. Accurate central ray centering on a lateral sacral projection is accomplished by centering the central ray to the _____ (A) plane located 3 to 4 inches (7.5 to 10 cm) posterior to the elevated _____ (B).

112. Which anatomic structures are included on a lateral sacrum projection with accurate positioning?

_____

_____

113. Describe how the gonads of male and female patients can be protected when a lateral sacrum projection is taken.

_____

_____

For the following descriptions of lateral sacrum projections with poor positioning, state how the patient would have been mispositioned for such a projection to be obtained.

114. The greater sciatic notches are demonstrated without superimposition, the median sacral crest is not in profile, and the inferiorly located femoral head is rotated posteriorly.

_____

115. The L5-S1 intervertebral disk space is closed, the fifth lumbar vertebra and sacrum are foreshortened, and the greater sciatic notches are demonstrated without superimposition.

_____

For the following lateral sacrum projections with poor positioning, state which anatomic structures are misaligned and how the patient should be repositioned for an optimal projection to be obtained.

Figure 9-24

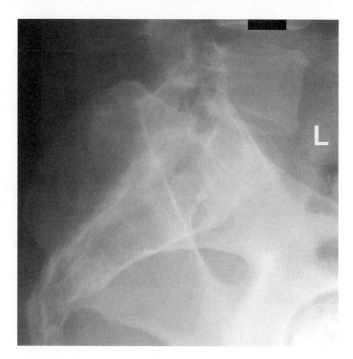

116. Figure 9-24: _____

_____

_____

_____

Figure 9-25

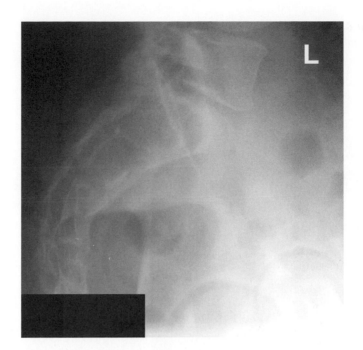

117. Figure 9-25: _____

_____

_____

_____

Figure 9-26

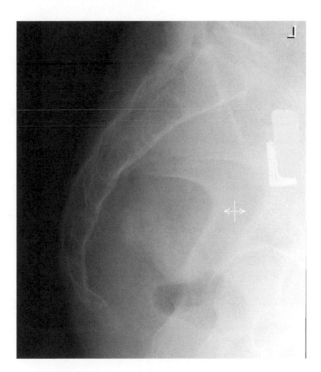

118. Figure 9-26: _____

_____

_____

_____

Coccyx: Anteroposterior Axial Projection

119. Identify the labeled anatomy in Figure 9-27.

Figure 9-27

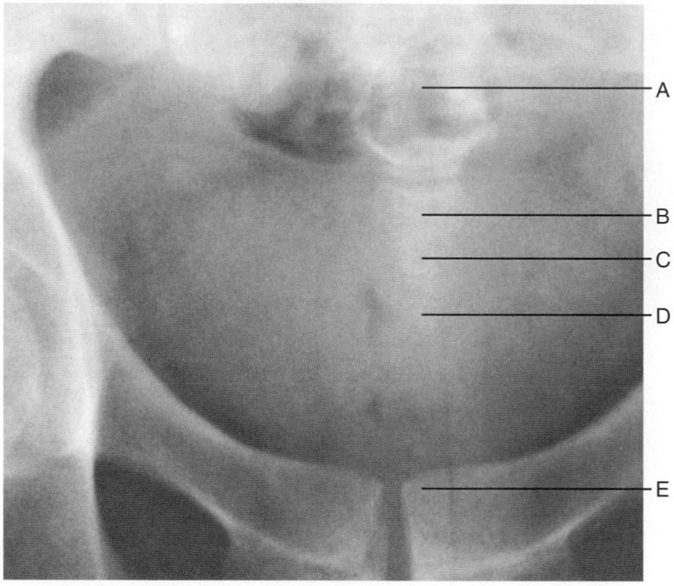

A. _____

B. _____

C. _____

D. _____

E. _____

120. Complete the statements below referring to AP axial coccyx projection analysis criteria.

Anteroposterior Axial Coccyx Projection Analysis Criteria
• There is no evidence of urine, gas, or fecal material superimposed over the coccyx.
• The coccyx is aligned with the _____ (A) and is at equal distances from the lateral walls of the _____ (B).
• The first through _____ (C) coccygeal vertebrae are seen without foreshortening and without symphysis pubis superimposition.

121. How much can the transverse field be safely collimated and still include the required anatomic structures for an AP coccyx projection?

_____

122. Where is the marker placed on an AP coccyx projection that is collimated to a 6-inch (15-cm) field size?

_____

123. Why is the patient instructed to empty the bladder and colon before an AP coccyx projection is taken? _____

_____

124. How can patient positioning be evaluated to ensure that pelvic rotation is not present on an AP coccyx projection?

_____

_____

125. When a patient is rotated for an AP coccyx projection, the coccyx rotates in the _____ (opposite/same)

(A) direction as the symphysis pubis and is positioned next to the lateral pelvic wall situated _____ (closer/farther) (B) to/from the IR.

126. How must the patient and central ray be positioned for an AP coccyx projection to demonstrate the coccyx without foreshortening?

_____

127. What is the curvature of the coccyx? _____

128. Accurate central ray centering on an AP coccyx projection is accomplished by positioning the central ray to the

_____ (A) plane at a level 2 inches (5 cm) superior to the _____ (B).

129. Which anatomic structures are included on an AP coccyx projection with accurate positioning?

_____

130. Should the gonads of male and female patients be shielded for an AP coccyx projection?

A. _____ (Yes/No)

Defend your answer.

B. _____

_____

For the following descriptions of AP coccyx projections with poor positioning, state how the patient or central ray would have been mispositioned for such a projection to be obtained.

131. The urinary bladder is dense and creating a shadow over the coccyx.

_____

132. The coccyx is not aligned with the symphysis pubis but is situated closer to the left lateral pelvic wall.

_____

133. The symphysis pubis is superimposed over the coccyx, and the second and third coccygeal vertebrae are foreshortened.

_____

For the following AP coccyx projections with poor positioning, state which anatomic structures are misaligned and how the patient should be repositioned for an optimal projection to be obtained.

Figure 9-28

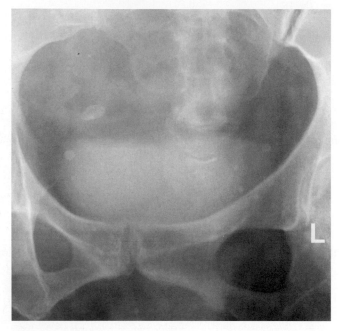

134. Figure 9-28: _____

_____

_____

_____

Figure 9-29

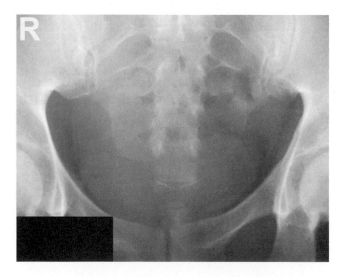

135. Figure 9-29: _____

_____

_____

_____

Coccyx: Lateral Projection

136. Identify the labeled anatomy in Figure 9-30.

Figure 9-30

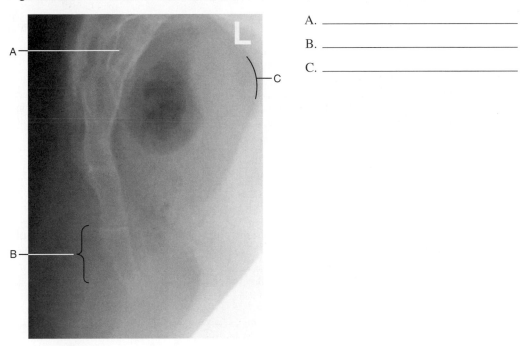

A. _____

B. _____

C. _____

137. Complete the statements below referring to lateral coccyx projection analysis criteria.

Lateral Coccyx Projection Analysis Criteria
• The median sacral crest is in _____ (A) and the greater sciatic notches are superimposed.
• The coccyx is seen without _____ (B).

138. List three methods of reducing the amount of scatter radiation that reaches the IR when a lateral coccyx projection is produced.

A. _____

B. _____

C. _____

139. How is the patient positioned to prevent rotation on a lateral coccyx projection?

_____

140. What is accomplished by placing a pillow or sponge between the patient's legs for a lateral coccyx projection?

_____

_____

141. How can rotation be detected on a rotated lateral coccyx projection?

_____

142. How is the patient positioned to prevent foreshortening of the coccyx on a lateral coccyx projection?

_____

_____

143. Accurate central ray centering on a lateral coccyx projection is accomplished by centering a perpendicular central ray approximately 3.5 inches (9 cm) _____ (A) and 2 inches (5 cm) _____ (B) to the _____ (C)

144. How tightly can one safely collimate on a lateral coccyx projection without fear of clipping any portion of the coccyx?

_____

145. Which anatomic structures are included on a lateral coccyx projection with accurate positioning?

_____

For the following description of a lateral coccyx projection with poor positioning, state how the patient would have been mispositioned for such a projection to be obtained.

146. The greater sciatic notches are demonstrated without superimposition, and the ischium is nearly superimposed over the third coccygeal segment.

_____

For the following lateral coccyx projection with poor positioning, state which anatomic structures are misaligned and how the patient should be repositioned for an optimal projection to be obtained.

Figure 9-31

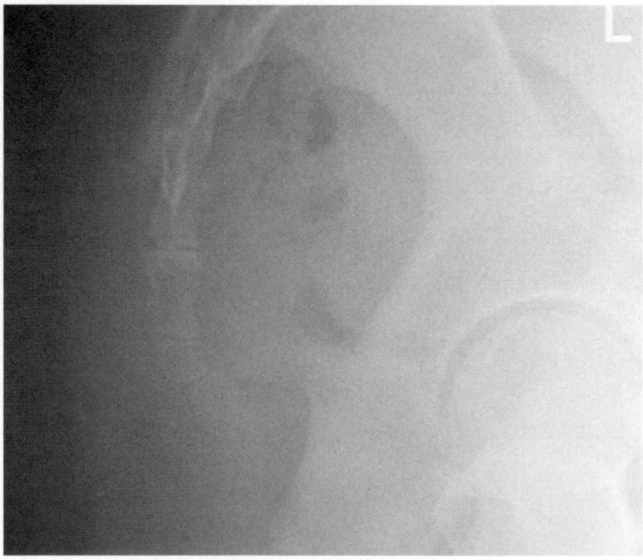

147. Figure 9-31: _____

_____

_____

_____

10 Sternum and Ribs

STUDY QUESTIONS

1. Describe how the following sternum and rib projections should be displayed on a view box or digital monitor.

   A. PA oblique sternum (RAO position): _____

   B. Lateral sternum: _____

   C. Left AP oblique rib (LPO position): _____

2. Complete Exercise 10-1.

EXERCISE 10-1 Sternum and Rib Technical Data			
Projection	kVp	Grid	SID
PA oblique (RAO position) sternum			
Lateral sternum			
AP or PA upper ribs			
AP or PA lower ribs			
AP oblique, upper ribs			
AP oblique, lower ribs			

Sternum: PA Oblique Projection (RAO Position)

3. Identify the labeled anatomy in Figure 10-1.

Figure 10-1

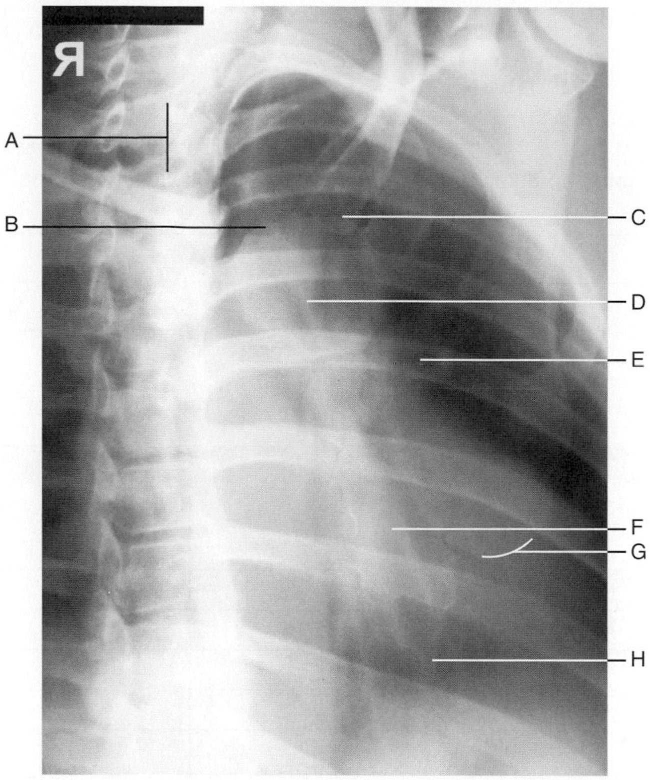

A. _____

B. _____

C. _____

D. _____

E. _____

F. _____

G. _____

H. _____

4. Define the following terms.

A. Homogeneous: _____

B. Costal breathing: _____

5. Complete the statements below referring to PA oblique sternum projection (RAO position) analysis criteria.

Posteroanterior Oblique Sternum Projection (RAO position) Analysis Criteria
• Sternum demonstrates homogeneous density.
• Sternum is demonstrated without motion or distortion. Ribs and lung markings are (A) _____, and the posterior ribs and (B) _____ are magnified.
• Manubrium, Sternoclavicular joints (SCs), sternal body, and xiphoid process are demonstrated within the heart shadow without (C) _____ superimposition.

6. Why is the PA oblique projection obtained in the RAO instead of the LAO position when imaging the sternum?

_____

7. Keeping the entire sternum within the heart shadow for the PA oblique projection (RAO position) provides a sternal projection that demonstrates density that is _____.

8. List four structures that overlie the sternum in a PA oblique sternal projection (RAO position).

   A. _____

   B. _____

   C. _____

   D. _____

9. Using a short SID will result in _____ (lower/higher) patient entrance skin dosage.

10. Using a long exposure time and (A) _____ breathing for the PA oblique sternal projection (RAO position) will (B) _____ the lung markings and (C) _____.

11. If the patient breathes deeply during the exposure for a PA oblique sternal projection (RAO position), the resulting image demonstrates a _____ sternum.

12. The sternum is rotated from beneath the thoracic vertebrae for a PA oblique sternal projection (RAO position) by rotating the patient until the (A) _____ plane is aligned (B) _____ degrees with the IR.

13. Any portion of the sternum that is positioned outside the heart shadow on a PA oblique sternal projection (RAO position) demonstrates _____ (more/less) density than that positioned within the heart shadow.

14. On a PA oblique sternal projection (RAO position) with accurate positioning, the _____ is centered within the collimated field.

15. Proper centering for a PA oblique sternal projection (RAO position) is accomplished by centering the central ray (A) _____ inches to the left of the (B) _____ and placing the top of the IR approximately 1½ inches superior to the (C) _____.

16. When the patient is rotated for a PA oblique sternal projection (RAO position), the (A) _____ (superior/inferior) portion of the sternum remains situated closer to the thoracic vertebrae than the (B) _____ (superior/inferior) portion.

17. Because the long axis of the sternum does not align with the long axis of the IR in the PA oblique sternal projection (RAO position), transverse collimation should be limited to the (A) _____ and (B) _____.

18. Adequate RAO obliquity is obtained on a PA oblique sternal projection (RAO position) when the (A) _____ and (B) _____ are no longer superimposed.

For the following description of a PA oblique sternal projections (RAO positions) with poor positioning, state how the patient would have been mispositioned for such a projection to be obtained.

19. The right SC joint and right side of the manubrium are superimposed by the thoracic vertebrae.

   _____

For the following PA oblique sternal projections (RAO positions) with poor positioning, state what anatomic structures are misaligned and how the patient should be repositioned for an optimal projection to be obtained.

Figure 10-2

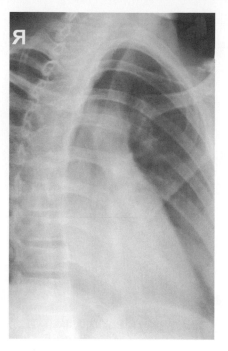

20. Figure 10-2: _____

_____

_____

_____

Figure 10-3

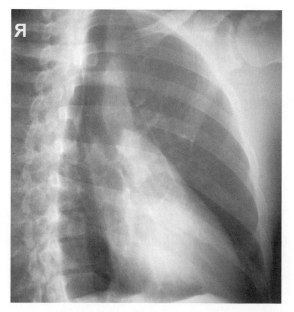

21. Figure 10-3: _____

_____

_____

_____

Sternum: Lateral Projection

22. Identify the labeled anatomy in Figure 10-4.

Figure 10-4

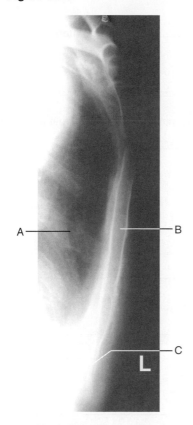

A. _____

B. _____

C. _____

23. Identify the labeled anatomy in Figure 10-5.

Figure 10-5

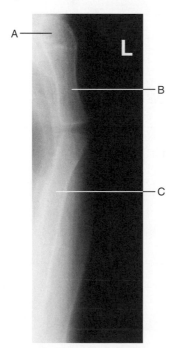

A. _____

B. _____

C. _____

24. Complete the statements below referring to lateral sternum projection analysis criteria.

> **Lateral Sternum Projection Analysis Criteria**
>
> • Sternum demonstrates homogeneous density.
>
> • Manubrium, sternal body, and xiphoid process are in (A) _____, and the anterior ribs are not superimposed over the sternum.
>
> • No superimposition of (B) _____ soft tissue over the sternum is present.

25. Why is it often difficult to demonstrate the superior and inferior sternum simultaneously on a lateral sternal projection?

_____

_____

26. List three methods of controlling the amount of scatter radiation that reaches the IR on a lateral sternal projection.

A. _____

B. _____

C. _____

27. How is rotation avoided when positioning the patient for a lateral sternal projection?

_____

_____

28. How is rotation identified on a lateral sternal projection? _____

_____

29. Describe how one can determine on a lateral sternal projection with poor positioning that the patient's right thorax is rotated anteriorly.

_____

_____

30. Deep suspended respiration draws the sternum away from the _____.

31. How is the patient positioned to prevent humeral soft tissue from superimposing the sternum? _____

_____

32. Accurate central ray centering on a lateral sternal projection is accomplished by placing the top edge of the IR

(A) _____ inches above the (B) _____ and aligning the receptor's long axis and a (C) _____ central ray to the midsternum.

33. Why is a 72-inch (180-cm) SID used for a lateral sternum projection?

_____

_____

34. What anatomic structures are included on a lateral sternal projection with accurate positioning?

_____

For the following descriptions of lateral sternal projections with poor positioning, state how the patient would have been mispositioned for such a projection to be obtained.

35. The anterior ribs are demonstrated without superimposition, the sternum is not in profile, and the superior heart shadow extends beyond the sternum and into the anteriorly situated lung.

_____

36. The anterior ribs are demonstrated without superimposition, the sternum is not in profile, and the superior heart shadow does not extend beyond the sternum.

_____

For the following lateral sternal projection with poor positioning, state what anatomic structures are misaligned and how the patient should be repositioned for an optimal projection to be obtained.

Figure 10-6

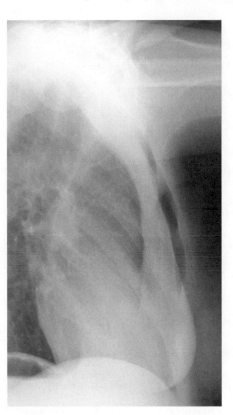

37. Figure 10-6: _____

_____

_____

_____

Ribs: AP or PA Projection

38. Identify the labeled anatomy in Figure 10-7.

Figure 10-7

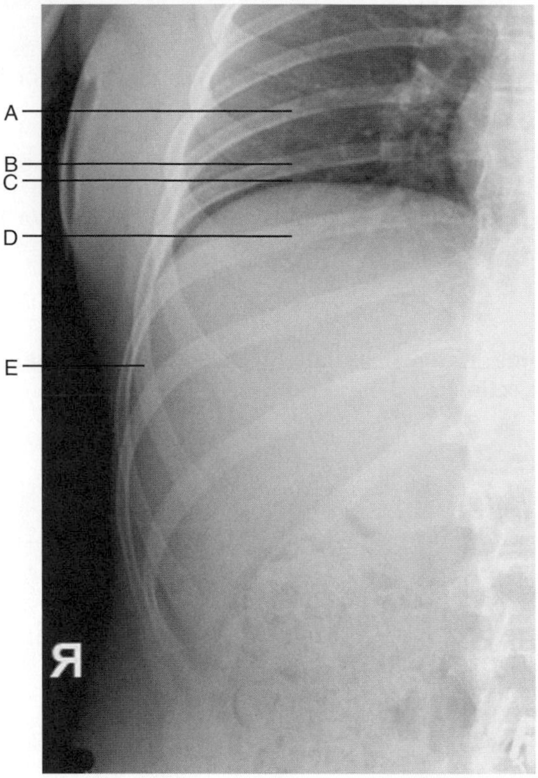

A. _____

B. _____

C. _____

D. _____

E. _____

39. Complete the statements below referring to AP/PA rib projection analysis criteria.

Anteroposterior or Posteroanterior Rib Projection Analysis Criteria
• Rib magnification is kept to a minimum.
• Thoracic vertebrae–rib head articulations are demonstrated, the sternum and (A) _____ are superimposed, and the distances from the (B) _____ to the sternal ends of the clavicles, when seen, are equal.
Above diaphragm:
• Scapulae are outside the lung field, and the chin does not obscure the (C) _____.
• (D) _____ posterior ribs are seen above the diaphragm.
Below diaphragm:
• (E) _____ through twelfth posterior ribs are demonstrated below the diaphragm.

40. Why do some facilities require the technologist to tape a rib marker (lead "BB") on the patient's skin near the area

where the ribs are tender? _____

_____

41. A. What patient respiration is used when imaging ribs located above the diaphragm?

    _____

    B. What patient respiration is used when imaging ribs located below the diaphragm?

    _____

42. Explain why a higher kVp is used when imaging below-diaphragm ribs versus above-diaphragm ribs?

    _____

    _____

43. What soft-tissue structures are evaluated for associated injury on the following rib projections?

    A. Upper ribs: _____

    _____

    B. Lower ribs: _____

    _____

44. If the patient complains of anterior rib pain, what projection of the ribs should be taken?

    A. _____ (AP/PA)

    When the patient indicates posterior rib pain, what projection of the ribs should be taken?

    B. _____ (AP/PA)

    If the opposite is taken for these two situations, what difference would result?

    C. _____

45. How is spinal scoliosis identified on PA and AP rib projections?

    _____

    _____

46. Describe how the patient is positioned to prevent thoracic rotation for the following projections of the ribs.

    A. AP: _____

    _____

    B. PA: _____

    _____

47. For each of the following projections, describe how the patient is positioned to obtain a projection of the ribs with the scapula placed outside the lung field.

    A. AP: _____

    _____

    B. PA: _____

48. If an AP or PA supine rib projection is taken in full suspended inspiration, how many ribs are demonstrated above the

    diaphragm? _____

49. What ribs are demonstrated below the diaphragm when an AP or PA rib projection is taken on expiration?

_____

50. Accurate central ray centering on an above-diaphragm AP or PA rib projection is accomplished on an AP projection by centering the central ray halfway between the (A) _____ and affected lateral body surface at a level halfway between the (B) _____ and (C) _____. This centering is accomplished on a PA projection by placing the central ray halfway between the (D) _____ and lateral rib surface at the level of the (E) _____.

51. What anatomic structures are included on an above-diaphragm AP or PA rib projection with accurate positioning?

_____

52. Accurate central ray centering on a below-diaphragm AP or PA rib projection is accomplished by placing the lower border of the IR at the (A) _____, centering a perpendicular central ray to the IR, and moving the patient side to side until the longitudinal collimator light line is aligned halfway between the (B) _____ and lateral body surface.

How should this centering be adjusted for a hypersthenic patient?

C. _____

53. What anatomic structures are included on an AP or PA below-diaphragm rib projection with accurate positioning?

_____

For the following descriptions of AP or PA rib projections with poor positioning, state how the patient would have been mispositioned for such a projection to be obtained.

54. The sternum and SC joints are demonstrated to the left of the patient's vertebral column on an AP projection taken because of left rib pain.

_____

55. The left scapula is superimposed over the upper lateral rib field on a PA projection.

_____

56. The tenth through twelfth posterior ribs are demonstrated below the diaphragm on a below-diaphragm projection.

_____

For the following AP or PA rib projections with poor positioning, state what anatomic structures are misaligned and how the patient should be repositioned for an optimal projection to be obtained.

Figure 10-8

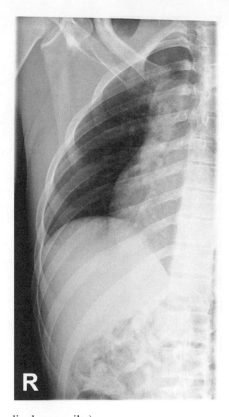

57. Figure 10-8 (AP projection, above-diaphragm ribs): _____

_____

_____

_____

Figure 10-9

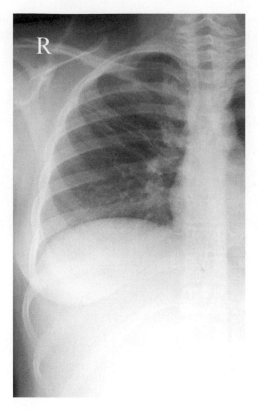

58. Figure 10-9 (AP projection, above-diaphragm ribs): _____

_____

_____

_____

Figure 10-10

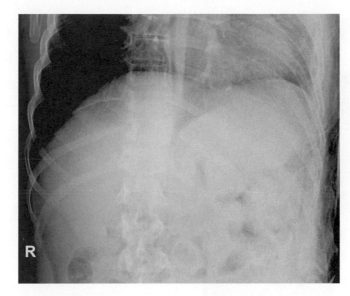

59. Figure 10-10 (AP projection, below-diaphragm ribs): _____

_____

_____

_____

Ribs: AP Oblique Projection (RPO and LPO Positions)

60. Identify the labeled anatomy in Figure 10-11.

Figure 10-11

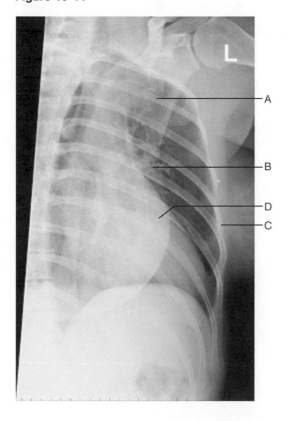

A. _____

B. _____

C. _____

D. _____

61. Identify the labeled anatomy in Figure 10-12.

Figure 10-12

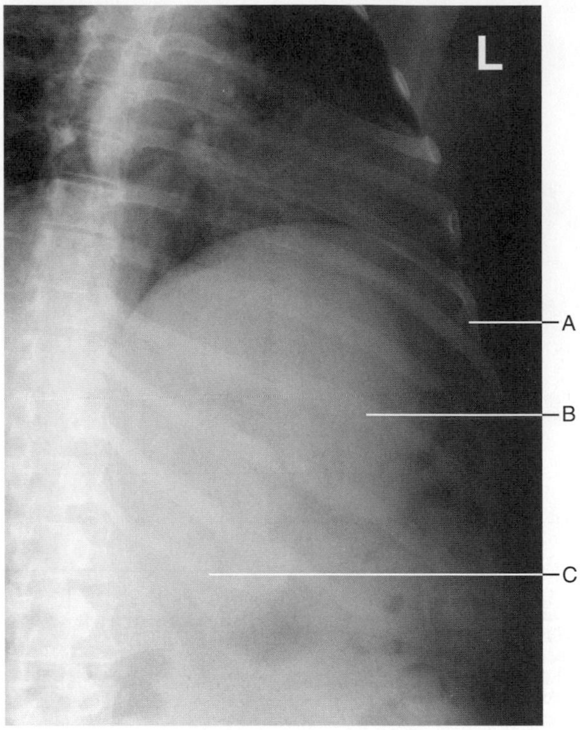

A. _____

B. _____

C. _____

62. Complete the statements below referring to AP oblique rib projection analysis criteria.

Anteroposterior Oblique Rib Projection (RPO or LPO Position) Analysis Criteria

- Rib magnification is kept to a minimum.
- (A) _____ is located halfway between the lateral rib surface and the vertebral column, and the axillary ribs are free of superimposition.
- (B) _____ are demonstrated without superimposition and are located in the center of the collimated field, and the anterior ribs are located at the lateral edge.

Above diaphragm:

- (C) _____ axillary ribs are demonstrated above the diaphragm.

Below diaphragm:

- (D) _____ through twelfth axillary ribs are demonstrated below the diaphragm.

63. Which oblique position demonstrates the sharper axillary rib details?

A. _____ (AP/PA)

Defend your answer.

B. _____

64. What degree of patient rotation is used for AP oblique rib projections?

A. _____

What body plane is used to align this angle?

B. _____

65. For the following projections, state whether the patient is rotated toward or away from the affected side to demonstrate the axillary ribs in the AP oblique projection.

A. AP oblique: _____

B. PA oblique: _____

66. How can one determine from an AP oblique rib projection if the patient has been rotated 45 degrees?

_____

67. What patient respiration is used when imaging ribs located above the diaphragm?

_____

68. What patient respiration is used when imaging ribs located below the diaphragm?

_____

69. Accurate central ray centering on an above-diaphragm AP oblique rib projection is accomplished by centering a

(A) _____ central ray halfway between the midsagittal plane and (B) _____, at a level

halfway between the (C) _____ and (D) _____.

70. What anatomic structures are included on an above-diaphragm AP oblique rib projection with accurate

positioning?_____

_____

71. Accurate central ray centering on a below-diaphragm AP oblique rib projection is accomplished by positioning the

lower IR border at the patient's (A) _____ and centering the central ray halfway between the (B)

_____ and lateral rib surface.

72. What anatomic structures are included on a below-diaphragm AP oblique rib projection?

_____

For the following descriptions of AP oblique rib projections with poor positioning, state how the patient would have been mispositioned for such a projection to be obtained.

73. The axillary ribs demonstrate increased self-superimposition, and the sternum is rotated toward the patient's left side on a projection taken for right side rib pain.

_____

74. The sternal body is demonstrated adjacent to the vertebral column.

_____

75. An above-diaphragm AP oblique rib projection demonstrates the first through seventh posterior ribs above the diaphragm.

_____

For the following AP and PA oblique rib projections with poor positioning, state what anatomic structures are misaligned and how the patient should be repositioned for an optimal projection to be obtained.

Figure 10-13

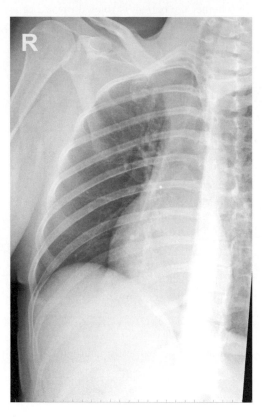

76. Figure 10-13 (AP oblique projection): _____

_____

_____

_____

Figure 10-14

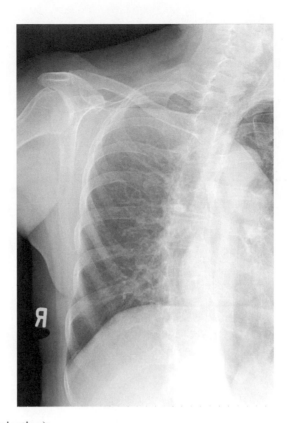

77. Figure 10-14 (PA oblique projection): _____

_____

_____

_____

11 Cranium

STUDY QUESTIONS

1. Describe how the following images should be displayed on a view box or digital monitor.

    A. Anteroposterior cranial projection:

    _____

    B. Parietoacanthial sinuses projection (Waters method): _____

    _____

    C. Submentovertex mandibular projection (Schueller method):

    _____

    D. AP axial cranial projection (Caldwell method): _____

    _____

2. Complete Exercise 11-1.

EXERCISE 11-1 Cranium, Facial Bones, Sinuses, and Mandible Technical Data					
Projection	**Structure**	**kVp**	**Grid**	**AEC Chamber (s)**	**SID**
AP or PA	Cranium				
	Mandible				
PA axial (Caldwell method)	Cranium				
	Facial bones				
	Sinuses				
AP axial (Towne method)	Cranium				
	Mandible				
Lateral	Cranium				
	Facial bones				
	Sinuses				
	Nasal bones				
Submentovertex (Schueller method)	Cranium				
	Mandible				
	Sinuses				
	Zygomatic arches				
Parietoacanthial (Waters method)	Facial bones				
	Sinuses				
Tangential (Superoinferior)	Nasal bones				

AEC, Automatic exposure control; *kVp*, kilovoltage peak; *SID*, source–image receptor distance.

Cranium and Mandible: Posteroanterior or Anteroposterior Projection

3. Identify the labeled anatomy in Figure 11-1.

Figure 11-1

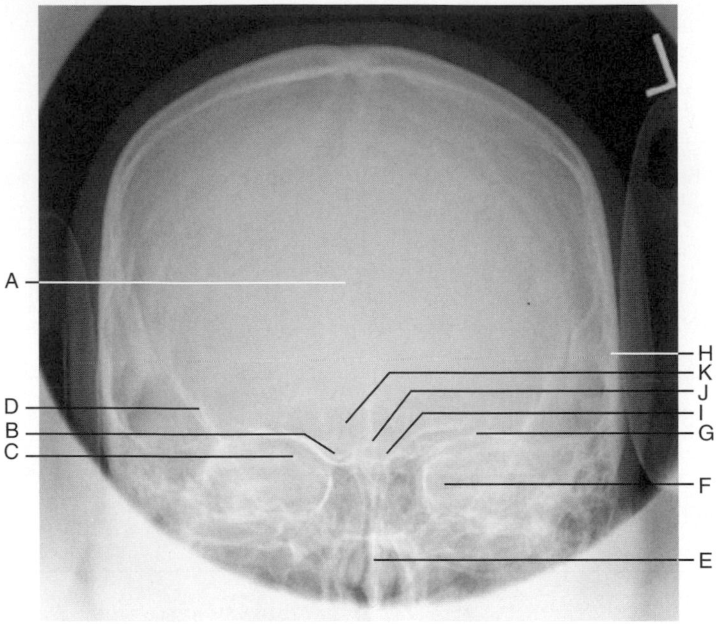

A. _____

B. _____

C. _____

D. _____

E. _____

F. _____

G. _____

H. _____

I. _____

J. _____

K. _____

4. Define the following terms.

A. OML: _____

_____

B. Glabella: _____

_____

5. Complete the statements below referring to PA cranial and mandible projection analysis criteria.

Posteroanterior Cranium and Mandible Projection Analysis Criteria
• The distances from the lateral margin of orbits to the lateral cranial _____ (A) from the crista galli to the lateral cranial cortices, and from the mandibular rami to the lateral cervical vertebrae on both sides are equal.
• The anterior clinoids and dorsum sellae are seen superior to the _____ (B).
• The petrous ridges are superimposed over the _____ (C), and the internal acoustic meatus and visualized horizonally through the center of the orbits.
• Mandible: The mouth is closed, with the teeth together.
• The crista galli and _____ (D) are aligned with the long axis of the exposure field, and the supraorbital margins and the temporomandibular joints are demonstrated on the same horizontal plane.

6. The midsagittal plane is positioned _____ (A) to the image receptor (IR) for a PA cranial

projection to prevent rotation. How is this positioning best accomplished? _____

_____ (B)

7. How is cranial rotation identified on a rotated PA skull projection?

_____

8. How is the patient's head position adjusted to prevent rotation on an AP skull projection taken in a patient with a suspected cervical injury?

_____

9. PA and AP skull projections demonstrate different magnified anatomic structures. Which of these projections demonstrates the greater orbital magnification?

A. _____

Which projection demonstrates the greater parietal bone magnification?

B. _____

10. What patient positioning line is used to obtain an accurate PA projection? _____ (A) How is this line positioned with respect to the imaging table? _____ (B)

11. If the patient is unable to position the line indicated in question 10 to the IR accurately for a PA cranial projection, how is the central ray adjusted to compensate?

_____

12. When the patient's chin is tucked for a PA cranial projection, in which direction will the supraorbital margins move with respect to the petrous ridges? _____ (inferiorly/superiorly)

13. If the patient is unable to adjust the degree of chin elevation for an AP trauma cranial projection, how is the central ray used to compensate?

_____

14. A PA skull projection with poor positioning demonstrates approximately 1 inch (2.5 cm) of space between the petrous ridges and supraorbital margins. The ridges are inferior. Where are the dorsum sellae and anterior clinoids demonstrated with respect to the ethmoid sinuses on this image?

_____

15. On a trauma AP cranial projection with poor positioning, the petrous ridges are demonstrated superior to the supraorbital margins. The distance between them is approximately 0.5 inch (1.25 cm). Will there be an increase or decrease in the amount of dorsum sella and anterior clinoid superimposition above the ethmoid sinuses on this image?

_____

16. Which two anatomic structures are aligned with the long axis of the image if the patient's midsagittal plane is accurately aligned with the collimated field on a PA or AP cranial projection?

A. _____

B. _____

17. On a PA or AP cranial projection with accurate positioning, the _____ (A) is centered within the collimated field. This centering is obtained when the central ray is centered to the _____ (B).

18. Which anatomic structures are included on a PA or AP cranial projection with accurate positioning?

_____

19. On a PA or AP mandible projection with accurate positioning, the _____ _____ (A) is centered within the collimated field. This centering is obtained when the central ray is centered to _____ (B).

20. Which anatomic structures are included on a PA or AP mandibular projection with accurate positioning?

_____

For the following descriptions of PA and AP cranial projections with poor positioning, state how the patient or central ray would have been mispositioned for such an image to be obtained.

21. The distance from the lateral orbital margins to the lateral cranial cortex and from the crista galli to the lateral cranial cortex on the left side is greater than on the right side.

_____

22. The petrous ridges are demonstrated inferior to the supraorbital margins, and the dorsum sellae and anterior clinoids are superimposed over the ethmoid sinuses. How was the patient mispositioned?

A. _____

If this were a trauma AP projection, how would the central ray have been mispositioned?

B. _____

23. The petrous ridges are demonstrated superior to the supraorbital margins. How was the patient mispositioned?

A. _____

If this were a trauma AP projection, how would the central ray have been mispositioned?

B. _____

For the following PA and AP cranial projections with poor positioning, state which anatomic structures are misaligned and how the patient should be repositioned for an optimal image to be obtained.

Figure 11-2

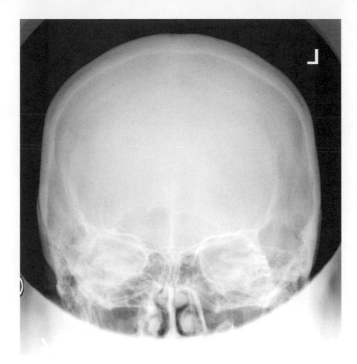

24. Figure 11-2 (PA projection): _____

_____

_____

_____

Figure 11-3

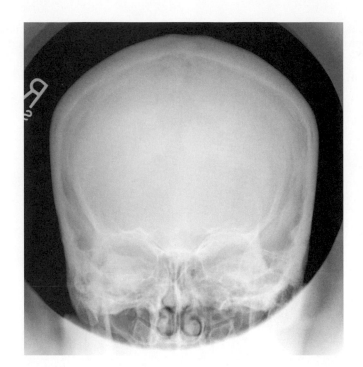

25. Figure 11-3 (PA projection): _____

_____

_____

_____

Figure 11-4

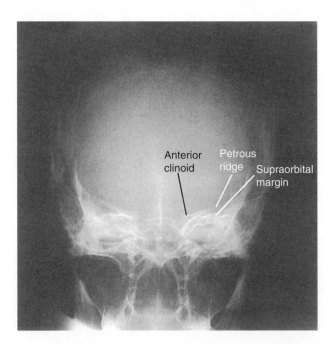

Anterior
clinoid

Petrous
ridge

Supraorbital
margin

26. Figure 11-4 (PA projection): _____

_____

_____

_____

Figure 11-5

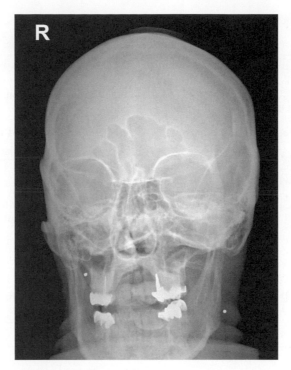

27. Figure 11-5 (AP projection, trauma): _____

_____

_____

_____

Cranium, Facial Bones, and Sinuses: Posteroanterior Axial Projection (Caldwell Method)

28. Identify the labeled anatomy in Figure 11-6.

Figure 11-6

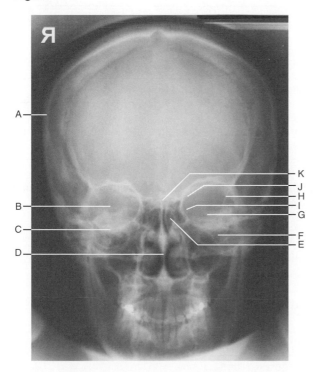

A. _____

B. _____

C. _____

D. _____

E. _____

F. _____

G. _____

H. _____

I. _____

J. _____

K. _____

29. Complete the statements below referring to PA axial cranium, facial bones, and sinuses projection analysis criteria.

Posteroanterior Axial Cranium, Facial Bones, and Sinuses Projection (Caldwell Method) Analysis Criteria

- The distances from the lateral orbital margins to the lateral cranial cortices on both sides and from the crista galli to the lateral cranial cortices on both sides are equal.

- The petrous ridges are demonstrated horizontally through the lower third of the _____ (A), the petrous pyramids are superimposed over the _____ (B), and the superior orbital fissures are seen within the orbits.

- The _____ (C) and nasal septum are aligned with the long axis of the exposure field, and the supraorbital margins are demonstrated on the same horizontal plane.

---

30. Describe how the patient is positioned to prevent rotation on a PA axial projection.

_____

_____

31. Which plane is positioned perpendicular to the IR for a PA axial projection?

_____

32. When rotation is present on a PA axial projection, the patient's face is rotated _____ (toward/away from) (A) the side of the cranium that demonstrates the greater distance. On an AP axial projection, the patient's face is rotated _____ (toward/away from) (B) the side of the cranium that demonstrates the greater distance.

33. Why are the orbits more magnified on an AP axial projection of the cranium than on a PA axial projection?

A. _____

_____

Which projection demonstrates less parietal magnification?

B. _____

_____

34. What are the degree and direction of the central ray angulation used on a PA axial projection of the cranium?

_____

35. What are the degree and direction of the central ray angulation used on an AP axial projection of the cranium when the patient is capable of adequately positioning the head?

_____

36. Accurate positioning for a PA or AP axial cranial projection is obtained when the _____ line is aligned perpendicular to the IR.

37. How is the central ray angulation determined for a PA axial cranial projection of a patient who is unable to accurately position the head? _____

_____

38. What is the central ray angulation for a PA axial projection of the cranium for a patient who can tuck the chin only enough to place the orbitomeatal line (OML) at a 10-degree cephalad angle with the IR?

_____

39. What is the central ray angulation for an AP axial projection of the cranium for a patient who can tuck the chin only enough to place the OML at a 5-degree caudal angle with the IR?

_____

40. How is the patient positioned to align the crista galli and nasal septum with the long axis of the collimated field?

_____

_____

41. On a PA and AP axial projection with accurate positioning, the _____ (A) are centered within

the collimated field. This is accomplished by centering the central ray to _____ (B).

42. Describe the location of the nasion. _____

_____

43. Which anatomic structures are included on a PA or AP axial projection of the cranium with accurate positioning?

A. _____

On an image of facial bones or sinuses?

B. _____

For the following descriptions of PA axial cranial projections with poor positioning, state how the patient or central ray would have been mispositioned for such an image to be obtained.

44. The distance from the lateral orbital margin to the lateral cranial cortex on the left side is greater than that on the right side. Will the distance from the left or right side of the crista galli to the lateral cranial cortex demonstrate the smaller distance on this image?

A. _____

How was the patient mispositioned for this image?

B. _____

45. The petrous ridges are demonstrated inferior to the inferior orbital margins. How was the patient mispositioned for such an image to be obtained if the central ray was accurately angled?

A. _____

How was the central ray mispositioned for such an image to be obtained if the patient was accurately positioned?

B. _____

46. The petrous ridges and pyramids are superior to the supraorbital margins, and the internal auditory canals are distorted. How was the patient mispositioned for such an image to be obtained if the central ray was accurately angled?

A. _____

How was the central ray mispositioned for such an image to be obtained if the patient was accurately positioned?

B. _____

For the following PA and AP axial cranial projections with poor positioning, state which anatomic structures are misaligned and how the patient should be repositioned for an optimal image to be obtained.

Figure 11-7

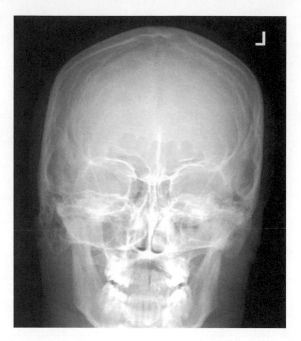

47. Figure 11-7 (PA axial projection): _____

_____

_____

_____

Figure 11-8

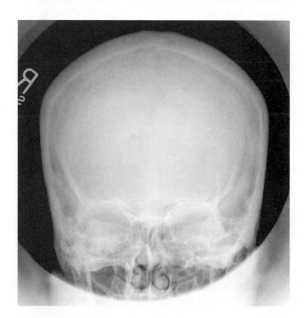

48. Figure 11-8 (PA axial projection): _____

_____

_____

_____

Figure 11-9

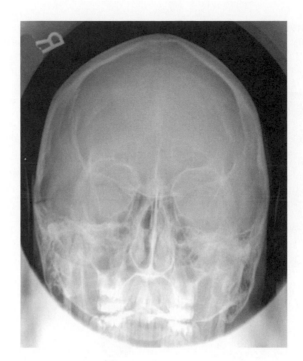

49. Figure 11-9 (PA axial projection): _____

_____

_____

_____

Figure 11-10

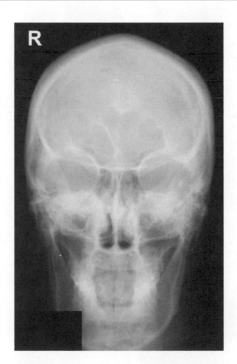

50. Figure 11-10 (AP axial projection, trauma): _____

_____

_____

_____

51. Identify the labeled anatomy in Figure 11-11.

Figure 11-11

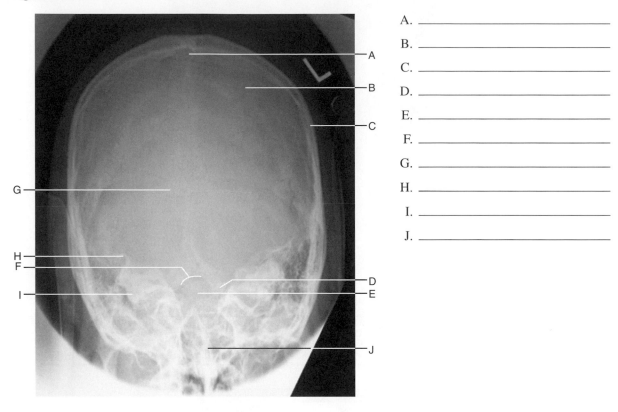

A. _____

B. _____

C. _____

D. _____

E. _____

F. _____

G. _____

H. _____

I. _____

J. _____

52. Identify the labeled anatomy in Figure 11-12.

Figure 11-12

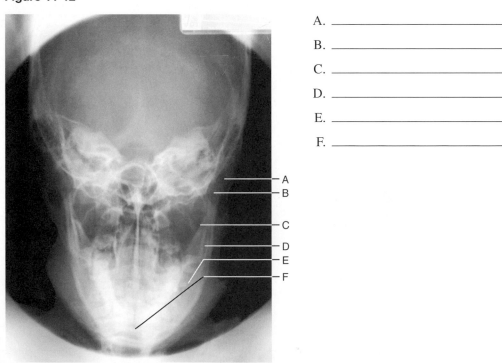

A. _____

B. _____

C. _____

D. _____

E. _____

F. _____

53. Complete the statements below referring to AP axial cranium and mandible projection analysis criteria.

Anteroposterior Axial Cranium and Mandible Projection (Towne Method) Analysis Criteria

- The distances from the posterior clinoid process to the lateral borders of the _____ (A) on both sides and the mandibular necks to the lateral cervical vertebrae on both sides are equal, the petrous ridges are symmetrical, and the dorsum sellae is centered within the _____ (B).

- Cranium: The dorsum sellae and _____ (C) are seen within the foramen magnum without foreshortening or superimposition of the atlas's posterior arch.

- Mandible: The dorsum sellae and posterior clinoids are at the level of the _____ (D) foramen magnum and the mandibular condyles and fossae are clearly demonstrated, with minimal mastoid superimposition.

- The _____ (E) and nasal septum are aligned with the long axis of the exposure field.

---

54. Define *infraorbitomeatal* line. _____

_____

55. How is the patient positioned to prevent rotation on an AP axial projection of the cranial with accurate positioning?

_____

_____

56. State two methods for identifying rotation on an AP axial projection of the cranial.

A. _____

_____

B. _____

_____

57. The _____ (A) plane is positioned _____ (B) to the IR to prevent rotation on an AP axial projection.

58. When rotation is present on an AP axial projection, the side demonstrating less distance between the posterior clinoid process and the lateral border of the foramen magnum is the side _____ (toward/away from) where the patient's face is rotated.

59. When the correct central ray angulation and head position are used on an AP axial projection, the _____ (A) and posterior clinoids are demonstrated within the _____ (B).

60. What are the degree and direction of the central ray angulation used on an AP axial projection of the cranium and mandible?

_____

61. What positioning line is aligned perpendicular to the IR for an AP axial projection of the cranium?

_____

62. How is the central ray angulation determined for an AP axial projection of the cranium in a patient who is unable to accurately position the head?

_____

63. Which two anatomic structures are aligned with the long axis of the IR if the patient's midsagittal plane is accurately aligned with the collimated field on an AP axial projection?

A. _____

B. _____

64. Which anatomic structures are included on an AP axial projection of the cranium with accurate positioning?

_____

_____

For the following descriptions of AP axial projections of the cranium with inaccurate positioning, state how the patient or central ray would have been mispositioned for such an image to be obtained.

65. The distance from the posterior clinoid process to the lateral foramen magnum on the patient's left side is less than that on the patient's right side.

_____

66. The dorsum sellae and anterior clinoids are demonstrated superior to the foramen magnum. How would the patient have been mispositioned for such an image to be obtained if the central ray was accurately angled?

A. _____

How would the central ray have been mispositioned for such an image to be obtained if the patient was accurately positioned?

B. _____

67. The dorsum sella is foreshortened and superimposed over the atlas's posterior arch. How would the patient have been mispositioned for such an image to be obtained if the central ray was accurately angled?

A. _____

How would the central ray have been mispositioned for such an image to be obtained if the patient was accurately positioned?

B. _____

For the following AP axial projections of the cranium and mandible with poor positioning, state which anatomic structures are misaligned and how the patient should be repositioned for an optimal image to be obtained.

Figure 11-13

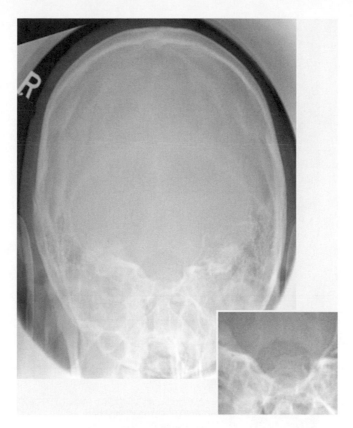

68. Figure 11-13:_____

_____

_____

_____

Figure 11-14

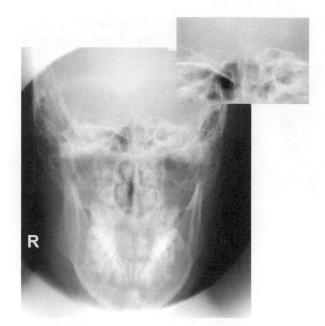

69. Figure 11-14: _____

_____

_____

_____

Figure 11-15

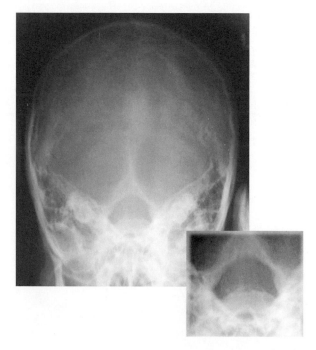

70. Figure 11-15: _____

_____

_____

_____

Cranium, Facial Bones, Nasal Bones, and Sinuses: Lateral Projection

71. Identify the labeled anatomy in Figure 11-16.

Figure 11-16

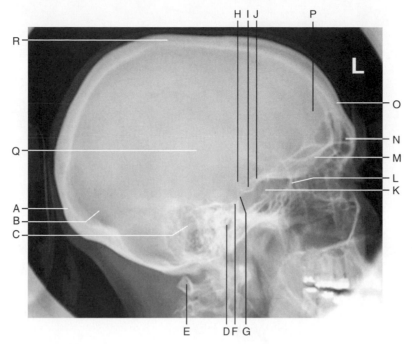

A. _____

B. _____

C. _____

D. _____

E. _____

F. _____

G. _____

H. _____

I. _____

J. _____

K. _____

L. _____

M. _____

N. _____

O. _____

P. _____

Q. _____

R. _____

72. Identify the labeled anatomy in Figure 11-17.

Figure 11-17

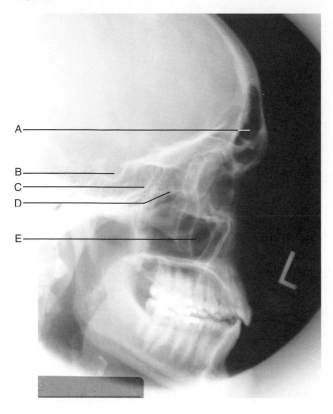

A. _____

B. _____

C. _____

D. _____

E. _____

73. Identify the labeled anatomy in Figure 11-18.

Figure 11-18

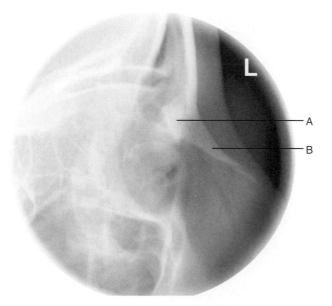

A. _____

B. _____

74. Complete the statements below referring to lateral cranium, facial and nasal bones, and sinuses projection analysis criteria.

Lateral Cranium, Facial and Nasal Bones, and Sinuses Projection Analysis Criteria
• When visualized, the sella turcica is seen in _____ (A). The orbital roofs, mandibular rami, greater wings of the sphenoid, external acoustic canals, zygomatic bones, and cranial cortices are superimposed.
• Cranium: The posteroinferior occipital bones and _____ (B) of the atlas are free of superimposition.

75. Define the following terms.

A. Interpupillary line: _____

_____

B. Outer canthus: _____

C. EAM: _____

76. Which sinuses are demonstrated on a lateral projection of the sinuses when adequate contrast and density have been obtained?

_____

77. Why is it best to take a lateral sinus projection with the patient in an upright position?

_____

78. What plane is used to position the patient to prevent rotation and tilting on a lateral cranial projection?

A. _____

How is it aligned with the IR?

B. _____

How does this positioning align the interpupillary (IP) line with the IR?

C. _____

79. How is the patient or IR positioned to include the occipital bone for a lateral cranial image of a recumbent patient without cervical trauma?

A. _____

Of a recumbent patient with cervical trauma?

B. _____

80. How can cranial tilting be distinguished from rotation on a lateral cranial projection? _____

_____

_____

81. How is the patient positioned to ensure that the posteroinferior occipital bone and posterior arch of the atlas are free of superimposition?

_____

82. On a lateral cranial projection with accurate positioning, the central ray is centered 2 inches (5 cm) _____ (A) to the _____ (B).

83. Which anatomic structures are included on a lateral cranial projection with accurate positioning?

_____

84. On a lateral sinus projection with accurate positioning, the _____ (A) are centered within the collimated field. This is accomplished by centering the central ray halfway between the _____ (B) and _____ (C).

85. Which anatomic structures are included on a lateral sinus projection with accurate positioning?

_____

86. On a lateral nasal projection with accurate positioning, the _____ (A) are centered within the collimated field. This is accomplished by centering the central ray 0.5 inch (1.25 cm) _____ (B) to the nasion.

87. Which anatomic structures are included on a lateral nasal bone projection with accurate positioning?

_____

_____

For the following descriptions of lateral cranial projections with poor positioning, state how the patient would have been mispositioned for such an image to be obtained.

88. The greater wings of the sphenoid and the anterior cranial cortices are demonstrated without superimposition. One of each corresponding structure is demonstrated anterior to the other.

_____

89. The orbital roofs, external auditory meatus, and inferior cranial cortices are demonstrated without superimposition. One of each corresponding structure is demonstrated superior to the other and the posterior arch is seen in profile.

_____

For the following lateral cranial projections with poor positioning, state which anatomic structures are misaligned and how the patient should be repositioned for an optimal image to be obtained.

Figure 11-19

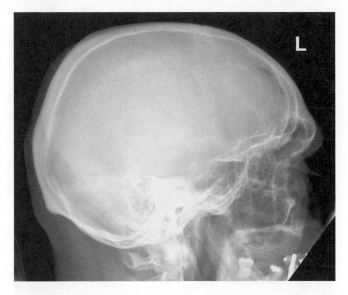

90. Figure 11-19: _____

_____

_____

_____

Figure 11-20

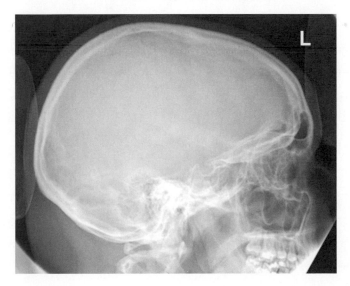

91. Figure 11-20: _____

_____

_____

_____

92. Identify the labeled anatomy in Figure 11-21.

Figure 11-21

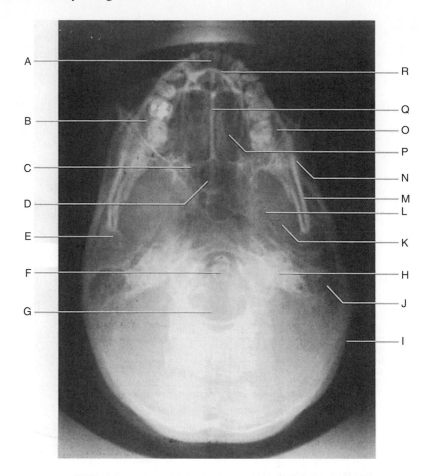

A. _____   J. _____

B. _____   K. _____

C. _____   L. _____

D. _____   M. _____

E. _____   N. _____

F. _____   O. _____

G. _____   P. _____

H. _____   Q. _____

I. _____   R. _____

93. Complete the statements below referring to submentovertex cranium, mandible, and sinuses projection analysis criteria.

Submentovertex Cranium, Mandible, and Sinuses Projection (Schueller Method) Analysis Criteria
• The mandibular mentum and nasal fossae are demonstrated just anterior to the _____ (A).
• The distances from the mandibular ramus and body to the lateral cranial cortex on both sides are equal.
• The vomer, bony nasal septum, and _____ (B) are aligned with the long axis of the exposure field.

94. Accurate mandibular mentum and nasal fossae positioning on a submentovertex cranial projection is obtained when the _____ (A) positioning line is aligned _____ (B) with the IR.

95. Which structures are obscured on a submentovertex cranial projection if the patient's neck is not adequately extended?

    A. _____

    B. _____

    C. _____

    D. _____

96. How is the positioning setup adjusted for a submentovertex cranial projection in a patient who is unable to extend the neck as far as needed?

    _____

97. How is cranial tilting identified on a tilted submentovertex cranial projection?

    A. _____

    _____

    How is the patient positioned to prevent tilting on a submentovertex cranial projection?

    B. _____

98. How is the patient positioned to align the vomer, bony nasal septum, and dens with the long axis of the collimated field on a submentovertex projection?

    A. _____

    Will rotation of the head affect any anatomic relationships on a submentovertex projection?

    B. _____ (Yes/No)

99. On a submentovertex cranial projection with accurate positioning, the _____ (A) is centered within the collimated field. This is accomplished when the central ray is centered to the _____ (B) plane at a level _____ inch (C) anterior to the level of the _____ (D).

100. Which anatomic structures are included on a submentovertex cranial projection with accurate positioning?

_____

_____

101. On a submentovertex sinus and mandible projection with accurate positioning, the _____ (A) are cen-

tered within the collimated field. This is accomplished by centering the central ray to the _____ (B)

plane at a level _____ inches (C) inferior to the _____ (D).

102. Which anatomic structures are included on a submentovertex sinus and mandible projection with accurate

positioning? _____

_____

For the following descriptions of submentovertex cranial projections with poor positioning, state how the patient or central ray would have been mispositioned for such an image to be obtained.

103. The mandibular mentum is demonstrated too far anterior to the ethmoid sinuses.

_____

104. The mandibular mentum is demonstrated posterior to the ethmoid sinuses. How would the patient have been mispositioned?

A. _____

_____

How would the central ray have been mispositioned?

B. _____

105. The distance from the left mandibular ramus and body to its corresponding lateral cranial cortex is greater than the distance from the right mandibular ramus and body to its corresponding lateral cranial cortex.

_____

For the following submentovertex cranial, facial bone, and sinus projections with poor positioning, state which anatomic structures are misaligned and how the patient should be repositioned for an optimal image to be obtained.

Figure 11-22

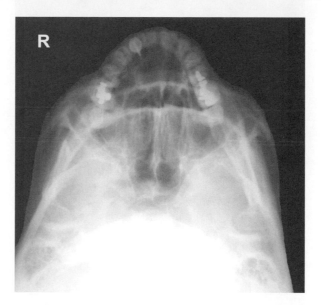

106. Figure 11-22: _____

_____

_____

_____

Figure 11-23

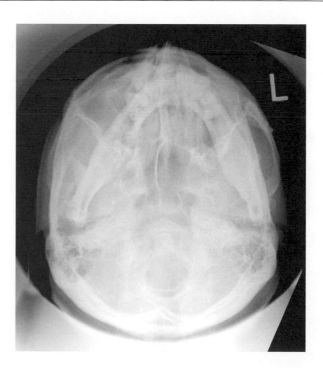

107. Figure 11-23: _____

_____

_____

_____

Figure 11-24

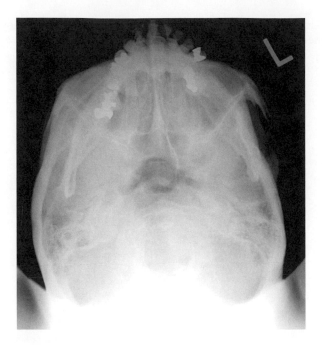

108. Figure 11-24: _____

_____

_____

_____

Facial Bones and Sinuses: Parietoacanthial and Acanthioparietal Projection (Waters and Open-Mouth Waters Methods)

109. Identify the labeled anatomy in Figure 11-25.

Figure 11-25

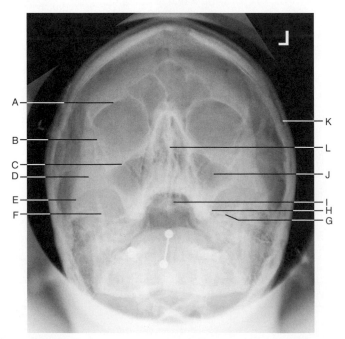

A. _____

B. _____

C. _____

D. _____

E. _____

F. _____

G. _____

H. _____

I. _____

J. _____

K. _____

L. _____

110. Complete the statements below referring to parietoacanthial and acanthioparietal facial bones and sinuses projection analysis criteria.

Parietoacanthial and Acanthioparietal Facial Bones and Sinuses Projection (Waters Method) Analysis Criteria
• The distances from the lateral orbital margin to the lateral cranial cortex and the distance from the bony nasal septum to the lateral cranial cortex on both sides are equal.
• The petrous ridges are demonstrated _____ (A) to the maxillary sinuses and extend _____ (B) from the posterior maxillary alveolar process.
• The bony nasal septum is aligned with the long axis of the exposure field, and the infraorbital margins are demonstrated on the same horizontal plane.

111. Define *mentomeatal* line. _____

_____

112. What sinuses are demonstrated on an open-mouth parietoacanthial projection that are not demonstrated on a closed-mouth parietoacanthial projection? _____

113. Describe how the patient is positioned to prevent rotation on a parietoacanthial sinus projection.

_____

_____

114. Cranial rotation results when the distances stated in question 113 are no longer equal. When rotation is present on a parietoacanthial projection, the patient's face is rotated _____ (toward/away from) (A) the side of the cranium that demonstrates the greatest distance. If an acanthioparietal projection is taken, the patient's face is rotated _____ (toward/away from) (B) the side of the cranium that demonstrates the greatest distance.

115. Why are the orbits more magnified on an acanthioparietal projection of the cranium than on a parietoacanthial projection?

A. _____

Which projection demonstrates the least parietal magnification?

B. _____

116. How is the patient positioned to accurately demonstrate the petrous ridges inferior to the maxillary sinuses on a parietoacanthial projection?

_____

117. How is the patient positioned for a parietoacanthial projection to align the bony nasal septum with the long axis of the collimated field?

_____

118. What are the results of cranial tilting on a parietoacanthial projection?

A. _____

B. _____

119. On a parietoacanthial projection with accurate positioning, the _____ (A) is centered within the collimated field. This is accomplished by centering the central ray to the _____ (B).

120. Which anatomic structures are included on a parietoacanthial projection with accurate positioning?

_____

_____

For the following descriptions of parietoacanthial cranial projections with poor positioning, state how the patient would have been mispositioned for such an image to be obtained.

121. The distances from the lateral orbital margin to the lateral cranial cortex and from the bony nasal septum to the lateral cranial cortex on the left side of the patient are greater than the distances on the right side.

_____

122. The petrous ridges are demonstrated within the maxillary sinuses and superior to the posterior maxillary alveolar process.

_____

123. The petrous ridges are inferior to the maxillary sinuses and posterior maxillary alveolar process.

_____

For the following parietoacanthial projections with poor positioning, state which anatomic structures are misaligned and how the patient should be repositioned for an optimal image to be obtained.

Figure 11-26

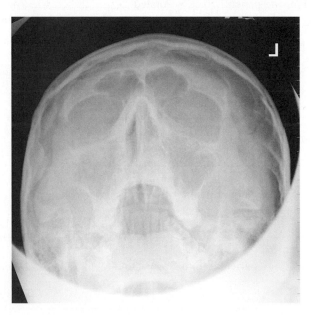

124. Figure 11-26: _____

_____

_____

_____

Figure 11-27

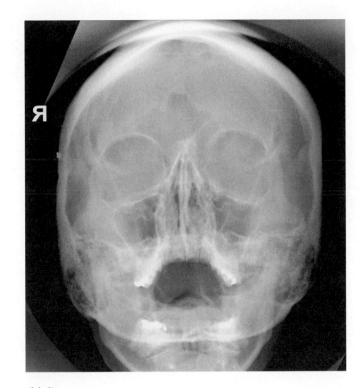

125. Figure 11-27 (parietocanthial): _____

_____

_____

_____

Figure 11-28

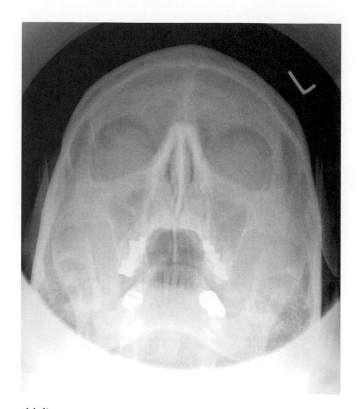

126. Figure 11-28 (parietocanthial): _____

_____

_____

_____

Nasal Bones: Tangential Projection (Superoinferior Projection)

127. Identify the labeled anatomy in Figure 11-29.

Figure 11-29

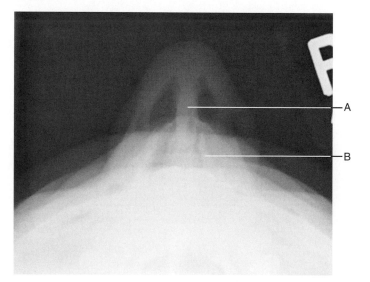

A. _____

B. _____

128. Complete the statements below referring to tangential nasal bones projection analysis criteria.

Tangential Nasal Bones (Superoinferior) Projection Analysis Criteria
• Equal amounts of soft tissue are seen from the nasal bones to the lateral soft tissue on both sides.
• The petrous ridges are seen inferior to the _____ and extend laterally from the posterior maxillary alveolar process.

129. Define *glabelloalveolar* line. _____

_____

130. To obtain a tangential nasal bone projection with accurate positioning, the glabelloalveolar line is aligned

_____ (A) to the IR and the _____ (B) plane is aligned perpendicular to the IR.

131. The petrous ridges are accurately positioned on a tangential nasal bones projection when the _____
is aligned perpendicular to the IR.

132. On a tangential nasal bone projection with accurate positioning, the _____ (A) are centered within the

collimated field. This is accomplished by centering the central ray to the _____ (B).

133. Which anatomic structures are included on a tangential nasal bone projection with accurate positioning?

_____

_____

For the following descriptions of tangential nasal bones projections with poor positioning, state how the patient would have been mispositioned for such an image to be obtained.

134. More soft tissue width is demonstrated from the nasal bones to the lateral soft tissue on right side than on the left side.

_____

135. The posterior nasal bones are superimposed by the glabella.

_____

12 Digestive System

STUDY QUESTIONS

1. How is the patient instructed to dress before upper and lower gastrointestinal examinations?

_____

_____

2. List the patient preparation procedure for the following examinations.

A. Esophagus: _____

_____

B. Stomach: _____

_____

C. Small intestine: _____

_____

_____

D. Large intestine: _____

_____

_____

3. Why are short exposure times needed when imaging the digestive system?

_____

_____

4. Define *peristalsis*, and state how it is recognized on stomach and large and small intestine projections.

_____

_____

_____

_____

5. Complete Exercise 12-1.

EXERCISE 12-1 Digestive System Technical Data				
Projection	**kVp**	**Grid**	**AEC**	**SID**
UPPER GASTROINTESTINAL SYSTEM				
PA oblique (RAO position), esophagus	SC =			
Lateral, esophagus	SC =			
AP or PA, esophagus	SC =			
PA oblique (RAO position), stomach	SC =			
	DC =			
PA, stomach	SC =			
	DC =			
Right lateral, stomach	SC =			
	DC =			
AP oblique (LPO position), stomach	SC =			
	DC =			
AP projection, stomach	SC =			
	DC =			
SMALL INTESTINE				
PA or AP	SC =			
Large intestine				
AP	SC =			
	DC =			
Lateral (rectum)	SC =			
	DC =			
AP or PA (lateral decubitus position)	SC =			
	DC =			
PA oblique (RAO position)	SC =			
	DC =			
PA oblique (LAO position)	SC =			
	DC =			
PA axial or PA axial oblique (RAO position)	SC =			
	DC =			

AEC, Automatic exposure control; *DC*, double contrast; *kVp*, kilovoltage peak; *LPO*, left posterior oblique; *RAO*, right anterior oblique; *SC*, single contrast; *SID*, source–image receptor distance.

6. State the size, shape, and placement in the abdominal cavity of the stomach for the following types of habitus.

   A. Hypersthenic: _____

   _____

   _____

   B. Asthenic: _____

   _____

   _____

   C. Sthenic: _____

   _____

   _____

7. State the position of the lower intestine within the abdominal cavity for the following types of habitus.

   A. Hypersthenic: _____

   _____

   _____

   B. Asthenic: _____

   _____

   _____

   C. Sthenic: _____

   _____

   _____

8. How many posterior ribs are demonstrated superior to the diaphragm dome when an upper or lower gastrointestinal projection is obtained after full expiration, and why is this important?

   _____

   _____

UPPER GASTROINTESTINAL SYSTEM

Esophagram

9. What barium weight or volume suspension is used for esophagus projections? _____

   _____

10. When might the patient be asked to swallow cotton balls soaked in barium, barium-filled gelatin capsules, or barium tablets for an esophagram?

   _____

   _____

Esophagram: Posteroanterior Oblique Projection (Right Anterior Oblique Position)

11. Identify the labeled anatomy in Figure 12-1.

Figure 12-1

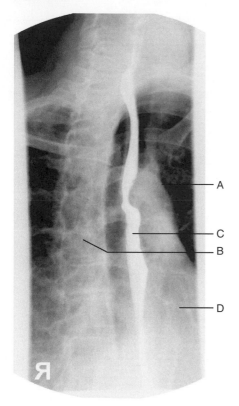

A. _____

B. _____

C. _____

D. _____

12. An adequately rotated PA oblique esophagram projection (RAO position) will demonstrate the esophagus between

the _____ (A) and _____ (B) and approximately _____ inch (C) of the right sternoclavic-

ular end to the left of the vertebrae, and is accomplished by rotating the patient _____ degrees (D).

13. On a PA oblique esophagram projection (RAO position) with accurate positioning, the _____ (A) is
centered within the collimated field. This centering is obtained when a perpendicular central ray is centered 3 inches

to the left of the _____ (B) and _____ inches (C) inferior to the jugular notch.

14. Which anatomic structures are included on a PA oblique esophagram projection (RAO position) with accurate
positioning?

_____

**For the following descriptions of PA oblique esophagram projections (RAO positions) with poor positioning, state
how the patient or central ray would have been mispositioned for such a projection to be obtained.**

15. The superior and inferior ends of the esophagus are not filled with barium.

_____

16. The vertebrae are superimposed over the right sternoclavicular end and a portion of the esophagus.

_____

For the following PA oblique esophagram projections (RAO positions) with poor positioning, state which anatomic structures are misaligned and how the patient should be repositioned for an optimal projection to be obtained.

Figure 12-2

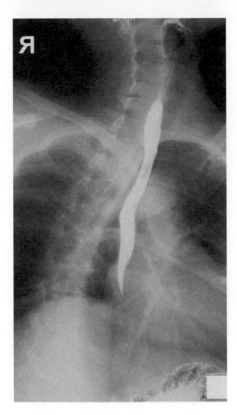

17. Figure 12-2: _____

_____

_____

_____

Figure 12-3

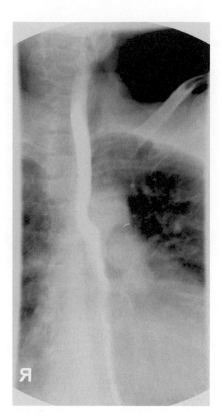

18. Figure 12-3: _____

_____

_____

_____

Esophagram: Lateral Projection

19. Identify the labeled anatomy in Figure 12-4.

Figure 12-4

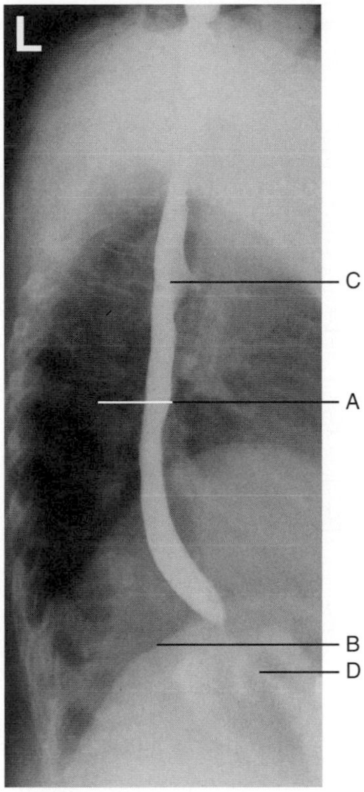

A. _____

B. _____

C. _____

D. _____

20. A lateral projection of the esophagus is obtained when the esophagus is demonstrated anterior to the thoracic vertebrae, the _____ (A) surfaces of each vertebral body are superimposed and no more than _____ (B) inch of space is seen between the _____ (C).

21. How should the patient be positioned to prevent rotation on a lateral esophagram projection?

_____

_____

22. How are the patient's shoulders and humeri positioned to place them away from the esophagus on a lateral projection? _____

_____

_____

23. On a lateral esophagram projection with accurate positioning the _____ (A), at the level of _____ (B), is centered within the collimated field. This centering is obtained when a perpendicular central ray is centered 2 to 3 inches inferior to the _____ (C).

24. Which anatomic structures are included on a lateral esophagram projection with accurate positioning?

_____

_____

For the following description of a lateral esophagram projection with poor positioning, state how the patient or central ray would have been mispositioned for such a projection to be obtained.

25. The posterior ribs demonstrate more than 0.5 inch (1.25 cm) of space between them.

_____

Esophagram: PA Projection

26. Identify the labeled anatomy in Figure 12-5.

Figure 12-5

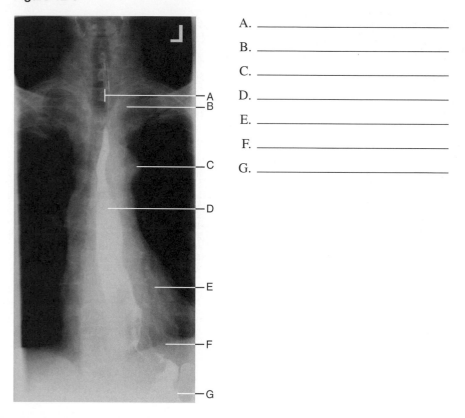

A. _____

B. _____

C. _____

D. _____

E. _____

F. _____

G. _____

27. The distances from the _____ (A) to the _____ (B) are equal, and the vertebrae are superimposed over the esophagus on a nonrotated PA esophagram projection.

28. How is the patient positioned to obtain a nonrotated PA esophagram projection?

_____

_____

29. How should a patient who has had one breast removed be positioned differently?

_____

30. On a PA esophagram projection with accurate positioning the _____ (A), at the level of _____ (B), is centered within the collimated field. This centering is obtained when a perpendicular central ray is centered 2 to 3 inches superior to the _____ (C).

31. Which anatomic structures are included on a lateral esophagram projection with accurate positioning?

_____

For the following description of a PA esophagram projection with poor positioning, state how the patient or central ray would have been mispositioned for such a projection to be obtained.

32. The esophagus is to the right of the vertebrae, and the right sternal clavicular end is demonstrated without vertebral column superimposition.

_____

For the following PA esophagram with poor positioning, state which anatomic structures are misaligned and how the patient should be repositioned for an optimal projection to be obtained.

Figure 12-6

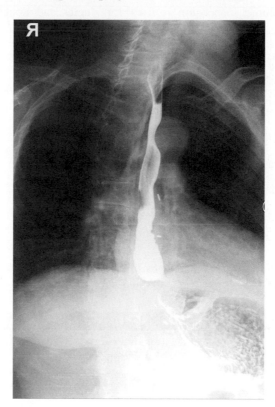

33. Figure 12-6: _____

_____

_____

_____

34. What is the goal of the following upper gastrointestinal studies.

    A. Single contrast: _____

    _____

    B. Double contrast: _____

    _____

35. What barium weight or volume suspension is used for single- and double-contrast upper gastrointestinal projections?

    A. Single contrast: _____

    B. Double contrast: _____

36. The negative contrast used in a double-contrast study is mostly commonly _____ (A)

    and is used to provide _____ (B).

37. The barium in a double-contrast study provides the thin coating that covers the (A) _____.

    How is adequate barium coating of the stomach and duodenum achieved? _____

    _____

    _____

38. List the stomach and duodenum structures that are barium-filled and air-filled for a double-contrast study when the patient is placed in the following positions by completing Exercise 12-2.

EXERCISE 12-2 Double-Contrast Filling of Upper Gastrointestinal System		
Stomach	**Barium-Filled Structures**	**Air-Filled Structures**
PA oblique projection (RAO position)		
PA projection		
Right lateral projection		
AP oblique projection (LPO position)		
AP projection		

LPO, Left posterior oblique; *RAO*, right anterior oblique.

39. The quality of the mucosal coating depends on:

    A. _____

    B. _____

    C. _____

    D. _____

Stomach and Duodenum: Posteroanterior Oblique Projection (Right Anterior Oblique Position)

40. Identify the labeled anatomy in Figure 12-7.

Figure 12-7

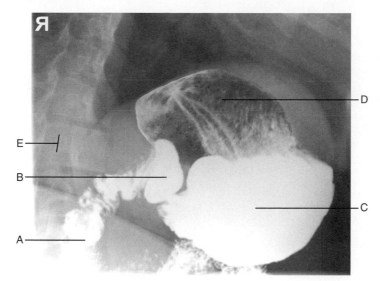

A. _____

B. _____

C. _____

D. _____

E. _____

41. Identify which body type is being represented in the PA oblique stomach and duodenal projections (RAO positions) indicated below, and state the degree of patient obliquity required to obtain the projection.

A. Figure 12-7: _____

Figure 12-8

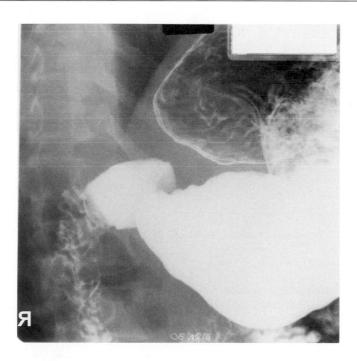

B. Figure 12-8: _____

Figure 12-9

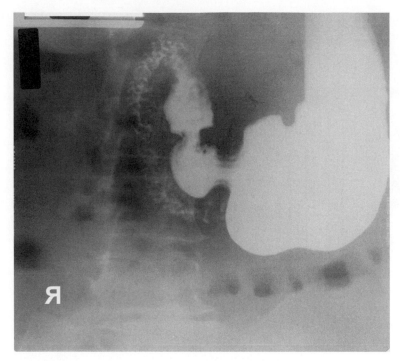

C. Figure 12-9: _____

42. An adequately rotated hypersthenic PA oblique stomach and duodenal projection (RAO position) will demonstrate the left zygapophyseal joints in the _____ (A) of the vertebral body, the duodenal bulb and _____ (B) duodenum in profile, and the long axis of the stomach demonstrating foreshortening with a _____ (C) lesser curvature.

43. An adequately rotated sthenic PA oblique stomach and duodenal projection (RAO position) demonstrates the left zygapophyseal joints at the _____ (A) of the vertebral body, the duodenal bulb and _____ (B) duodenum in profile, and the long axis of the stomach demonstrating partial foreshortening with a partially closed _____ (C).

44. An adequately rotated asthenic PA oblique stomach and duodenal projection (RAO position) demonstrates the left zygapophyseal joints in the _____ (A) of the vertebral bodies, the duodenal bulb and _____ (B) duodenum in profile, and the long axis of the stomach demonstrated without foreshortening; the _____ (C) is open.

45. Explain why it is necessary to rotate the patient differing amounts for a PA oblique stomach and duodenal projection (RAO position) to demonstrate the duodenal bulb and descending duodenum in profile.

_____

_____

46. On a PA oblique stomach and duodenal projection (RAO position) with accurate positioning, the _____ (A) is centered within the collimated field. This centering is obtained on the sthenic patient when a perpendicular central ray is centered halfway between the _____ (B) and _____ (C) of the elevated side, at a level 1 to 2 inches (2.5 to 5 cm) _____ (D) to the inferior rib margin.

47. State how the central ray position is adjusted from the sthenic patient for a PA oblique stomach and duodenal projection (RAO position) for the following habitus.

A. Hypersthenic: _____

_____

B. Asthenic: _____

_____

48. Which anatomic structures are included on a PA oblique stomach and duodenal projection (RAO position) with accurate positioning?

_____

Stomach and Duodenum: Posteroanterior Projection

49. Identify the labeled anatomy in Figure 12-10.

Figure 12-10

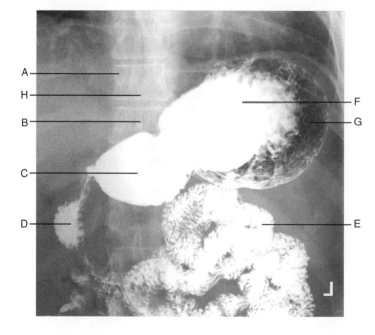

A. _____

B. _____

C. _____

D. _____

E. _____

F. _____

G. _____

H. _____

50. Identify which body type is being represented in the following PA stomach and duodenal projections.

A. Figure 12-10: _____

Figure 12-11

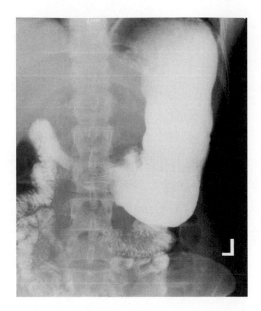

B. Figure 12-11: _____

Figure 12-12

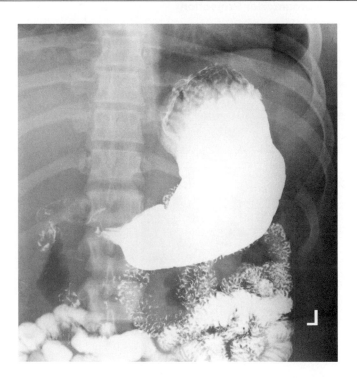

C. Figure 12-12: _____

51. An optimal PA stomach and duodenal projection has been obtained when the spinous processes are aligned with the _____ (A) of the vertebral bodies and the distances from the pedicles to the _____ (B) are equal on both sides.

52. A hypersthenic PA stomach and duodenal projection will demonstrate the stomach aligned almost _____ (A) with the duodenal bulb at the level of the _____ (B) thoracic vertebrae. The lesser and greater curvatures are demonstrated almost on end, with the greater curvature being more _____ (C) situated and the _____ (D) almost on end.

53. A sthenic PA stomach and duodenal projection will demonstrate the stomach aligned almost _____ (A), with the duodenal bulb at the level of the _____ (B) lumbar vertebrae. The lesser and greater curvature, esophagogastric junction, pylorus, and duodenal bulb are in _____ (C).

54. An asthenic PA stomach and duodenal projection will demonstrate the stomach aligned _____ (A), with the duodenal bulb at the level of the _____ lumbar vertebrae (B). The stomach is _____ -shaped (C), and its long axis is demonstrated without foreshortening; the _____, _____, _____, and _____ (D) are in profile.

55. On a PA stomach and duodenal projection with accurate positioning, the _____ (A) is centered within the collimated field. For the sthenic patient, this centering is obtained when a perpendicular central ray is centered halfway between the _____ (B) and _____ (C) at a point approximately 1 to 2 inches (2.5 to 5 cm) _____ (D) to the lower rib margin.

56. State how the central ray position is adjusted from the sthenic patient for a PA stomach and duodenal projection for the following types of habitus.

A. Hypersthenic: _____

_____

B. Asthenic: _____

_____

57. Which anatomic structures are included on a PA stomach and duodenal projection with accurate positioning?

_____

For the following descriptions of PA stomach and duodenal projections with poor positioning, state how the patient or central ray would have been mispositioned for such a projection to be obtained.

58. The stomach demonstrates a blotchy appearance within the barium. The stomach contains residual food particles.

_____

59. The distance from the right pedicles to the spinous processes is greater than the distance from the left pedicles to the spinous processes.

_____

Stomach and Duodenum: Lateral Projection (Right Lateral Position)

60. Identify the labeled anatomy in Figure 12-13.

Figure 12-13

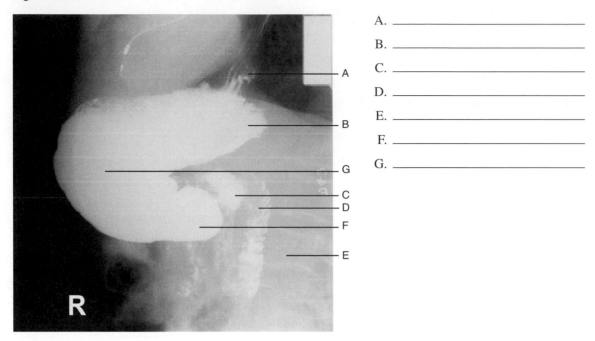

A. _____

B. _____

C. _____

D. _____

E. _____

F. _____

G. _____

61. Identify which body type is being represented in the lateral stomach and duodenal projections indicated below.

A. Figure 12-13: _____

Figure 12-14

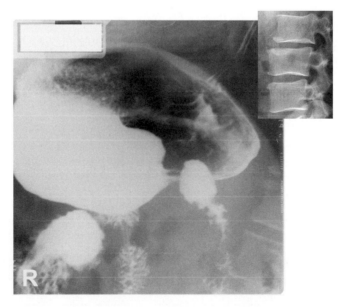

B. Figure 12-14: _____

Figure 12-15

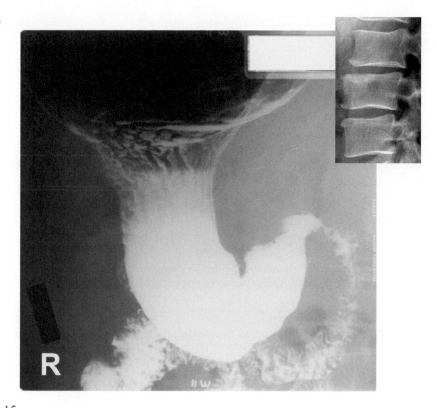

C. Figure 12-15: _____

62. An optimal right lateral stomach and duodenal projection has been obtained when the _____ (A) surfaces of the thoracic and lumbar vertebrae are superimposed and the _____ (B) space is demonstrated.

63. A hypersthenic lateral stomach and duodenal projection demonstrates the _____ (A) and _____ (B) in profile, and the long axis of the stomach demonstrates foreshortening with a _____ (C) lesser curvature.

64. A sthenic lateral stomach and duodenal projection demonstrates the _____ (A) and _____ (B) in profile, and the long axis of the stomach is _____ (C) foreshortened, with a _____ (D) lesser curvature.

65. An asthenic lateral stomach and duodenal projection demonstrates the _____ (A) and _____ (B) in profile, and the long axis of the stomach is demonstrated _____ (C) foreshortening, with an _____ (D) lesser curvature.

66. On a lateral stomach and duodenal projection with accurate positioning, the _____ (A) is centered within the collimated field. For the sthenic patient, this centering is obtained when a perpendicular central ray is centered halfway between the _____ (B) and _____ (C) at the level of the _____ (D).

67. State how the central ray position is adjusted from the sthenic patient for a lateral stomach and duodenal projection for the following habitus.

A. Hypersthenic: _____

_____

B. Asthenic: _____

_____

68. Which anatomic structures are included on a lateral stomach and duodenal projection with accurate positioning?

_____

For the following description of a lateral stomach and duodenal projection with poor positioning, state how the patient or central ray would have been mispositioned for such a projection to be obtained.

69. The descending duodenum is partially superimposed over the duodenal bulb and vertebrae, and the posterior surfaces of the thoracic and lumbar vertebrae are not superimposed.

_____

Stomach and Duodenum: Anteroposterior Oblique Projection (Left Posterior Oblique Position)

70. Identify the labeled anatomy in Figure 12-16.

Figure 12-16

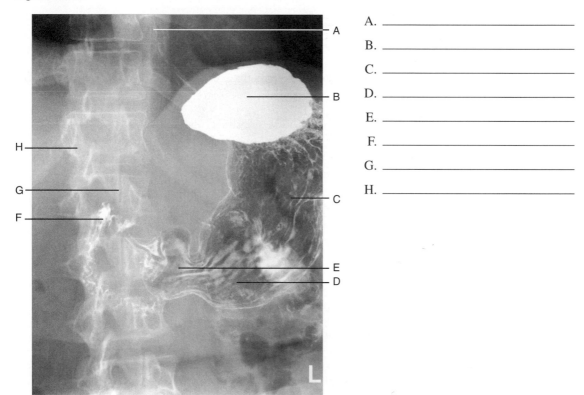

A. _____

B. _____

C. _____

D. _____

E. _____

F. _____

G. _____

H. _____

71. Identify which body type is being represented in the following AP oblique stomach and duodenal projections (LPO positions), and state the degree of patient obliquity required to obtain the projection.

A. Figure 12-16: _____

Figure 12-17

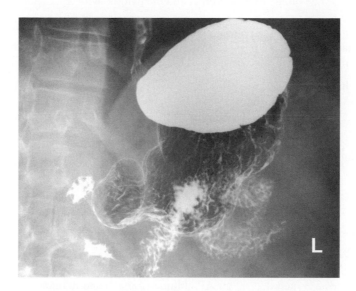

B. Figure 12-17: _____

Figure 12-18

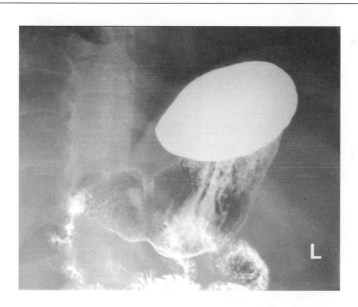

C. Figure 12-18: _____

72. An adequately rotated hypersthenic AP oblique stomach and duodenal projection (LPO position) will demonstrate the left zygapophyseal joints in the _____ (A) of the vertebral body, the duodenal bulb and _____ (B) duodenum in profile, and the pylorus superimposed over the _____ (C).

73. An adequately rotated sthenic AP oblique stomach and duodenal projection (LPO position) demonstrates the left zygapophyseal joints at the _____ (A) of the vertebral body, the duodenal bulb and _____ (B) duodenum in profile, and the pylorus with _____ (C) vertebral superimposition.

74. An adequately rotated asthenic AP oblique stomach and duodenal projection (LPO position) demonstrates the left zygapophyseal joints in the _____ (A) of the vertebral bodies, the duodenal bulb and _____ (B) duodenum in profile, and the pylorus with _____ (C) vertebral superimposition.

75. On an AP oblique stomach and duodenal projection (LPO position) with accurate positioning, the _____ (A) is centered within the collimated field. This centering is obtained on the sthenic patient when a perpendicular central ray is centered halfway between the _____ (B) and _____ (C), at a level _____ (D) between the xiphoid process and inferior rib margin.

76. State how the central ray position is adjusted from the sthenic patient for an AP oblique stomach and duodenal projection (LPO position) for the following type of habitus.

A. Hypersthenic: _____

_____

B. Asthenic: _____

_____

77. Which anatomic structures are included on an AP oblique stomach and duodenal projection (LPO position) with accurate positioning?

_____

Stomach and Duodenum: Anteroposterior Projection

78. Identify the labeled anatomy in Figure 12-19.

Figure 12-19

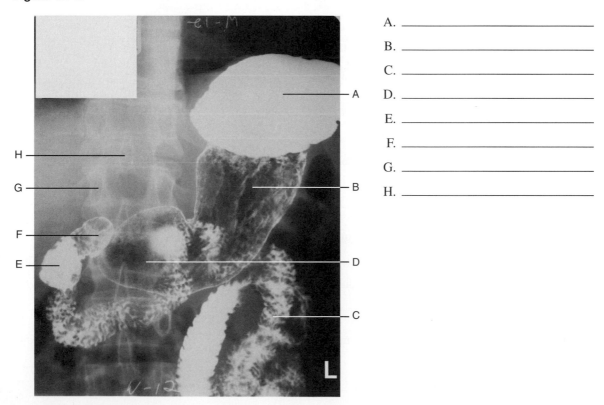

A. _____

B. _____

C. _____

D. _____

E. _____

F. _____

G. _____

H. _____

79. Identify which body type is being represented in the following AP stomach and duodenal projections.

A. Figure 12-19: _____

Figure 12-20

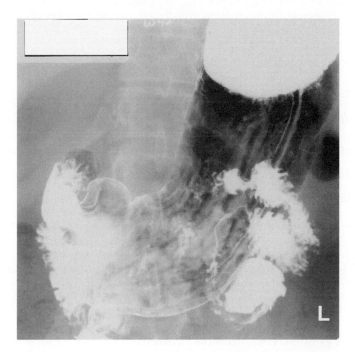

B. Figure 12-20: _____

Figure 12-21

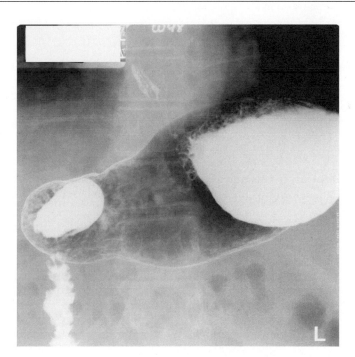

C. Figure 12-21: _____

80. An optimal AP stomach and duodenal projection has been obtained when the spinous processes are aligned with the

_____ (A) of the vertebral bodies and the distances from the pedicles to the _____ (B) are equal on each side.

81. A hypersthenic AP stomach and duodenal projection will demonstrate the stomach aligned almost _____ (A) with the duodenal bulb at the level of the _____ (B) thoracic vertebrae. The lesser and greater curvatures are demonstrated almost on end, with the greater curvature being more _____ (C) situated and the _____ (D) almost on end.

82. A sthenic AP stomach and duodenal projection will demonstrate the stomach aligned almost _____ (A), with the duodenal bulb at the level of the _____ (B) lumbar vertebrae. The lesser and greater curvature, esophagogastric junction, pylorus, and duodenal bulb are in _____ (C).

83. An asthenic AP stomach and duodenal projection will demonstrate the stomach aligned _____ (A) with the duodenal bulb at the level of the _____ (B) lumbar vertebrae. The stomach is _____ -shaped (C), and its long axis is demonstrated without foreshortening; the _____, _____, _____, and _____ (D) are in profile.

84. On an AP stomach and duodenal projection with accurate positioning, the _____ (A) is centered within the collimated field. For the sthenic patient, this centering is obtained when a perpendicular central ray is centered halfway between the _____ (B) and _____ (C) at a level _____ (D) between the xiphoid process and inferior rib margin.

85. State how the central ray position is adjusted from the sthenic patient for an AP stomach and duodenal projection for the following habitus.

    A. Hypersthenic: _____

    _____

    B. Asthenic: _____

    _____

86. Which anatomic structures are included on an AP stomach and duodenal projection with accurate positioning?

    _____

For the following description of an AP stomach and duodenal projection with poor positioning, state how the patient or central ray would have been mispositioned for such a projection to be obtained.

87. The distance from the left pedicles to the spinous processes is greater than the distance from the right pedicles to the spinous processes.

    _____

    _____

Small Intestine: Posteroanterior Projection

88. Identify the labeled anatomy in Figure 12-22.

Figure 12-22

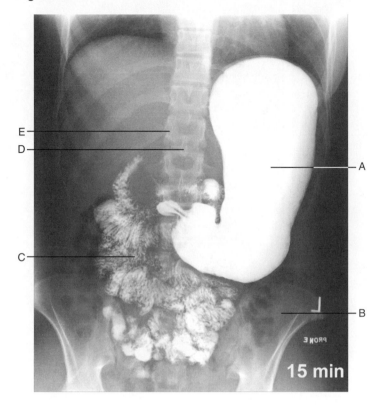

A. _____

B. _____

C. _____

D. _____

E. _____

89. How are PA small intestine projections marked?

_____

_____

90. What is the typical timing sequence for a small intestine series?

_____

91. A nonrotated PA small intestine projection demonstrates the spinous processes aligned with the _____
    (A) and symmetrical _____ (B).

92. Why is the prone position chosen over the supine position for the small intestine series?

_____

93. Compare Figures 12-23 and 12-24. State which projection was taken earlier in the series, and explain how you know this.

Figure 12-23

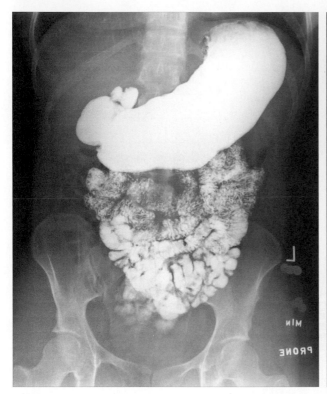

Figure 12-24

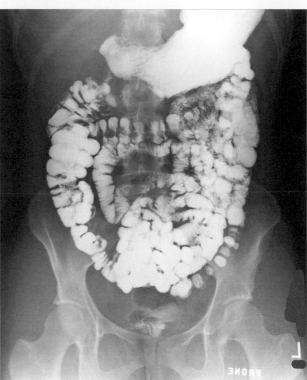

_____

_____

_____

_____

94. Figure 12-25 demonstrates the last projection that was taken in a small bowel series. Based on this projection, should the patient wait longer and have another projection obtained? Why or why not?

Figure 12-25

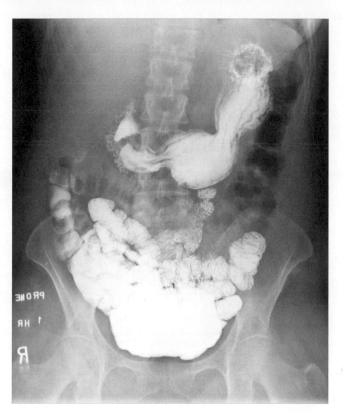

_____

_____

_____

_____

95. On a PA small intestine projection with accurate positioning, the _____ (A) is centered within the

collimated field. Early in the series, a perpendicular central ray is centered to the _____

(B) at a level 2 inches (5 cm) _____ (C) to the iliac crest. Later in the series, the central ray is centered

at the level of the _____ (D).

96. State why the central ray is centered in different locations when a projection is obtained early versus late in the series.

_____

_____

97. Which anatomic structures are included on a PA small intestine projection with accurate positioning? _____

_____

_____

98. Optimal double-contrast coating has been obtained when the lumina are distended, without _____ (A), the mucosal surface demonstrates a thin coating of barium, and barium pooling is limited to _____ (B).

99. What is the purpose of the barium pool? _____

100. State whether air or barium will be within the indicated structure by completing Exercise 12-3 for the positions listed.

EXERCISE 12–3 Double-Contrast Filling of Large Intestinal Structures		
Large Intestine	**AP Projection (Supine Position)**	**PA Projection (Prone Position)**
Cecum		
Ascending colon		
Acending limb right colic (hepatic) flexure		
Descending limb right colic (hepatic) flexure		
Transverse colon		
Ascending limb left colic (splenic) flexure		
Descending limb left colic (splinic) flexure		
Descending colon		
Sigmoid colon		
Rectum		

101. How is poor gaseous distention identified on a large intestine projection?

_____

_____

102. How is poor barium coating identified on a large intestine projection?

_____

_____

Large Intestine: Posteroanterior or Anteroposterior Projection

103. Identify the labeled anatomy in Figure 12-26.

Figure 12-26

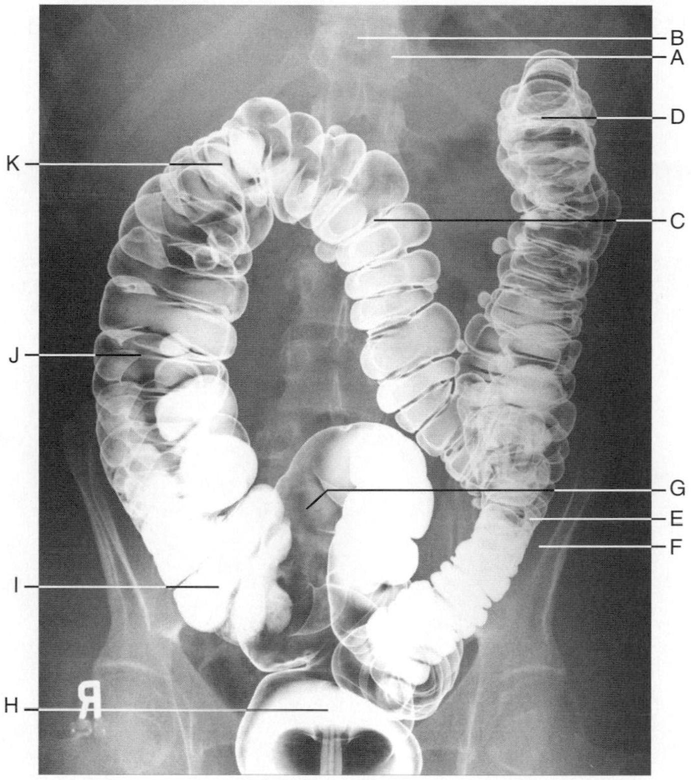

A. _____

B. _____

C. _____

D. _____

E. _____

F. _____

G. _____

H. _____

I. _____

J. _____

K. _____

104. A nonrotated PA or AP large intestine projection is demonstrated when the spinous processes are aligned with the

_____ (A) of the vertebral bodies, the distance from the pedicles to the _____ (B)

is the same on both sides, and the iliac ala arc _____ (C). The ascending and descending limbs

of the _____ (D) demonstrate some degree of superimposition.

105. To obtain a nonrotated PA or AP large intestine projection the _____ (A) and _____ (B) are
positioned at equal distances from the imaging table.

106. The side demonstrating the greater distance from the pedicles to the spinous processes, wider iliac ala, and colic
flexure with the greater ascending and descending limb superimposition is the side positioned _____
from the IR on a rotated PA large intestine projection.

107. The iliac ala on an AP large intestine projection are _____ (wider/narrower) than on a PA projection.

108. On an AP or PA large intestine projection with accurate positioning, the _____ (A)
is centered within the collimated field. This centering is obtained by centering a perpendicular central ray with the

patient's _____ (B) plane at the level of the _____ (C) for a PA large intestine
projection obtained with a 14- × 17-inch lengthwise image receptor (IR).

109. For an AP or PA large intestine projection obtained on a hypersthenic patient when two 14- × 17-inch IRs are used,

the first projection is obtained with the central ray centered to the _____ (A) at a level

halfway between the _____ (B) and _____ (C) for the lower projection.

110. Which anatomic structures are included on an AP or PA large intestine projection with accurate positioning?

_____

_____

111. Compare the projections in Figures 12-27 and 12-28. State the projection used to obtain each projection, and explain how you know this.

Figure 12-27   **Figure 12-28**

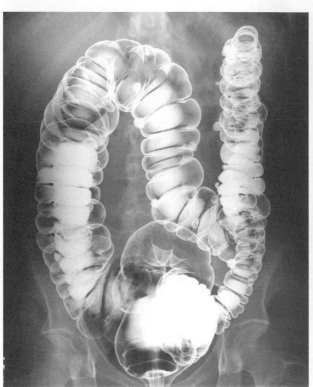   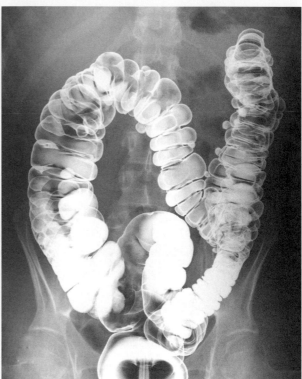

_____

_____

_____

_____

For the following descriptions of AP or PA large intestine projections with poor positioning, state how the patient or central ray would have been mispositioned for such a projection to be obtained.

112. AP projection: The right iliac ala is narrow and the left wide, the distance from the right pedicles to the spinous processes is narrower than the same distance on the left side, and the left colic (splenic) flexure demonstrates greater ascending and descending limb superimposition.

_____

113. PA projection: The left colic (splenic) flexure and part of the transverse colon are not included on the projection.

_____

_____

_____

For the following AP or PA large intestine projections with poor positioning, state which anatomic structures are misaligned and how the patient should be repositioned for an optimal projection to be obtained.

Figure 12-29

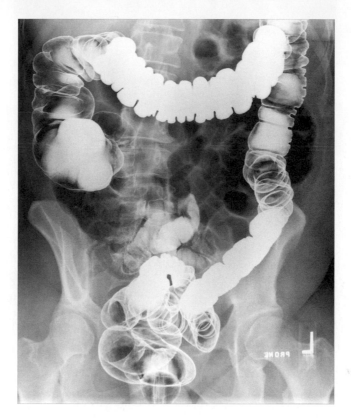

114. Figure 12-29: _____

_____

_____

_____

Figure 12-30

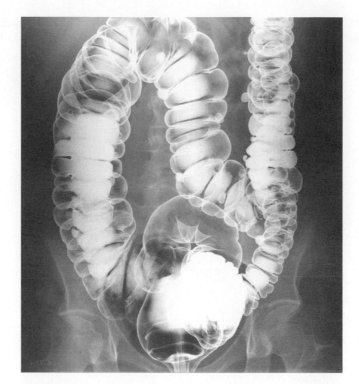

115. Figure 12-30: _____

_____

_____

_____

Large Intestine (Rectum; Lateral Projection)

116. Identify the labeled anatomy in Figure 12-31.

Figure 12-31

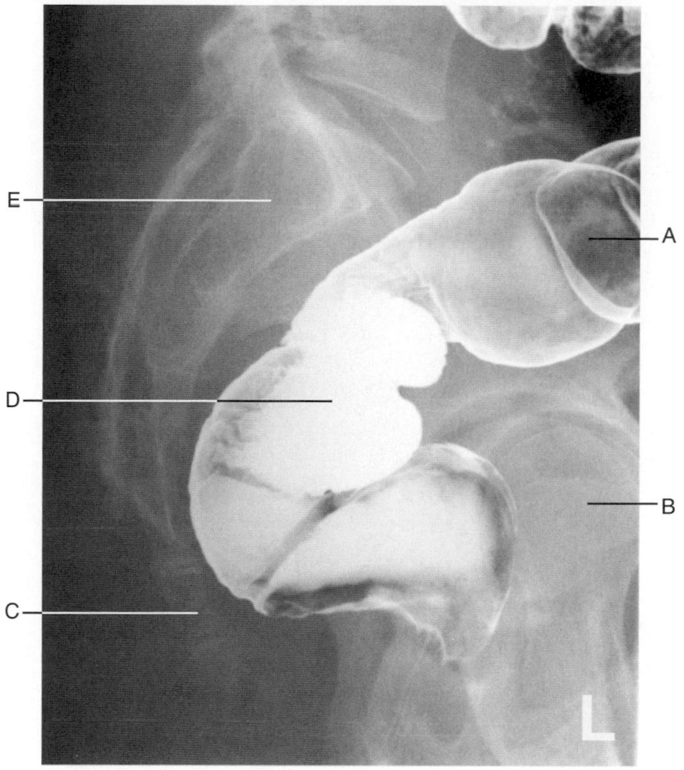

A. _____

B. _____

C. _____

D. _____

E. _____

117. How is scatter radiation controlled for a lateral large intestine (rectum) projection?

_____

118. A lateral rectum projection with accurate positioning is demonstrated when the sacral medium sacral crest is in

_____ (A) and the _____ (B) are superimposed.

119. On a lateral rectum projection with accurate positioning, the _____ (A) is centered within the collimated field. This centering is obtained by centering a perpendicular central ray with the patient's

_____ (B) plane at the level of the _____ (C).

120. Which anatomic structures are included on a lateral rectum projection with accurate positioning? _____

_____

For the following description of a lateral rectum projection with poor positioning, state how the patient or central ray would have been mispositioned for such a projection to be obtained.

121. The femoral heads are not superimposed; the right femoral head is rotated anterior to the left femoral head.

_____

For the following lateral rectum projections with poor positioning, state which anatomic structures are misaligned and how the patient should be repositioned for an optimal projection to be obtained.

Figure 12-32

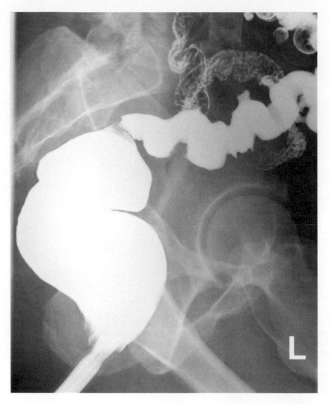

122. Figure 12-32:_____

_____

_____

_____

Figure 12-33

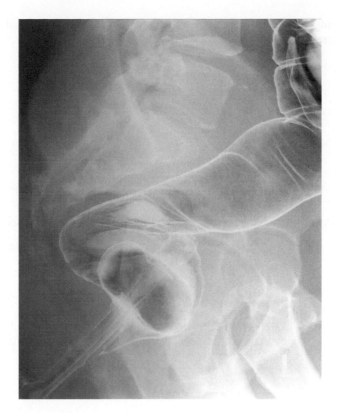

123. Figure 12-33: _____

_____

_____

_____

Large Intestine: Anteroposterior or Posteroanterior Projection (Lateral Decubitus Position)
124. Identify the labeled anatomy in Figure 12-34.

Figure 12-34

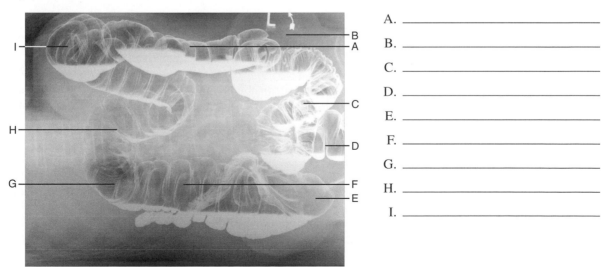

A. _____

B. _____

C. _____

D. _____

E. _____

F. _____

G. _____

H. _____

I. _____

125. How is uniform density obtained across the abdomen when imaging a patient with excessive abdominal soft tissue that drops toward the imaging table for an AP or PA large intestine projection (lateral decubitus position)?

_____

_____

_____

126. A nonrotated AP projection (lateral decubitus) is obtained when the spinous processes are aligned with the midline of

the_____(A), the distances from the pedicles to the_____

(B) are the same on both sides, and the _____ (C) are symmetrical.

127. The side demonstrating the smaller distance from the pedicles to the spinous processes, narrower iliac ala, and colic

flexure with less ascending and descending limb superimposition is the side positioned _____ from the
IR on a rotated AP decubitus large intestine projection.

128. The iliac ala on a PA large intestine projection (lateral decubitus) are _____ (wider/narrower) than on
an AP projection (lateral decubitus).

129. Why is the patient elevated on a radiolucent sponge or hard surface for a decubitus large intestine projection?

_____

_____

130. The _____ (A) is centered within the collimated field for a PA/AP large intestine
projection (lateral decubitus). This centering is obtained by centering a perpendicular central ray with the patient's

_____ (B) plane at the level of the _____ (C).

131. For a PA-AP large intestine projection (lateral decubitus) of a hypersthenic patient in which two 14- × 17-inch IRs

are used, the first projection is obtained with the central ray centered to the _____ (A) plane at a level

halfway between the _____ (B) and _____ (C) for the lower projection.

132. Which anatomic structures are included on a PA-AP large intestine projection (lateral decubitus) with accurate positioning?

_____

_____

For the following descriptions of AP or PA large intestine projections (lateral decubitus position) with poor positioning, state how the patient or central ray would have been mispositioned for such a projection to be obtained.

133. Artifact lines are superimposing over the left lateral abdomen region.

_____

134. AP projection: The distances from the right pedicles to the spinous processes are less than the distances from the left pedicles to the spinous processes, the right iliac ala is narrower than the left, and the ascending and descending limbs of the left colic (splenic) flexure demonstrate increased superimposition.

_____

For the following AP-PA large intestine projections (lateral decubitus position) with poor positioning, state which anatomic structures are misaligned and how the patient should be repositioned for an optimal projection to be obtained.

Figure 12-35

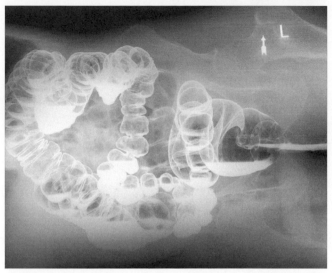

135. Figure 12-35 (AP projection): _____

_____

_____

_____

Figure 12-36

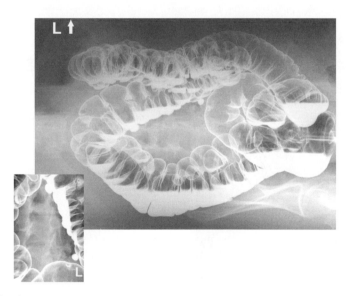

136. Figure 12-36 (AP projection): _____

_____

_____

_____

Figure 12-37

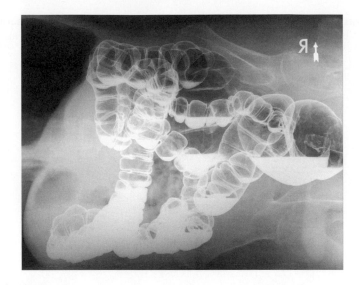

137. Figure 12-37 (PA projection): _____

_____

_____

_____

Large Intestine: Posteroanterior Oblique Projection (Right Anterior Oblique Position)

138. Identify the labeled anatomy in Figure 12-38.

Figure 12-38

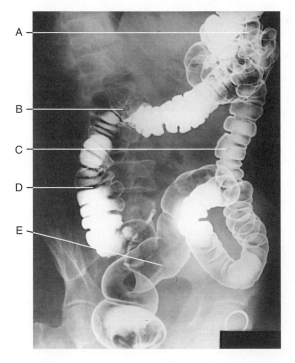

A. _____

B. _____

C. _____

D. _____

E. _____

139. A PA oblique large intestine projection (RAO position) with accurate positioning demonstrates decreased ascending and descending limb superimposition of the _____ (A) when compared with the PA projection, whereas the limbs of the _____ (B) demonstrate increased superimposition. The _____ (right/left) (C) iliac ala is narrower than the opposite ala.

140. To obtain an accurate PA oblique large intestine projection (RAO position), position the midcoronal plane _____ (A) degrees with the IR. Rotating the patient toward the right side moves the _____ (ascending/descending) (B) right colic (hepatic) flexure from beneath the _____ (ascending/descending) (C) right colic flexure and the distal sigmoid from beneath the _____ (D).

141. On a PA oblique large intestine projection (RAO position) with accurate positioning, the _____ (A) is centered within the collimated field. This centering is obtained by centering a perpendicular central ray approximately 1 to 2 inches (2.5 to 5 cm) to the _____ (right/left) (B) of the midsagittal plane at the level of the _____ (C).

142. Which anatomic structures are included on a PA oblique large intestine projection (RAO position) with accurate positioning?

_____

For the following description of a PA oblique large intestine projection (RAO position) with poor positioning, state how the patient or central ray would have been mispositioned for such a projection to be obtained.

143. The ascending and descending limbs of the right colic (hepatic) flexure and the rectum and distal sigmoid, respectively, demonstrate increased superimposition. The iliac ala are uniform in width.

_____

Large Intestine: Posteroanterior Oblique Projection (Left Anterior Oblique Position)
144. Identify the labeled anatomy in Figure 12-39.

Figure 12-39

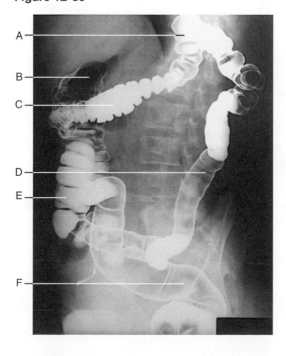

A. _____

B. _____

C. _____

D. _____

E. _____

F. _____

145. The ascending and descending limbs of the _____ (right/left) (A) colic flexure are demonstrated with decreased superimposition when compared with the PA projection and the _____ (right/left) (B) iliac ala is narrower on a PA oblique large intestine projection with accurate positioning.

146. To obtain an accurate PA oblique large intestine projection (LAO position), position the midcoronal plane _____ degrees (A) with the IR. Rotating the patient toward the left side moves the _____ (ascending/descending) (B) left colic (hepatic) flexure from beneath the _____ (ascending/descending) (C) left colic flexure.

147. On a PA oblique large intestine projection (LAO position) with accurate positioning, the _____ (A) is centered within the collimated field. This centering is obtained by centering a perpendicular central ray approximately 1 to 2 inches (2.5 to 5 cm) to the _____ (right/left) (B) of the midsagittal plane at the level 1 to 2 inches (2.5 to 5 cm) superior to the _____ (C).

148. Which anatomic structures are included on a PA oblique large intestine projection (LAO position) with accurate positioning?

_____

Large Intestine: Posteroanterior Axial and Posteroanterior Axial Oblique (Right Anterior Oblique Position)

149. Identify the labeled anatomy in Figure 12-40.

Figure 12-40

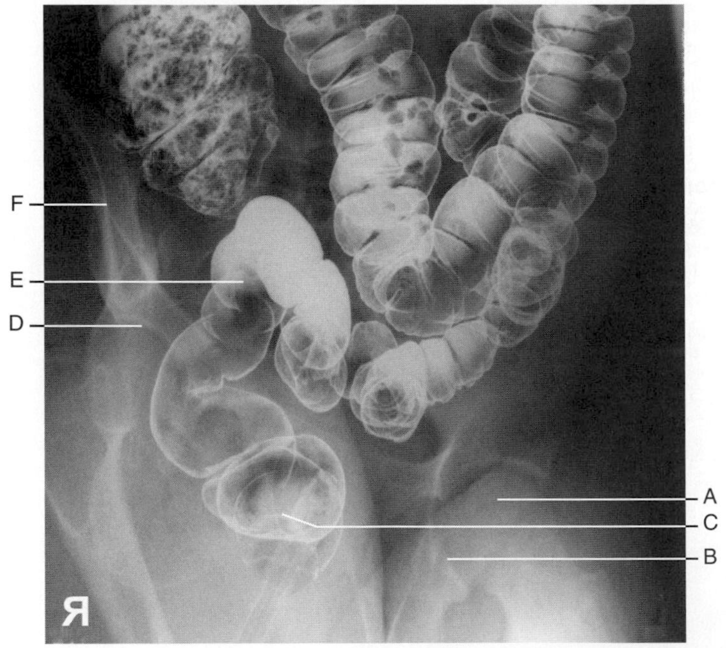

A. _____

B. _____

C. _____

D. _____

E. _____

F. _____

150. _____ (A) are demonstrated without transverse superimposition, the right sacroiliac (SI) joint is shown just _____ (B) to the anterior inferior spine, and the _____ (right/left) (C) obturator foramen is open.

151. To achieve accurate PA axial oblique large intestine positioning (RAO position), the patient is rotated toward the _____ (A) side until the _____ (B) plane is at a 35- to 45-degree angle with the imaging table.

152. A PA axial large intestine projection with accurate positioning demonstrates _____ iliac ala and obturator foramen.

153. The rectosigmoid segment is demonstrated without _____ (A) superimposition, the pelvis demonstrates elongation, and the left inferior acetabulum is at the level of the _____ (B) when the central ray is accurately angled _____ degrees (C) _____ (caudally/cephalically) (D) for a PA axial and PA axial oblique large intestine projection.

154. On PA axial and PA axial oblique (RAO) large intestine projections with accurate positioning, the _____ (A) is centered within the collimated field. This centering is obtained for a PA axial projection by centering to exit at the level of the _____ (B) and midsagittal plane. This centering is obtained for a PA axial oblique projection by centering the central ray to exit at the _____ (C) and 2 inches (5 cm) to the _____ (right/left) (D) of the spinous processes.

155. Which anatomic structures are included on a PA axial and PA axial oblique large intestine projection with accurate positioning?

_____

For the following descriptions of PA axial oblique large intestine projections (RAO positions) with poor positioning, state how the patient or central ray would have been mispositioned for such a projection to be obtained.

156. The right SI joint is obscured, and the left obturator foramen is closed.

_____

157. The inferior aspect of the left acetabulum is demonstrated superior to the distal rectum.

_____

For the following PA axial oblique large intestine projections (RAO positions) with poor positioning, state which anatomic structures are misaligned and how the patient should be repositioned for an optimal projection to be obtained.

Figure 12-41

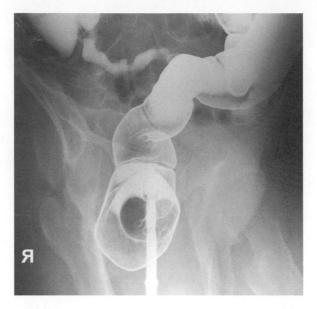

158. Figure 12-41: _____

_____

_____

_____

Figure 12-42

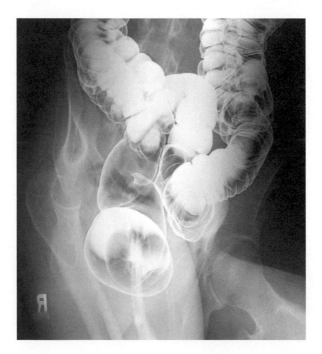

159. Figure 12-42: _____

_____

_____

_____

Study Question Answers

CHAPTER 1   IMAGE ANALYSIS GUIDELINES

1. A. Demographic information (patient and facility name, time, date)
   B. Correct markers in the appropriate position without superimposing anatomy of interest
   C. Desired anatomic structures in accurate alignment with each other
   D. Maximum geometric integrity
   E. Appropriate radiation protection
   F. Best possible density, contrast, and gray scale with minimal noise
   G. No preventable artifacts.
2. A. Midcoronal
   B. Anterior
   C. Posterior
   D. Superior
   E. Inferior
   F. Anterosuperior
   G. Posteroinferior
3. Anterolateral
4. Posteromedial
5. Anterosuperior
6. Mediolateral
7. A. Midsagittal
   B. Lateral
   C. Medial
   D. Inferolateral
   E. Superolateral
8. A. Proximal
   B. Distal

9.

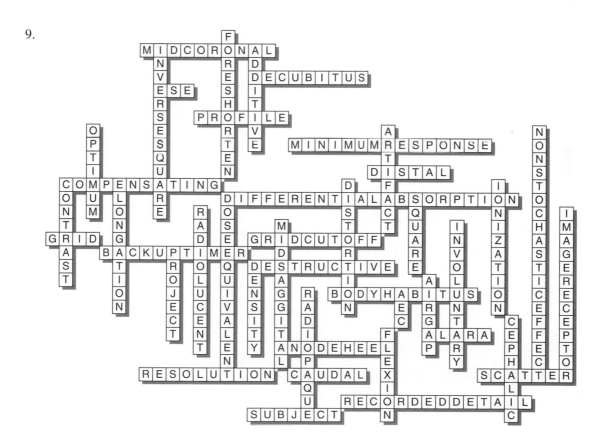

10. A. Source-object distance
    B. Object–image receptor distance
    C. Source–image receptor distance
11. A. 1 and 3
    B. 2
    C. 1
    D. 1 and 3
    E. 4
    F. 4
    G. 1 and 5
    H. 1 and 5
    I. 1 and 5
    J. 1 and 5
    K. 6
    L. 1
    M. 1
12. A. The knee image is accurately displayed. The marker is correct and it is accurately displayed as if hanging from the patient's hip.
    B. The marker is reversed, indicating that the image needs to be flipped horizontally. The image is accurately displayed by the fingertip.
    C. The marker is reversed, indicating that the image needs to be flipped horizontally. The image is accurately displayed, as if the patient were in an upright position.
    D. Forearm images should be displayed as if hanging by the fingertips and not the elbow. The image is horizontally displayed correctly, as indicated by the correctness of the marker.
    E. Lateral feet projections should be displayed as if hanging from the patient's hip. The image should be moved 90 degrees counterclockwise. The marker is also reversed and should be correct for a lateral foot projection. Flip the image horizontally.
    F. The marker is reversed and should be correct for AP oblique projections. The image should be flipped horizontally, with the left marker positioned on the viewer's right side. The image is accurately displayed as if the patient were in an upright position.
13. Left
14. A. Facility's name
    B. Patient's name
    C. Patient's age or birth date
    D. Hospital identification number
    E. Date of examination
    F. Time of examination
15. A. Place it outside the collimated field whenever possible.
    B. Position it away from the direction in which the central ray is angled.
    C. Position it next to the narrowest anatomic structure.
16. A. Right
    B. Laterally, adjacent to the patient's right side
17. A. Right
    B. Anteriorly

18. A. The marker is situated too medially, superimposing anatomic structures of interest. It should remain within the collimated field but be moved as far laterally as possible.
    B. The marker is situated at the midsagittal plane. It should be placed on the left side of the vertebral column as far laterally as possible while staying within the collimated field.
    C. The marker is superimposed on the shoulder anatomy of interest. Move the marker as far laterally as possible while staying within the collimated field.
    D. The marker is placed to the right of the vertebral column. It should be placed on the left side of the vertebral column as far laterally as possible while staying within the collimated field.
    E. The marker is only partially demonstrated. Move the marker completely within the collimated field.
19. A. Lead
    B. Radiopaque
20. Closer to
21.

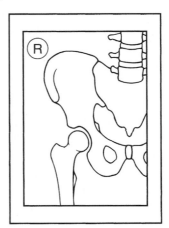

22.

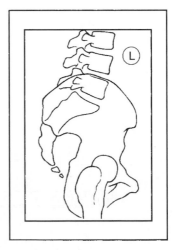

23. Mark the side that is positioned closer to the IR, and place a face-up marker laterally, adjacent to that side.

24. Circle the marker and restate the information that it displays next to it for hard copy images, or add a marker next to the original during postprocessing for digital systems.

25. A. 4
    B. 1
    C. 1
    D. 1
    E. 4
    F. 3
    G. 1
    H. 4
    I. 1
    J. 4

26. A. Hyposthenic
    B. Hypersthenic
    C. Hypersthenic
    D. Hyposthenic

27. Needed to prevent the off-centered joint(s) from being projected off the IR; they will move in the direction that the diverged x-ray beams used to record them on the image are moving.

28. The ankle joint has been projected off the IR, whereas more of the distal femur is included than needed. The lower leg was not centered correctly on the IR. Palpate the joints to determine accurate centering.

29. The IR is too small to accommodate both hand images and the two images are overlapping in the center. Choose a larger IR and position the images evenly on each side of the IR with an unexposed space between them, or put both images on separate image receptors.

30. A. Decrease
    B. Increase
    C. Scatter radiation

31. Make an imaginary X diagonally connecting the corners of the collimated field. The center of the X indicates where the central ray was centered. The central ray was centered to the T9-10 intervertebral disk space.

32. A. Larger
    B. The x-ray beams continue to diverge as they move through the patient to the IR.

33. A. Too much of the patient's abdominal structures have been included and the lateral collimation borders are not within 0.5 inch (1.25 cm) of the skin line. The superior aspect of the chest is not included. The central ray is centered too inferiorly to collimate tightly.
    B. The posterior and superior collimation borders are within 0.5 inch (1.25 cm) of the skin line, but the anterior and inferior borders are too wide. The central ray is centered too anteroinferiorly to be collimated tightly.
    C. The central ray was centered anterior to the foot instead of on the tarsal bones and the foot was aligned diagonally instead of with the long axis of the exposure field, preventing the collimation borders from being within 0.5 inch (1.25 cm) from the skin line.

D. The central ray was centered to the upper cervical vertebrae region instead of to the center of the skull, preventing the shoulder and cervical vertebrae from being collimated off the image, and the collimation borders are not within 0.5 inch (1.25 cm) of the skull skin line.

34. The marker should be placed on the IR so that it is 2 inches (5 cm) from the lateral edge of the cassette and 1 inch (2.5 cm) from the bottom edge of the IR.

35. A. A
    B. B
    C. The clavicular image A demonstrates grid cutoff, which occurs when the central ray and grid are not properly aligned.

36. Use palpable anatomic structures located around the area of interest.

37. A. It would superimpose it.
    B. (1) Proximal
       (2) No
       (3) Because letter A is farther from the IR, it will be projected farther proximally than letter B.
    C. (1) Distally
       (2) Letter A would be projected even more distally.
    D. Possibly superimposed over it or positioned only slightly distal or proximal to it, depending on the SID used. The placement would vary depending on the SID, because the angle used to record A and B could be perpendicular or proximal if a short SID were used and caudal if a long SIS were used.

38. A.

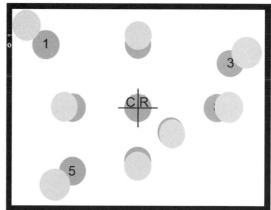

B.

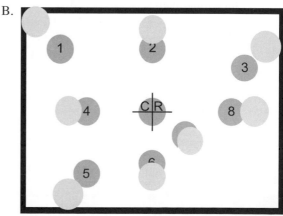

39. A. The SC joints would be projected to the right of the vertebral column.
    B. The SC joints are currently at the level of the third thoracic vertebra. The 10-degree cephalic angle would project the SC joints superior to this position.
    C. The answers would be the same, although the amount of movement to the right for A and superiorly for B would be less because the x-rays recording the structures would be less diverged.
    D. The answers would be the same, although the amount of movement would be less because the heart shadow is not as far away from the IR as the SC joints.
40. A. Parallel
    B. Perpendicular
41. A. Elongation
    B. Foreshortening
42. Elongation
43. A. Foreshortening
    B. Elongation
    C. Elongation
44. A. Magnification—proportional magnification of proximal, distal, and midshaft of humerus
    B. Foreshortening. The proximal humerus was placed farther from the IR, as demonstrated by the increased magnification of the proximal humerus when compared with the distal humerus.
    C. Elongation. The distal humerus was placed farther from the IR, as demonstrated by the increased magnification of the distal humerus when compared with the proximal humerus.
45. Image 2
46. Image 2
47. Close to
48. A. Increase the OID.
    B. Decrease the SOD or SID.
49. A. Use identifiable structures that surround the identical structures.
    B. Use surrounding bony projections.
    C. Identify expected magnification.
50. A. Adjust the patient half the distance demonstrated between the two structures that should be superimposed.
    B. Adjust the patient the entire distance between the structures that should be superimposed.
51. A. 0
    B. 68
    C. 45
    D. 23
    E. 90
52. A. 45
    B. 45
    C. 30
    D. 105

53.

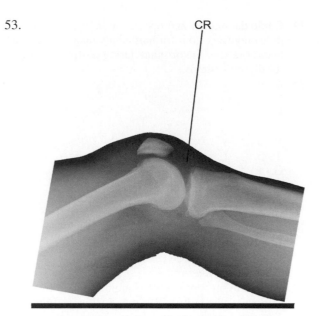

54. A. Fully extend the patient's finger.
    B. Align the central ray parallel with the IP joint or perpendicular to the phalange of interest. For this examination, the central ray would have needed to be angled proximally until it was parallel with the joint of interest.
55. A. Farther from
    B. Closer to
56. A. Internally rotate the hand 0.5 inch (1.25 cm).
    B. Direct the central ray anteriorly to move the second metacarpal toward the fifth metacarpal. Because the physical distance between the second and fifth metacarpals is 2.5 inches (0.6 cm) and a 5-degree angle will move the second metacarpal 0.5 inch (1.25 cm) for this amount of physical separation, and the amount of mispositioning is off by 1 inch (2.5 cm), a 10-degree angle should be placed on the central ray.
57. A. Externally rotate the leg 1 inch (2.5 cm).
    B. Direct the central ray anteriorly to move the medial condyle toward the lateral condyle. Because the physical distance between the condyles is approximately 2.5 inches (6.25 cm), a 5-degree angle will move the medial condyle 0.25 inch (0.6 cm) for this amount of physical separation, and because the condyles are mispositioned by 2 inches (5 cm), a 40-degree angle should be placed on the central ray.
58. A. Internally rotate the leg 0.125 inch (0.3 cm).
    B. Direct the central ray posteriorly to move the medial talar dome toward the lateral dome. Because the physical distance between the talar domes is 1 inch (2.5 cm), a 5-degree angle will move the medial condyle 0.25 inch (0.6 cm) for this amount of physical separation, and because the domes are mispositioned by 0.25 inch (0.6 cm), a 5-degree angle should be placed on the central ray.

59. A. Small
    B. Smaller
60. A. Explain the examination to the patient.
    B. Make the patient comfortable.
    C. Keep the exposure time short.
    D. Use positioning devices.
61. When patient is unable to control the motion
62. Use a short exposure time.
63. Voluntary motion demonstrates blurred gastric patterns and bony cortical outlines, whereas involuntary motion demonstrates blurred gastric patterns and sharp cortical outlines.
64. A. Involuntary
    B. Involuntary
65. A double-exposed image will demonstrate two cortical outlines of each anatomic structure and unexplainable overexposure.
66. A. Double-exposure
    B. Motion
    C. Double-exposure (noticeable at the proximal forearm)
67. Motion will demonstrate blur throughout the radiograph, whereas poor screen-film contact will demonstrate blur only where the film and screen are not in direct contact.
68. Image 2
69. A. When gonads are within 2 inches (5 cm) of the primary x-ray beam.
    B. If the patient is of reproductive age
    C. If the gonadal shield does not cover information of interest
70. Ovaries, uterine tubes, and uterus
71.

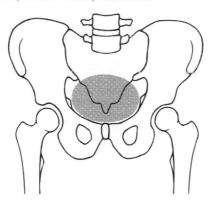

72. Place the narrow end of the shield superior to the palpable symphysis pubis and determine side-to-side centering by placing the shield at equal distances from the anterior superior iliac spines.
73. The shield is placed at a large OID and will greatly magnify, possibly covering needed information.
74. A. Testes within scrotal pouch
    B. Along midsagittal plane, inferior to the symphysis pubis
75. 1 to 1.5 inches (2.5 to 4 cm) inferior to the symphysis pubis

76.

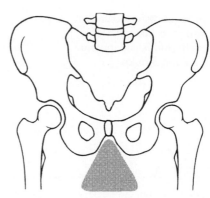

77. This is a male shield used on a female patient. It covers too much of the sacrum and does not cover the required gonadal organs. The shield is situated too superiorly and is not the correct shape.
78. The shield is poorly shaped for a male and does not cover the gonadal organs. The shield should be moved superiorly.
79. The shield is slightly off-centered to the left and is smaller than the inlet pelvis.
80. Palpate the patient's coccyx and elevated anterior superior iliac spine (ASIS). Draw an imaginary line connecting the coccyx with a point 1 inch (2.5 cm) posterior to the ASIS. Position the flat contact shield against this imaginary line.
81. A. Breasts
    B. Eyes
    C. Thyroid
    D. Gonads
    E. 2 inches (5 cm)
82. A. Anatomic artifact
    B. Use positioning devices such as sponges and sandbags to help the patient hold position.
83. The technologist must maintain a source-skin distance (SSD) of at least 12 inches (30 cm) to prevent an unacceptable entrance skin dose. The SID should be elevated at least 2 inches (5 cm).
84. Milliampere-seconds
85. The cortical outlines will still be visible on an underexposed image but not on an underpenetrated image.
86. 30%
87. Decrease by 3 to 4 times
88. A. 3 to 4 times too dark
    B. Contrast is acceptable.
    C. Penetration is acceptable.
    D. 73 kVp at 5 mAs
89. A. 3 to 4 times too light
    B. Contrast is acceptable.
    C. Penetration is acceptable.
    D. 53 kVp at 32 mAs
90. A. 2 times (100%) too light
    B. Contrast is acceptable.
    C. Penetration is acceptable.
    D. 73 kVp at 100 mAs

91. A. 2 times (100%) too dark
    B. Contrast is acceptable.
    C. Penetration is acceptable.
    D. 60 kVp at 3 mAs

92. Kilovoltage
93. A. Increased
    B. 15
94. Additive

95.

	Technical Adjustment	Additive or Destructive
A. Ascites	+50% mAs	Additive
B. Emphysema	−8% kVp	Destructive
C. Pleural effusion	+35% mAs	Additive
D. Osteoporosis	−8% kVp	Destructive
E. Osteoarthritis	+8% kVp	Additive
F. Pneumothorax	−8% kVp	Destructive
G. Pneumonia	+50% mAs	Additive
H. Bowel obstruction	−8% kVp	Destructive
I. Osteochondroma	+8% kVp	Additive
J. Rheumatoid arthritis	−8% kVp	Destructive
K. Pulmonary edema	+50%	Additive
L. Cardomegaly	+50%	Additive

96. A. T
    B. F
    C. T
    D. F
    E. T
    F. T
    G. F
    H. T
    I. T
    J. T
    K. F
    L. F
97. A. The AEC should not have been used when hardware or a prosthetic device is included in the exposure field.
    B. The center cell was used on this chest image. The center cell was positioned beneath a structure that has much greater atomic density than the structures of interest (lungs).
    C. The outside cells were chosen and the central ray was centered too high, positioning part of the cells beneath the lung fields. The lungs have a much smaller atomic density than the abdominal structures.
98. 125 mAs
99. A. Amount of scatter produced and directed toward the IR
    B. Degree of OID.

100. A. 23
     B. 57
     C. 91
     D. 114
     E. 107
     F. 40
101. A. Increase by 50%; new mAs to use is 4.5
     B. There is no need to increase the mAs for the second image. The kVp is low enough that few of the scatter photons are being diverged at a narrow angle with the IR so density is not affected by increasing collimation.
102. The density is not even from the toes to the metacarpals, demonstrating increased density at the distal metacarpals. The filter needs to be moved approximately 1 inch (2.5 cm) proximally.
103. A. F
     B. T
     C. F
     D. T
     E. F
104. A. Atomic density
     B. Atomic number
     C. Thickness
105. A. H
     B. H
     C. L
     D. L

E. L

F. L

G. L

106. A. 72

B. 80

107. A. Use a grid.

B. Use tight collimation.

C. Place a flat contact shield or edge of an apron along the appropriate collimated border.

108. Place the straight edge of a lead apron along the anterior collimation border.

109. A. An anatomic structure within a collimated field that could have been removed

B. Two exposures are taken on the same IR without processing being done between them

C. Patient and hospital belongings that are found outside the patient's body that could have been removed but were not and are demonstrated on the image

D. Objects located within the patient's body that cannot be removed and are demonstrated on the image

E. Artifacts that are caused by the imaging equipment

F. Artifacts that are caused by the processor or the way the IR was handled or stored

110. A. External artifact

B. Anatomic artifact

C. Internal artifact

D. Equipment-related artifact

E. Improper film handling or processor artifact

111. A. Inverted or off-focused

B. Off-center

112. A. Toward

B. Increase

C. Higher

113. When the artifact can be eliminated and is obscuring a portion of the area of interest

114. An optimal image is perfect in all aspects, whereas an acceptable image does not have to be repeated but has aspects that could be improved.

115. The goal of mobile and trauma imaging is to demonstrate accurate relationships between the anatomic structures for the projection or position imaged, without further patient injury and with minimal discomfort.

116. A. Midcoronal plane

B. Line connecting the humeral epicondyles

C. Midcoronal plane

D. Line connecting the femoral epicondyles

E. Orbitomeatal line (OML)

117.

	kVp adjustment	mAs adjustment
A. Small to medium plaster cast	+5–7	+50%–60%
B. Fiberglass cast	No adjustment	No adjustment
C. Wood backboard	+5	+ 25%–30%
D. Postmortem imaging of head, thorax, and abdomen	Not recommended	+ 35%–50%
E. Upper airway obstruction	−15%–20%	Not recommended
F. Wood sliver embedded in soft tissue	−15%–20%	Not recommended

118. A. 20

B. 30

119. There is a distal ulnar fracture and the wrist is not in a lateral projection. When the patient is unable to place both joints in the true position at the same time the joint closest to the injury should be in the true position.

120. A. T

B. T

C. T

D. T

E. T

F. F

G. T

H. F

I. T

J. T

1.

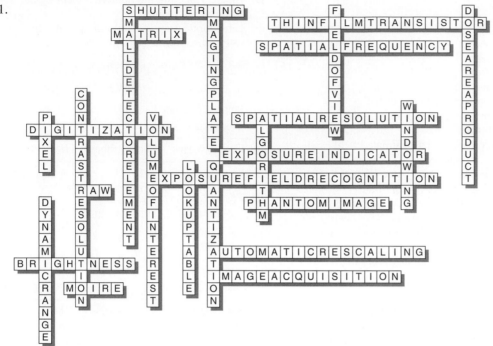

2. Increased, 15
3. Energy
4. Analog-to-digital converter (ADC)
5. More
6. To ensure that the histogram generated from the image data is shaped correctly and the VOI is accurately identified before automatic rescaling of the data occurs.
7. A. Pixel values
   B. Number of pixels with that brightness value
8. Minimal
9. A. 5
   B. 2
   C. 1
   D. 4
   E. 3
10. A. Poor positioning
    B. Poor collimation
    C. Poor alignment of part on IR
    D. Unusual pathologic conditions
    E. Artifacts
    F. Include anatomy not normally included
    G. Excessive scatter fogging
11. A. 120
    B. 60
12. At the midpoint of defined VOI (halfway between S1 and S2)
13. Electrical signals of varying intensity.
14. Where the technologist collimates to
15. Before
16. Only the pixels receiving exposure will send signals to the computer for processing.

17. Near the x-ray source, below the collimator and before the patient
18. False
19. True
20. Better detail to make an optimal diagnosis
21. A. Overexposure
    B. Brightness
    C. Contrast concerns
21. 80 kVp at 48 mAs
23. Underexposure (blotchy, mottled appearance)
24. Double exposure (image of an AP pelvis and an AP L-spine)
25. Figure 2-5, *A*: abdomen; Figure 2-5, *B*: chest
26. Central ray centering not over photocell (part not over photocell)
27. A. Inverted grid
    B. Grid tilted
    C. Grid cut off, grid was not removed before exposure
28. Moiré effect
29. Phantom image
30. Back of IR toward source
31. A. 3
    B. 2
    C. 4
32. X-ray taken and central ray directed toward the cassettes in the metal basket
33. The computer uses the collimated borders. It is best to have four collimated borders shown at an equal distance from the edges of the IR.
34. 30%

1. A. As if the patient were in an upright position; marker is reversed.
   B. As if the patient were in an upright position; marker is correct.
   C. As if the patient were in an upright position; marker is correct.
   D. As if the patient were in an upright position; marker is reversed.
   E. Display so that side of the patient that was positioned upward when the image was exposed is upward on the displayed image; marker is correct for AP projection and reversed for PA projection.

2. A. Halt patient respiration.
   B. Halt body movements.
   C. Use a short object–image receptor distance (OID).
   D. Use a 72-inch (183-cm) SID.

3. Vascular lung markings and fluid levels or air within the pleural cavity

4. A. Thoracic vertebrae
   B. Posterior ribs

5.

ADULT AND PEDIATRIC CHEST TECHNICAL DATA				
Projection	kVp	Grid	AEC Chamber(s)	SID
ADULT CHEST TECHNICAL DATA				
PA	110	Grid	Both outside	72 inches (183 cm)
Lateral	125	Grid	Center	72 inches (183 cm)
AP mobile	80 – 95	Nongrid		48 – 50 inches (120 cm)
AP supine in Bucky	80 – 100	Grid	Both outside	48 – 50 inches (120 cm)
AP-PA (lateral decubitus)	125	Grid	Center	72 inches (183 cm)
AP-PA axial (lordotic)	125	Grid	Both outside	72 inches (183 cm)
AP-PA oblique	125	Grid	Over lung of interest	72 inches (183 cm)
PEDIATRIC CHEST TECHNICAL DATA				
Neonate: AP	65 – 70			40 - 48 inches (100 – 120 cm)
Infant: AP	70 – 75			40 – 48 inches (100 – 120 cm)
Child: PA	75 – 80	Grid (if measures 4 inches or larger)		72 inches (183 cm)
Child: AP	70 – 75			40 – 48 inches (100 – 120 cm)
Neonate: Cross-table lateral	65 – 70			40 – 48 inches (100 – 120 cm)
Infant: Cross-table lateral	75 – 80			40 – 48 inches (100 – 120 cm)
Child: Lateral	75 – 80	Grid (if measures 4 inches or larger)		72 inches (180 cm)
Neonate: AP (lateral decubitus)	65 – 70			40 – 48 inches (100 – 120 cm)
Infant: AP (lateral decubitus)	70 – 75			40 – 48 inches (100 – 120 cm)
Child: AP (lateral decubitus)	75 – 80			72 inches (183 cm)

6. A. T
   B. T
   C. F
   D. T
   E. T
   F. F
   G. T
   H. T
   I. T
   J. T
   K. F
   L. T
   M. T
   N. F
   O. T
   P. T
   Q. T

7. A. Pleural drainage tube
   B. Central venous catheter
   C. Pulmonary artery catheter (external electrocardiogram leads are also demonstrated)
   D. Automatic implantable cardioverter defibrillator

8. A. 4
   B. 6
   C. 5
   D. 3
   E. 2
   F. 7
   G. 1

9. A. Should be placed in an upright position
   B. Should be horizontal

10. A. Pleural effusion
    B. Pneumothorax
    C. Pneumectomy

11. A. Seventh
    B. Costophrenic angle
    C. Equal
    D. Horizontal
    E. Outside
    F. Fourth thoracic
    G. 10 or 11
12. A. Right lung apex
    B. Clavicle
    C. Fourth thoracic vertebra
    D. Scapula
    E. Fourth anterior rib
    F. Diaphragm
    G. Costophrenic angle
    H. Heart shadow
    I. Lung
    J. Hilum
    K. Seventh posterior rib
    L. Aortic arch
    M. Superior manubrium
    N. Left SC joint
    O. Air-filled trachea
13. A. Transversely
    B. Anteroposteriorly
    C. Vertically
14. Vertical
15. Disease processes, advanced pregnancy, excessive obesity, slouching patient, or confining clothing
16. A. Hypersthenic
    B. Short and wide
17. A. Asthenic and hyposthenic
    B. Long and narrow
18. Place a hand along the patient's sides at the level of costophrenic angles. Ask the patient to inhale and observe whether your hands remain within the IR's boundaries.
19. Place the patient's shoulders and arms at equal distances from the IR.
20. A. Scoliosis
    B. No
    C. On a rotated patient, the distances will be uniform down the length of the lung field, but with scoliosis, the vertebral column to lateral lung edge distance will vary down the length of the each lung and between each lung.
21. The shoulders are depressed.
22. Place hands on hips and rotate elbows and shoulders anteriorly.
23. A. Midcoronal
    B. Fourth
    C. 1 inch (2.5 cm)
24. A. If the patient's shoulders are not depressed
    B. If the patient's upper midcoronal plane is leaning toward the IR
25. The diaphragm is allowed to move to its lowest position.
26. A. Placing the patient in an upright position
    B. Having the patient perform a deep inspiration
27. It coaxes the patient into a deeper inspiration.

28. A. Pneumothorax
    B. Foreign body
29. A. Higher
    B. Nine
    C. Broader
    D. Shorter
    E. Lighter
30. A. Horizontal or perpendicular
    B. Midsagittal
    C. Vertebral prominens
31. The apices, lateral lungs, and costophrenic angles
32. Rotated into an RAO position
33. The shoulders were not depressed.
34. The right elbow and shoulder were not rotated anteriorly.
35. The patient's upper midcoronal plane was tilted toward the IR.
36. The patient's upper midcoronal plane was tilted away from the IR.
37. The image was taken on expiration.
38. Eight posterior ribs are demonstrated above the diaphragm, and the clavicles are not on the same horizontal plane. Expose the image after coaxing the patient into a deeper inspiration and depress the shoulders.
39. The vertebral column is superimposed over the right sternal clavicular end, and the left inferior posterior ribs are longer than the right. Rotate the patient toward the left side until the shoulders are at equal distances from the IR.
40. The scapulae are demonstrated in the superolateral lung field, the third thoracic vertebra is superimposed over the manubrium, and the inferior tip of the costophrenic angles is not included in the collimation field. Rotate the shoulders and elbows anteriorly, tilt the patient's upper midcoronal plane toward the IR until it is parallel with the IR, and move the central ray and IR inferiorly by 0.5 inch (1.25 cm).
41. Less than 1 inch (2.5 cm) of the lung field is seen above the clavicles and the manubrium is at the level of third thoracic vertebra. Tilt the upper midcoronal plane toward the IR until it is parallel with the IR.
42. The fifth thoracic vertebra is superimposed over the manubrium, only a portion of the tenth posterior rib is seen above the diaphragm, and the right sternal clavicular end is superimposed by the vertebral column. Tilt the upper midcoronal plane away from the IR until it is parallel with the IR, expose the image after coaxing the patient into a deeper inspiration, and rotate the patient toward the left side until the shoulders are at equal distances from the IR.
43. More than 1 inch (2.5 cm) of the lung field is demonstrated above the clavicles, the manubrium is at the level of the fifth thoracic vertebra, and the scapulae are in the superolateral lung field. Tilt the upper midcoronal plane away from the IR until it is parallel with the IR and rotate the shoulders and elbows anteriorly. Increase collimation on all sides.

44. A. Lung apex
    B. Scapulae
    C. Thoracic vertebra
    D. Intervertebral foramen
    E. Posterior ribs
    F. Intervertebral disk space
    G. Costophrenic angles
    H. Diaphragm
    I. Heart shadow
    J. Sternum
    K. Hili
    L. Esophagus
    M. Trachea
45. A. Eighth
    B. 0.5 inch (1 cm)
    C. Hemidiaphragms
    D. Anterior
    E. Eleventh
46. Align the shoulders, posterior ribs, and posterior pelvic wings perpendicular to the IR holder.
47. A. Right
    B. It is situated farther from the IR, so diverged x-rays will cause it to magnify.
48. By evaluating the degree of posterior rib superimposition
49. A. Find the gastric air bubble, which is located beneath the left hemidiaphragm.
    B. Outline the heart shadow, which is located within the left hemidiaphragm.
50. Beneath the left hemidiaphragm
51. Left
52. Rotate the left side of the patient anteriorly approximately 1 inch (2.5 cm), or rotate the right side of the patient posteriorly approximately 1 inch (2.5 cm).
53. The anterior ribs will be superimposed, whereas the posterior ribs will demonstrate differing degrees of separation.
54. The midsagittal plane is parallel to the IR.
55. Right
56. A. The heart shadow will be more magnified on the right lateral chest projection.
    B. The left hemidiaphragm will project lower than the right hemidiaphragm on a right lateral chest projection.
57. A. Right lateral
    B. Left lateral
    C. Left lateral
58. Position the humeri vertically.
59. Anteroinferior
60. The eleventh thoracic vertebra will be superimposed by the lung field.
61. A. Take the exposure after the second full inspiration.
    B. Take the exposure with the patient in an upright position.
62. Twelfth
63. A. Midcoronal
    B. Inferior

64. The lung apices, sternum, posterior ribs, diaphragm, and costophrenic angles
65. The patient's humeri were not positioned vertically.
66. The left thorax was rotated anteriorly.
67. If no medical indication explains this relationship, the patient's lower thorax was situated closer to the IR than the upper thorax (midsagittal plane was not parallel with IR).
68. Image A: More than 0.5 inch (1.25 cm) of separation is present between the posterior ribs. The inferior heart shadow projects into the inferiorly and anteriorly located lung field. Rotate the patient's right side anteriorly approximately 0.5 inch (1.25 cm).
    Image B: The right and left posterior ribs are separated by more than 0.5 inch (1.25 cm), indicating that the chest was rotated. The superior heart shadow does not extend beyond the sternum and the gastric air bubble is demonstrated adjacent to the posteriorly situated lung, verifying that the right lung is situated anterior to the sternum, and the left lung posteriorly. Rotate the patient's right side posteriorly approximately 0.5 inch (1.25 cm).
69. The humeral soft tissue shadows are superimposed over the anterior lung apices. Position the patient's humeri vertically.
70. The hemidiaphragms cover only to the ninth thoracic vertebra, and the humeral soft tissue shadows are superimposed over the anterior lung apices. Take the exposure after coaxing the patient into taking a deeper inspiration and position humeri vertically.
71. A. The manubrium is at the level of the third thoracic vertebra. Tilt the upper midcoronal plane toward the IR until the midcoronal plane is parallel with the IR.
    B. This image reflects accurate positioning. One might conclude that the left hemidiaphragm is too superior and that the patient's midsagittal plane was tilted, but by evaluating the PA image, it can be determined that because the left hemidiaphragm is situated higher than the right on this patient, this positioning is accurate.
72. A. Right apex
    B. Right SC joint
    C. Scapula
    D. Fifth posterior rib
    E. Medial scapular border
    F. Diaphragm
    G. Costophrenic angle
    H. Heart shadow
    I. Aortic arch
    J. Manubrium
    K. Third thoracic vertebra
73. A. Seventh
    B. Sternal clavicular ends
    C. Manubrium
    D. Clavicles
    E. Horizontal
    F. Scapulae
    G. 9 to 10

74. So the reviewer knows which image was taken first if more than one were taken on the same day

75. So the reviewer will know the accuracy of the air-fluid levels demonstrated

76. The fluid is evenly spread throughout the lung field, so no definite air-fluid line is visible.

77. Kilovoltage

78. A. The vertical dimension does not fully expand in the recumbent or seated position.
    B. Because a low SID is used, resulting in increased magnification

79. Place the shoulders and anterior superior iliac spines at equal distances from the IR and bed.

80. Rotation is evident when the distances from the sternoclavicular ends to the vertebral column and the lengths of the right and left corresponding posterior ribs are not equal.

81. Clavicles will be on the same horizontal plane.

82. Poor shoulder positioning will demonstrate the manubrium at the level of the fourth thoracic vertebra, whereas poor central ray alignment will demonstrate the manubrium at a level inferior to the fourth thoracic vertebra and an increased lung field superior to the clavicles.

83. Place back of patient's hands on hips and rotate elbows and shoulders anteriorly.

84. A. More than 1 inch (2.5 cm) of apices will be seen above the clavicles, and the posterior ribs will be vertically shaped.
    B. Less than 1 inch (2.5 cm) of the apices will be seen above the clavicles, and the posterior ribs will be horizontal.

85. Angle the central ray 5 to 10 degrees cephalically.

86. A. 5 degrees caudally
    B. To offset the upward lift of the manubrium, clavicles, and superior ribs

87. Pressure from the abdominal organs prevents the diaphragm from shifting to an inferior position.

88. Instruct the patient to take two full breaths before the image is exposed.

89. The high-frequency ventilator maintains the lung expansion at a steady mean pressure.

90. A. Midsagittal
    B. 4
    C. Jugular notch

91. The lung apices, lateral lungs, and costophrenic angles

92. The patient would have been in a left posterior oblique (LPO) position, or the central ray would have been angled toward the left side of the chest.

93. The central ray was angled too caudally.

94. The central ray was angled too cephalically.

95. The central ray was aligned perpendicular to the IR. It would be best to angle it 5 to 10 degrees cephalically.

96. Eight posterior ribs are demonstrated superior to the diaphragm, the clavicles are not horizontal, the left SC joint appears away from the vertebral column, and the left posterior ribs demonstrate greater length than the right. Expose the image after coaxing the patient into a greater inspiration, depress the shoulders, and place an elevating device beneath the left IR border to position the IR parallel with the bed or angle the central ray toward the right side of the patient until it is aligned perpendicular to the IR.

97. More than 1 inch (2.5 cm) of apical lung field is demonstrated above the clavicles, and the posterior ribs have a vertical contour. Angle the central ray cephalically until it is aligned perpendicular to the midcoronal plane.

98. The manubrium is superimposed over the third thoracic vertebra, less than 1 inch (2.5 cm) is demonstrated above the clavicles, and the right sternal clavicular end superimposes the vertebral column. Angle the central ray caudally until it is aligned perpendicular to the midcoronal plane and rotate the patient toward the right side until the shoulders are at equal distances from the IR.

99. A. Diaphragm
    B. Tenth posterior rib
    C. Heart shadow
    D. Lateral scapular border
    E. Clavicle

100. A. Up and away
     B. Seventh
     C. Vertebral column
     D. Outside the lung field
     E. Fourth thoracic
     F. Clavicle
     G. Diaphragm

101. A. Mark the side positioned away from the table with an R marker and an arrow pointing upward or with a word marker identifying the side of the patient positioned upward.
     B. Display so that lateral right side of the chest is upward.

102. A. Air
     B. Fluid

103. Within the side of the chest positioned closer to the table or cart

104. A. Left AP-PA (lateral decubitus)
     B. Left AP-PA (lateral decubitus)

105. A. Posterior ribs
     B. Shoulders
     C. Posterior pelvic wings

106. AP

107. Above the patient's head

108. A. Midcoronal
     B. Parallel

109. Elevate the patient on a radiolucent sponge or cardiac board.

110. The right side of chest was positioned closer to the IR than left side.
111. The left side of chest was positioned closer to the IR than right side.
112. The patient's upper midcoronal plane was tilted toward the IR.
113. The right sternoclavicular end is superimposed over the vertebral column, and the posterior ribs on the left side demonstrate greater length than those on the right. Rotate the left side away from the IR until the midcoronal plane and IR are parallel.
114. The manubrium is superimposed over the fifth thoracic vertebra. Tilt the upper midcoronal plane toward the IR until it and the IR are parallel.
115. A. Lung apex
     B. Posterior fourth rib
     C. Anterior fourth rib
     D. Superior scapular angle
     E. Lateral border scapula
     F. Medial clavicular end
     G. First thoracic vertebra
116. A. Superior
     B. Superior
     C. Horizontally
     D. Lateral
     E. Vertebral column
     F. Horizontal
117. Lung apices
118. A. Arch the patient's back until the midcoronal plane is at a 45-degree angle to the IR. A perpendicular central ray is used.
     B. Have the patient remain completely upright, and use a 45-degree cephalic central ray angle.
     C. The patient's back is arched as much as possible, and the central ray is angled cephalically in the amount necessary to equal 45 degrees.
119. A. Increase the degree of patient arch.
     B. Increase the degree of central ray angulation.
120. Place the back of the patient's hands on the hips and rotate the elbows and shoulders anteriorly.
121. When the SC joints are not at equal distances from the vertebral column
122. A. Midsagittal
     B. Manubrium
     C. Xiphoid
123. The clavicles, lung apices, and two thirds of the lung field
124. The midcoronal plane was at less than a 45-degree angle to IR or the central ray was angled cephalically less than needed.
125. The elbows and shoulders were not drawn anteriorly.
126. The patient was rotated in an LPO position.
127. The medial clavicular ends are superimposed over the lung apices, and the anterior ribs are demonstrated inferior to their corresponding posterior rib. Cephalically increase the central ray angulation or have the patient increase the amount of back arch until the angle of the midcoronal plane and IR is 45 degrees.

128. A. SC joints
     B. Air-filled trachea
     C. Principal bronchi
     D. Heart shadow
     E. Posterior heart shadow
129. A. Principal bronchi
     B. SC joints
     C. Twice
     D. Manubrium
     E. 10 or 11
130. Midcoronal
131. 60
132. A. Right
     B. Right
133. LAO
134. Vertebra prominens
135. The apices, costophrenic angles, and lateral chest walls
136. The patient was not rotated enough.
137. The patient was rotated too much.
138. The patient was not rotated enough.
139. Less than two times the lung field is demonstrated on the left side of this thorax than on the right side. Increase the degree of patient obliquity until the midcoronal plane is at a 45-degree angle to the IR.
140. Approximately three times the lung field is demonstrated on the right side of this thorax than on the left side, which indicates that the patient was rotated approximately 60 degrees. An LAO chest projection taken to evaluate the lung field should demonstrate only two times the lung field on the right side than the left and would demonstrate the vertebral column superimposed over the heart shadow. Decrease the degree of patient obliquity until the midcoronal plane is at a 45-degree angle to the IR.
141. Neonates and infants have fewer alveoli, causing the lungs to be denser.
142. Head rotation and cervical flexion and extension cause the ET tip to move superiorly and inferiorly, making it difficult for the reviewer to determine exactly where the tube is positioned.
143. A. Clavicle
     B. Right lung apex
     C. Diaphragm
     D. Costophrenic angle
     E. Heart shadow
     F. Anterior rib
     G. Fourth posterior rib
144. A. Fourth
     B. Equal
     C. Equal
     D. Downward
     E. Cephalically
     F. 8
     G. 9
     H. Chin
145. A. Midsagittal
     B. Mammary line
     C. Upper airway, lungs, mediastinal structures, and costophrenic angles

146. Shape
147. The dense substances of blood, pus, protein, and cells and the less dense air
148. A. After neonates take a deep breath, as observed by watching chest movements
    B. When the manometer's digital bar or analog needle moves to its highest position
    C. At any time
149. The patient is rotated toward the right side (RPO position).
150. The central ray was centered too inferiorly.
151. The image was exposed with the ventilator's manometer at a level lower than the highest point.
152. The chin was tucked toward the chest.
153. The left sternoclavicular end is not adjacent to the vertebral column, and the left posterior ribs demonstrate greater length than the right posterior ribs. Rotate the patient toward the right side until the midcoronal plane is parallel with the IR.
154. The anterior ribs are projecting upwardly, the posterior ribs are horizontal, the sixth thoracic vertebra is in the center of the image, and the right sternoclavicular end is not adjacent to the vertebral column. Center the central ray approximately 1 inch (2.5 cm) superiorly (at the mammary line) and rotate the patient toward the left side until the midcoronal plane is parallel with the IR.
155. The seventh posterior rib is demonstrated superior to the diaphragm, and the chin is superimposed over the lung apices. If possible, take the exposure after a deeper inhalation and elevate the chin until the cervical vertebrae are in a neutral position.
156. The right sternoclavicular end is not adjacent to the vertebral column, the right posterior ribs demonstrate greater length than the left posterior ribs, an excessive amount of the cervical vertebrae and face is included on image, and the third thoracic vertebra is in the center of the image. Rotate the patient toward the left side until the midcoronal plane is parallel with the IR, center 1 inch (2.5 cm) inferiorly and increase collimation.
157. A. Second anterior rib
    B. Sixth posterior rib
    C. Lung
    D. Diaphragm
    E. Costophrenic angle
    F. Heart shadow
    G. Hilum
    H. Superior manubrium
    I. Left sternoclavicular joint
    J. Right lung apex
158. The patient's left side is rotated toward the IR (LPO position).
159. The image was exposed on expiration.
160. The central ray was not perpendicular with the midcoronal plane but was angled caudally.
161. The patient's upper midcoronal plane was tilted away from the IR.
162. The shoulders were elevated.

163. The manubrium is at the level of the third thoracic vertebra, the right medial clavicular end is not adjacent to the vertebral column, and the right posterior ribs demonstrate greater length than the left posterior ribs. Tilt the upper midcoronal plane toward the IR until it is parallel with the IR and rotate the patient toward the left side until the midcoronal plane is parallel with the IR.
164. The manubrium is at the level of the fifth thoracic vertebra, and the right sternoclavicular end is visualized away from the vertebral column. Tilt the upper midcoronal plane away from the IR until it is parallel with the IR, and rotate the patient toward the right side until the IR and midcoronal plane are parallel.
165. Eight posterior ribs are demonstrated above the diaphragm, the right sternoclavicular end is visualized away from the vertebral column, and the right posterior ribs demonstrate greater length than the left. Coax the patient into a deeper inhalation and rotate the patient toward the right side until the IR and midcoronal plane are parallel.
166. The manubrium is at the level of the seventh thoracic vertebra, the posterior ribs are vertical, and the right sternoclavicular end is visualized away from the vertebral column. Angle the central ray cephalically and toward the left side or elevate the right side of the patient until the midcoronal plane and CR are perpendicular.
167. The manubrium is at the level of the second thoracic vertebra, the posterior ribs are horizontal, five posterior ribs are demonstrated above the diaphragm, and the patient is in a slight LPO position. Angle the central ray caudally until it is perpendicular to the midcoronal plane, coax the patient into a deeper inhalation, and rotate the patient toward the right side until the IR and midcoronal plane are parallel.
168. A. Intervertebral foramen
    B. Thoracic vertebra
    C. Intervertebral disk space
    D. Costophrenic angle
    E. Diaphragm
    F. Heart shadow
    G. Sternum
    H. Lung apex
169. A. Midcoronal
    B. Mammary line
    C. Apices, costophrenic angles, posterior ribs, and airway
170. A. Less disturbance to the sensitive neonate
    B. Will not result in compression of the lung adjacent to the IR and overinflation of the other lung
171. Perpendicular
172. The OID difference between the right and left lungs is minimal.
173. The patient's left side is rotated posteriorly, and the right side is rotated anteriorly.
174. The arms were not elevated to a position near the patient's head.

175. The chin was not tilted upward.
176. The image was taken on expiration.
177. The posterior ribs are demonstrated without super-imposition. The right lung is the posterior lung, as indicated by the heart shadow demonstrated in the anteriorly and inferiorly located lung. Rotate the right lung anteriorly until an imaginary line connecting the shoulders and the pelvic wings is perpendicular to the IR.
178. The hemidiaphragms demonstrate an exaggerated cephalic curvature, and the humeral soft tissue is superimposed over the anterior lung apices. Expose the image on full inspiration, and raise the arms until the humeri are next to the patient's head.
179. A. Lung apex
     B. Thoracic vertebra
     C. Posterior ribs
     D. Costophrenic angles
     E. Diaphragm
     F. Heart shadow
     G. Sternum
     H. Esophagus
     I. Trachea
180. The patient's left lung was rotated posteriorly.
181. The image was exposed on expiration.
182. The arms were not elevated.
183. A portion of the right lung is positioned posterior to the left, as indicated by the left side gastric air bubble located beneath the superiorly and anteriorly located left lung. Rotate the right side of the patient anteriorly until an imaginary line connecting the posterior shoulders and posterior iliac wings is aligned perpendicular to the IR.
184. The humeral soft tissue is superimposing the apical lung field. Elevate the humeri until they are positioned superior to the lung field.
185. A portion of the right lung is positioned posterior to the left and the soft tissue of the arms is obscuring the anterior lung apices. Rotate the right side of the patient anteriorly until an imaginary line connecting the posterior shoulder and posterior iliac wings is aligned perpendicular to the IR, and elevate the arms.
186. A. Clavicle
     B. Humerus
     C. Third anterior rib
     D. Sixth posterior rib
     E. Pleural drainage tube
     F. Heart shadow
     G. Diaphragm
187. A. Fourth
     B. Vertebral column
     C. Clavicles
     D. Downward
     E. Cephalically
     F. Eight
     G. Midsagittal
188. Up away from the bed or cart

189. Patient's bottom lip
190. Perpendicular
191. The patient was rotated toward the right side (RPO position).
192. The central ray was angled too cephalically.
193. The image was exposed on expiration.
194. The patient was not elevated on a radiolucent sponge.
195. The right arm was not elevated to a position near the patient's head.
196. The patient's left arm is superimposed over the apical lung region, and the right sternal clavicular end is visible away from the vertebral column. Elevate the left arm until it is next to the patient's head, above the lung field, and rotate the right side of the thorax away from the IR until the shoulders and posterior iliac wings are at equal distances from the IR.
197. The patient's right arm is superimposed over the apical lung region and the left arm and upper vertebral column are not on the elevating device, resulting in lateral tilting of the upper vertebral column. Elevate the patient's humeri, positioning them next to the head, and elevate the entire thorax on the elevating device, placing the upper vertebral column parallel with the device.
198. The upper vertebral column tilts laterally, the left sternal clavicular end is away from the vertebral column, and the left posterior ribs demonstrate greater length than the right posterior ribs. Elevate the patient's head and upper vertebral column until the midsagittal plane is aligned parallel with the bed, and rotate the right side toward the IR until the shoulders and iliac wings are at equal distances from the IR.
199. A. Heart shadow
     B. Diaphragm
     C. Eighth posterior rib
     D. Third anterior rib
200. The right side of the patient was positioned closer to the IR than the left side (RAO position).
201. The left side of the patient was positioned closer to the IR than the right side (LPO position).
202. The upper midcoronal plane was tilted posteriorly.
203. The right sternal clavicular end is superimposed over the vertebral column, the posterior ribs on the left side demonstrate the greater length, and the arm is obscuring a small portion of the right lateral lung apex. Rotate the patient's left side away from the IR, and elevate the right arm until it is positioned next to the patient's head.
204. The left diaphragm is not included in its entirety. Move the central ray and IR inferiorly approximately 2 inches (5 cm).
205. A. As if the patient were in an upright position; marker is correct.
     B. So that the right side of the patient is upward on the displayed image; marker is correct.

577

206. A. Patient breathing during exposure
   B. Patient moving during exposure
207. A. Explaining to the patient the importance of holding still
   B. Making the patient as comfortable as possible
   C. Using the shortest exposure time
208. Peristaltic activity
209. Use the shortest possible exposure time.
210. A. Involuntary motion; cortical outlines of ribs and bony structures are sharp.
   B. Voluntary motion; cortical outlines of ribs are blurry.
211. They are located lateral to the lumbar vertebrae, starting at the first lumbar vertebra and extending to the lesser trochanters.
212. A. They are located lateral to the vertebral column, with the upper poles at approximately the eleventh thoracic vertebra and the lower poles at approximately the third lumbar vertebra.
   B. Right
   C. It is located beneath the liver.
213. A. Psoas major muscle
   B. Kidneys
   C. Inferior ribs
   D. Lumbar transverse processes
214. A. 30% to 50% decrease
   B. 5% to 8% decrease
215. A. Obesity
   B. Bowel obstruction
   C. Soft tissue masses
   D. Ascites
216. A. Increase 30% to 50%.
   B. Increase 5% to 8%.
217. Diaphragm, bowel gas pattern, and faint outline of bony structures
218. Little intrinsic fat is present to outline the organs.

219.

ADULT AND PEDIATRIC ABDOMEN TECHNICAL DATA				
Projection	kVp	Grid	AEC Chamber(s)	SID
ADULT CHEST TECHNICAL DATA				
AP	70 – 80	Grid	All	40 – 48 inches (100 – 120 cm)
AP (lateral decubitus)	70 – 80	Grid	Center	40 – 48 inches (100 – 120 cm)
PEDIATRIC ABDOMINAL TECHNICAL DATA				
Neonate: AP	65 – 75			40 – 48 inches (100 – 120 cm)
Infant: AP	65 – 75			40 – 48 inches (100 – 120 cm)
Child: AP	70 – 80	Grid (if measures 4 inches [10 cm] or larger)		40 – 48 inches (100 – 120 cm)
Neonate: AP (lateral decubitus)	65 – 75			40 – 48 inches (100 – 120 cm)
Infant: AP (lateral decubitus)	65 – 75			40 – 48 inches (100 – 120 cm)
Child: AP (lateral decubitus)	70 – 80	Grid (if measures 4 inches [10 cm] or larger)		40 – 48 inches (100 – 120 cm)

220. A. Kidney
   B. Pedicle
   C. Third lumbar vertebral body
   D. Intestinal gas
   E. Anterior superior iliac spine (ASIS)
   F. Inlet pelvis
   G. Sacrum
   H. Iliac wing
   I. Iliac crest
   J. Spinous process
   K. Eleventh thoracic vertebra
221. A. Diaphragmatic dome
   B. Pedicle
   C. Inlet pelvis
   D. Sacrum
   E. Spinous process
   F. Twelfth vertebral body
   G. Gastric bubble
   H. Diaphragmatic dome
   I. Ninth thoracic vertebra
222. A. Vertebral bodies
   B. Symphysis pubis
   C. Ninth
   D. Fourth
   E. Third
223. Intraperitoneal air is located directly beneath each diaphragm dome.
224. Position the patient's shoulders and anterior superior iliac spines at equal distances from the IR.
225. A. 5 to 20 minutes
   B. It allows time for the air to rise to the level of the diaphragm.

226. A. Inferior
    B. Superior
    C. Eighth or ninth
    D. Ninth
227. A. Expiration
    B. Because less pressure is placed on the abdominal organs
228. A. Ensures that the kidneys, tip of liver, and spleen are included on the image
    B. Ensures that the inferior border of the peritoneal cavity is included on the image
229. Because the male patient's pelvis is longer
230. A. Two crosswise
    B. One lengthwise
    C. One lengthwise
231. A. The eleventh thoracic spinous process, lateral body soft tissue, iliac wings, and symphysis pubis
    B. The diaphragm, lateral body soft tissue, and iliac wings
232. The patient was rotated into an RPO position.
233. The upper abdomen was in an AP projection, whereas the pelvic area was rotated into an LPO position.
234. The central ray and IR were centered too superiorly.
235. The sacrum is not aligned with the symphysis pubis, the distance from the left pedicles to the spinous processes is less than the distance from the right pedicles to the spinous processes, and the lateral soft tissue is not included on the image. Rotate the patient toward the left side until the shoulders and anterior iliac spines are positioned at equal distances from the IR, and expose images of the abdomen using two crosswise IRs instead of one lengthwise.
236. The symphysis pubis is not included on the image. This is a male patient. Center the central ray 1 inch (2.5 cm) superior to the iliac crest and align the IR with the central ray.
237. The lateral soft tissue of the abdomen has been clipped on both sides. Use two crosswise images to include all lateral tissue.
238. The sacrum is not aligned with the symphysis pubis and the distance from the right pedicles to the spinous processes is greater than the distance from the left pedicles to the spinous processes. Rotate the patient toward the left side until the shoulders and anterior iliac spines are positioned at equal distances from the IR.
239. The right iliac wing is wider than the left, the distance from the right pedicles to the spinous processes is greater than the distance from the left pedicles to the spinous processes, the vertebral column is not aligned with the long axis of the IR, and the symphysis pubis is not included on the image. Rotate the patient toward the left side until the shoulders and anterior iliac spines are positioned at equal distances from the IR, align the

midsagittal plane with the long axis of the collimated light field, and move the central ray and IR inferior enough to include the symphysis pubis.
240. The domes of the diaphragm are not included on the image. Center the central ray and IR approximately 2 inches (5 cm) superiorly.
241. A. Iliac wing
    B. Intestinal gas
    C. Diaphragmatic dome
    D. Pedicle
    E. Vertebral body
    F. Spinous process
242. A. Vertebral bodies
    B. Spinous processes
    C. Ninth
    D. Third
243. Measure the patient, and increase the mAs 30% to 50% or the kVp 5% to 8% from the routine technique that would normally be used for this body measurement.
244. Place the thicker end of the filter toward the right side of the patient and the thinner end toward the left side.
245. A. Left
    B. This will position the gastric air bubble away from the abdominal area where the intraperitoneal air would be demonstrated.
246. Align the shoulders, posterior ribs, and posterior pelvic wings perpendicular to the imaging table or cart.
247. Forward rotation of the side positioned farther from the imaging table
248. A. 5 to 20
    B. To allow time for the air to move away from the soft tissue structures and rise to the level of the right diaphragm
249. Right hemidiaphragm
250. Patient with wide hips and narrow waist and thorax
251. Expiration
252. The right hemidiaphragm, ninth thoracic vertebra, right lateral soft tissue, and right iliac wing
253. A. If two crosswise IRs are used and the upper abdomen is being imaged
    B. All the time
254. The right side of the patient was positioned farther from the IR than the left side.
255. The thorax and upper abdominal region were positioned accurately, whereas the right side of the pelvis and lower abdomen are closer to the IR than the left side.
256. The IR and central ray were positioned too inferiorly.
257. The right iliac wing is narrower than the left iliac wing and the distance from the right pedicles to the spinous processes is less than the distance from the left pedicles to the spinous processes. Rotate the patient's right side toward the IR until the shoulders and the anterior superior iliac spines are positioned at equal distances from the IR.

258. A. Diaphragm
    B. Iliac wing
    C. Symphysis pubis
    D. Posterior ribs
259. A. Eighth
    B. Fourth lumbar
260. A. Midsagittal
    B. 2
    C. Superior
    D. Iliac crest
261. The central ray was centered too inferiorly.
262. The patient's upper thorax is laterally tilted toward the left side.
263. The patient is rotated toward the left side (LPO position).
264. The patient is rotated toward the right side (RPO position).
265. The image was exposed on inspiration.
266. The central ray is centered to the third lumbar vertebra, the symphysis pubis and lateral soft tissue are not included in the collimated field, the right posterior ribs demonstrate greater length than the left, and the right iliac wing demonstrates greater width than the left. Center the central ray 1 inch (2.5 cm) inferiorly, collimate to within 0.5 inch (1.25 cm) of the lateral skin line, and rotate the patient toward the left side until the shoulders and the iliac wings are at equal distances from the IR.
267. The left posterior ribs demonstrate greater length and the left iliac wing greater width than the right side, and the domes of the diaphragm are not included within the collimated field. Rotate the patient toward the right side until the shoulders and iliac wings are at equal distance from the IR, move the central ray 12 inch (1.25 cm) superiorly, and then open the longitudinally collimated field 0. 5 inch (1.25 cm).
268. A. Intestinal gas
    B. Inlet pelvis
    C. Obturator foramen
    D. Symphysis pubis
    E. Sacrum
    F. Iliac wing
    G. Spinous process
    H. Third lumbar vertebra pedicle
    I. Twelfth thoracic vertebra
269. The patient was rotated toward the right side (RPO position).
270. The patient was rotated toward the left side (LPO position).
271. Poor radiation protection practices have been followed. The patient's left arm has been included on the image, longitudinal collimation is inadequate, and the gonadal shield is positioned too superiorly and slightly too laterally. Move the central ray medially until it is positioned at the midsagittal plane, increase transverse collimation to within 0.5 inch (1.25 cm) of the skin line, longitudinally collimate to the symphysis pubis, and move the gonadal shield slightly inferiorly and medially.

272. The symphysis pubis is not included in the collimation field, the central ray is too superior, the right iliac wing is wider than the left, and the right posterior ribs are longer than the left posterior ribs. Center the central ray 2 inches (5 cm) inferiorly, and rotate the patient toward the left side until the shoulders and the iliac wings are at equal distances from the IR.
273. The diaphragm is not included within the collimated field. Move the central ray and IR superiorly approximately 2 inches (5 cm).
274. A. Symphysis pubis
    B. Iliac wing
    C. Posterior rib
    D. Diaphragm
    E. Lumbar vertebra
    F. Intestinal gas
275. To position the gastric bubble away from the elevated diaphragm, where free intraperitoneal air will migrate
276. A. Midsagittal
    B. 2
    C. Superior
    D. Iliac crest
277. The patient was rotated toward the right side (RPO position).
278. The central ray was centered too inferiorly.
279. The patient was rotated toward the right side (RPO position).
280. The diaphragm is not included within the collimated field, the posterior ribs on the right side are longer than those on the left, and the right iliac wing is wider than the iliac wing on the left side. Move the central ray superiorly enough to include a transverse level 1 inch (2.5 cm) inferior to the mammary line, and rotate the patient away from the IR until the shoulders and the iliac wings are at equal distances from the IR.
281. The diaphragm is demonstrated inferior to the ninth posterior rib, and the right posterior ribs are longer than the left. Expose the patient after exhalation, and rotate the right side toward the IR until the shoulders and the iliac wings are at equal distances from the IR.
282. A. Right ilium
    B. Spinous process
    C. Pedicle
    D. Second vertebral body
    E. Diaphragm
283. Free interperitoneal air under the right diaphragm
284. The image was exposed when the ventilator's manometer indicator was not at its highest level.
285. The patient was rotated toward the left side (LPO position).
286. The diaphragm is inferior to the ninth posterior rib, indicating that the exposure was taken on inspiration. Expose the image after the patient has exhaled. Free intraperitoneal air is demonstrated adjacent to the right hemidiaphragm.

287. The right iliac wing is wider than the left, and the right posterior ribs are longer than the left posterior ribs. Rotate the patient toward the left side until the shoulders and iliac wings are at equal distances from the IR.

CHAPTER 4   UPPER EXTREMITY

1. A. From the fingertips, with the marker correct
   B. From the fingertips, with the marker correct
   C. From the fingertips, with the marker correct
   D. From the fingertips, with the marker correct

E. From the shoulder, with the marker correct for lateromedial and reversed for mediolateral projection
2. A. Patient motion
   B. Explaining the procedure to the patient
   C. Making the patient comfortable
   D. Using a short exposure time
   E. Using immobilization props
3. A. High
   B. Low
4. A. Bony trabecular
   B. Cortical
5. A. 50-60
   B. 40-48 inches (100-200 cm)

6.

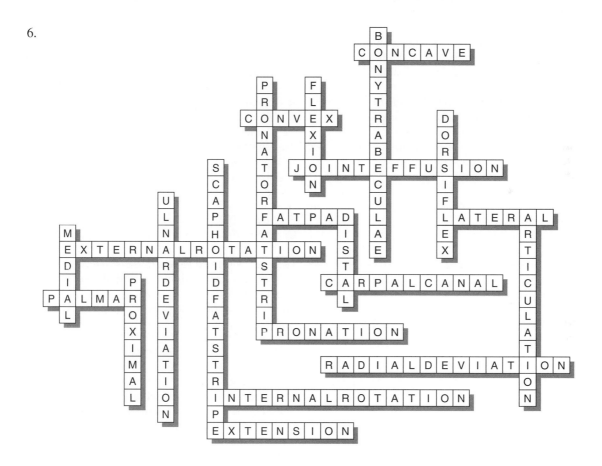

7. A. Distal phalanx
   B. Middle phalanx
   C. Interphalangeal joints
   D. Proximal phalanx
   E. Metacarpophalangeal joint
   F. Metacarpal head
8. A. Equal
   B. MP
   C. PIP
   D. Metacarpal

9. Shift the ring as far away from the affected area as possible. Note on the requisition that the patient was unable to remove the ring.
10. Flat
11. A. Externally into a medial oblique position
    B. The thumb prevents internal rotation.
12. A. Farther
    B. Greater
13. Second
14. Fifth

15. A. The collimator's light line
    B. Phalanx
    C. Metacarpal
16. Spread the fingers apart.
17. A. Parallel
    B. Perpendicular
18. A. Closed
    B. Foreshortened
19. A. Supinating
    B. Perpendicular
20. A. Perpendicular
    B. PIP
21. A. Phalanges
    B. Metacarpal
22. Within 0.5 inch (1.25 cm) of the finger skin line
23. The finger was internally rotated.
24. The finger was flexed.
25. Soft tissue width and concavity arc increased on the side of the finger facing the thumb. Rotate the hand and finger internally until they are flat against the IR.
26. The phalanges are foreshortened, the IP and MP joints are closed, and increased concavity is present on the side of the finger facing the third digit. Unflex the finger and internally rotate the hand until the finger and hand are flat against the IR.
27. A. Distal phalanx
    B. Middle phalanx
    C. Interphalangeal joints
    D. Proximal phalanx
    E. Metacarpophalangeal joint
    F. Metacarpal
28. A. Twice
    B. Concavity
    C. Open spaces
    D. PIP
29. A. Object-IR distance
    B. Proximal interphalangeal
    C. Interphalangeal
    D. Metacarpophalangeal
30. 45
31. A. Externally
    B. Internally or externally
    C. This rotation will result in the smallest OID.
32. So one can tightly collimate without clipping needed anatomic structures
33. To prevent soft tissue overlap from adjacent fingers
34. A. Extended
    B. Parallel
35. To prevent the finger from tilting toward the IR
36. A. Perpendicular
    B. PIP
37. The distal, middle, and proximal phalanges and half of the metacarpal
38. The finger was not rotated enough and was too close to a PA projection.
39. The finger was rotated closer to a lateral projection than a 45-degree PA oblique projection.
40. The fingers were not spread apart.
41. The finger was flexed or tilted toward the IR.
42. Phalangeal concavity and soft tissue width are equal on each side of the digit. Rotate the hand and finger externally until the finger is at a 45-degree angle to the IR.
43. The anterior aspects of the middle and proximal phalanges demonstrate midshaft concavity, whereas the posterior aspects of these phalanges demonstrate convexity. Internally rotate the hand until the finger is at a 45-degree angle to the IR. The fourth and fifth digits demonstrate superimposition. Separate the digits.
44. The phalanges are foreshortened, and the IP and MP joints are closed. The finger was allowed to bend down toward the IR. Fully extend the finger, using an immobilization prop if the patient is unable to maintain the position.
45. A. Distal phalanx
    B. Distal interphalangeal joint
    C. Middle phalanx
    D. Proximal interphalangeal joint
    E. Proximal phalanx
    F. Metacarpophalangeal joint
    G. Metacarpals
46. A. Anterior
    B. Posterior
    C. PIP joint
47. 90
48. A. Internally
    B. Internally
    C. Externally
    D. Externally
49. The hand is rotated to obtain the smallest OID.
50. Flex the hand into a tight fist, with the affected finger extended.
51. The distal, middle, and proximal phalanges and the metacarpal head
52. A device to extend the finger and move the proximal phalanx away from the other phalanges should not be used distal to a fracture, or displacement of the fracture may occur.
53. The hand was not flexed into a tight fist.
54. The finger was not in a lateral projection but was in a PA oblique projection.
55. The affected finger was allowed to tilt toward the IR.
56. Twice as much soft tissue and more phalangeal concavity are present on one side of the digit as on the other, there is soft tissue overlap of fourth and fifth fingers, and the DIP and PIP joints are closed. Flex the unaffected fingers into a fist, and increase the degree of external hand obliquity until the finger is in a lateral projection. Position the long axis of the finger parallel with the IR.
57. The unaffected fingers are superimposed over the proximal phalanx. Flex the unaffected fingers into a fist while the finger of interest remains extended. Use a positioning device if needed to help extend the finger if no proximal phalanx injury is suspected.

58. A. Distal phalanx
    B. Interphalangeal joint
    C. Proximal phalanx
    D. Metacarpophalangeal joint
    E. Metacarpal
    F. Carpometacarpal joint
    G. Carpal bone (trapezium)
59. A. Concavity
    B. Soft tissue
    C. Thumb
    D. Open spaces
    E. Medial palm
    F. MP joint
60. A. Internally
    B. Directly
61. Closer
62. To allow tight collimation without clipping the required anatomy
63. Extended
64. Draw the medial palm surface away from the thumb by using the opposite hand or a positioning device.
65. A. Perpendicular
    B. MP
66. Thumb
67. The distal and proximal phalanges, metacarpal, and CM joint
68. The hand was internally rotated more than needed to place the thumb in an AP projection.
69. The thumb was flexed.
70. The medial palm soft tissue was not drawn away from the proximal first metacarpal.
71. The medial palm soft tissue is superimposed over the proximal metacarpal and CM joint. Draw the medial palm away from the proximal metacarpal, using the opposite hand to maintain this positioning.
72. More soft tissue width and phalanx concavity are present on the side adjacent to the other digits, and the thumbnail is facing away from the second through fifth digits. Decrease the amount of internal rotation until the fingernail is flat against the IR.
73. A. Distal phalanx
    B. Interphalangeal joint
    C. Proximal phalanx
    D. Metacarpophalangeal joint
    E. First metacarpal
    F. Second metacarpal
    G. Carpometacarpal joint
74. A. Anterior
    B. Posterior
    C. Second
    D. MP joint
75. Flex
76. Align the long axis of the thumb with the collimator's longitudinal light line.
77. Align the thumb parallel with the IR.
78. Second proximal metacarpal
79. A. Perpendicular
    B. MP
    C. To the thumb

80. The distal and proximal phalanges, metacarpal, and CM joint
81. The hand was overflexed, and possibly the thumb was not in maximum abduction.
82. The patient's hand was not flexed enough, resulting in underrotation.
83. The proximal second and third metacarpals are superimposed over the proximal first metacarpal. Abduct the thumb and slightly decrease the amount of hand flexion while maintaining a lateral thumb.
84. Twice as much soft tissue and more phalangeal and metacarpal midshaft concavity are present on the side of the thumb facing the fingers. Increase the amount of hand flexion until the thumb is in a lateral projection.
85. A. Distal phalanx
    B. Interphalangeal joint
    C. Proximal phalanx
    D. Metacarpophalangeal joint
    E. First metacarpal
    F. Carpometacarpal joint
86. A. Twice
    B. Thumb
    C. First MP joint
87. 45
88. A. Extended
    B. Flat
89. The distal and proximal phalanges, metacarpal, and CM joint
90. 0.5 inch (1.25 cm) of skin line
91. The hand was not flat against the IR, causing the thumb to be rotated closer to a lateral projection.
92. The anterior aspect of the proximal phalanx and metacarpal demonstrates midshaft concavity, whereas the posterior aspect of the phalanx and metacarpal demonstrates slight convexity. Decrease the degree of hand flexion, positioning the hand flat against the IR.
93. The IP joint is closed and the distal phalanx is foreshortened. Extend the thumb until it is parallel with the IR.
94. A. Distal phalanx
    B. Interphalangeal joint
    C. Proximal phalanx
    D. Metacarpophalangeal joint
    E. Metacarpal
    F. Carpometacarpal joint
    G. Radius
    H. Ulna
    I. Carpals
    J. Carpometacarpal joint
    K. Metacarpal
    L. Metacarpophalangeal joint
    M. Proximal phalanx
    N. Proximal interphalangeal joint
    O. Middle phalanx
    P. Distal interphalangeal joint
    Q. Distal phalanx

95. A. Metacarpal heads
    B. Phalanges
    C. IP, MP, and CM
    D. Third MP
96. If it is around the area of interest, shift it as far away as possible. Note on the requisition that the patient was unable to remove the ring.
97. A. Pronate
    B. Flat
98. The thumb prevents this rotation.
99. The third digit and metacarpal should be aligned with the collimated field's long axis.
100. The joint spaces would be closed, and the phalanges and metacarpals would be foreshortened.
101. The thumb would move into a lateral projection.
102. The distal, middle, and proximal phalanges, metacarpals, and carpals and 1 inch (2.5 cm) of the forearm
103. The hand was externally rotated into a medial oblique position.
104. The fingers were not separated.
105. The fingers and hand were flexed.
106. The second through fifth metacarpal midshafts are more concave on one side than on the other, and the third through fifth metacarpal heads demonstrate slight superimposition. The IP joint spaces are closed, and the proximal and middle phalanges are foreshortened. Extend and internally rotate the hand, placing it flat against the IR.
107. The second through fifth phalanges are foreshortened, and the IP joint spaces are closed. Extend the hand and place it flat against the IR.
108. Angle the central ray distally until it is aligned perpendicular to the metacarpals. Prop the IR on an angled sponge until it is perpendicular to the central ray.
109. A. Interphalangeal joints
    B. Metacarpophalangeal joint
    C. Second metacarpal
    D. Radius
    E. Ulna
    F. Carpals
    G. Fifth metacarpal
    H. Phalanges
110. A. First and second
    B. Third through fifth
    C. Fourth and fifth
    D. Third MP joint
111. A. 45
    B. Externally
112. Because the wrist will demonstrate more obliquity than the hand when they are rotated
113. They must be extended so that they are aligned parallel with the IR.
114. A. Yes, the phalanges are not being evaluated.
    B. The reviewer already knows that no injury to the fingers is present, as long as no new injury has occurred.
115. The distal, middle, and proximal phalanges, metacarpals, and carpals and 1 inch (2.5 cm) of the forearm
116. The hand was not rotated 45 degrees but was closer to a PA projection.
117. The hand was rotated more than 45 degrees.
118. The fingers were flexed toward the IR.
119. The third through fifth metacarpal heads are demonstrated without superimposition, the phalanges are foreshortened, and the IP joints are closed. Externally rotate the hand until it forms a 45-degree angle with the IR, and elevate the distal fingers until they are aligned parallel with the IR.
120. The midshafts of the third through fifth metacarpals are superimposed. The phalanges are foreshortened, and the IP and MP joints are closed. Internally rotate the hand until it forms a 45-degree angle with the IR, and elevate the distal fingers until they are aligned parallel with the IR.
121. Angle the central ray perpendicular to the midcoronal plane and then adjust it 45 degrees medially. Prop the IR until it is aligned perpendicular to the central ray.
122. Angle the central ray perpendicular to the midcoronal plane and then adjust it 45 degrees medially. Prop the IR until it is aligned perpendicular to the central ray.
123. A. Distal phalanx
    B. Distal interphalangeal joint
    C. Middle phalanx
    D. Proximal interphalangeal joint
    E. Proximal phalanx
    F. Metacarpophalangeal joint
    G. Metacarpal
    H. Radius
    I. Ulna
    J. Carpals
    K. Metacarpals
    L. Metacarpophalangeal joint
124. A. Fifth
    B. Fifth
    C. MP joints
125. The thicknesses of the fingers and the metacarpals are so different in this position that uniform image density is difficult to obtain.
126. A. Anteriorly
    B. Posteriorly
127. PA projection to a slight PA oblique projection
128. A. Shortest
    B. Longest
129. Depress the thumb until it is parallel with the IR.
130. The distal, middle, and proximal phalanges, metacarpals, and carpals and 1 inch (2.5 cm) of the forearm
131. The patient's hand was externally rotated or supinated.
132. The patient's hand was internally rotated or pronated.

133. The patient's fingers were not fanned.
134. The second through fifth metacarpal midshafts are not all superimposed. The fifth metacarpal is demonstrated anteriorly. Internally rotate the hand until the metacarpals are superimposed.
135. The second through fifth metacarpal midshafts are demonstrated without superimposition. The second metacarpal is demonstrated anteriorly. Externally rotate the hand until the metacarpals are superimposed.
136. The second through fifth digits are extended and superimposed and the fifth metacarpal is slightly anterior to other metacarpals. Fan or spread the fingers as far apart as possible without superimposing the thumb and internally rotate the hand.
137. A. Trapezoid
    B. Trapezium
    C. Capitate
    D. Scaphoid
    E. Radial styloid
    F. Radius
    G. Ulna
    H. Ulnar styloid
    I. Lunate
    J. Triquetrum
    K. Pisiform
    L. Hamate
    M. Metacarpals
138. A. Scaphoid
    B. Radioulnar
    C. 0.25 inch
    D. Second through fifth
    E. Carpal bones
139. Convex in shape and located lateral to the scaphoid
140. A change in the convexity of this stripe may indicate joint effusion or fracture.
141. A. Lateral
    B. Parallel with the IR
142. A. Posterior
    B. Anterior
143. Slightly depress the proximal forearm.
144. Allow the proximal forearm to hang off the IR and table enough to depress the proximal forearm slightly.
145. Flex the hand until the metacarpals form a 10- to 15-degree angle with the IR.
146. A. Flexed
    B. Anteriorly
147. A. To prevent ulnar and radial deviation
    B. Half of the lunate will be distal to the radius
148. A. Anteriorly
    B. Foreshortened
    C. Medially
149. Posteriorly
150. Perpendicular
151. The carpal bones, one fourth of the distal ulna and radius, and half of the proximal metacarpals
152. The central ray centering should be the same, but the longitudinally collimated field should be opened to include the needed amount of forearm.

153. The patient's elbow was not in a lateral projection, and the humerus was not parallel with the IR.
154. The patient's wrist was externally rotated (to a PA oblique projection).
155. The patient's wrist was internally rotated (to a PA oblique projection).
156. The proximal forearm was elevated or central ray centered too proximally.
157. The patient's hand was extended, causing wrist flexion.
158. The patient's hand was overflexed, causing wrist extension.
159. The patient's wrist was radial deviated.
160. The patient's wrist was ulnar deviated.
161. The laterally located carpals and metacarpals are superimposed, and the radioulnar articulation is closed. Externally rotate the hand and wrist into a PA projection.
162. The medially located carpals and metacarpals are superimposed, and the radioulnar articulation is closed. Internally rotate the hand and wrist into a PA projection. The carpals are not centered in the collimated field. Move the central ray proximally 1 inch (2.5 cm).
163. The scaphoid is elongated, and the second through fourth CM joints are closed. Decrease hand flexion until the metacarpals are at a 10- to 15-degree angle with the IR.
164. The scaphoid is foreshortened, and the third metacarpal and midforearm are not aligned. Ulnar-deviate until the third metacarpal and midforearm are aligned.
165. A. Capitate
    B. Hamate
    C. Pisiform
    D. Triquetrum
    E. Lunate
    F. Ulnar styloid
    G. Ulna
    H. Radius
    I. Radial styloid
    J. Scaphoid
    K. Trapezoid
    L. Trapezium
    M. Carpometacarpal joint
    N. First metacarpal
    O. Trapeziotrapezoidal joint
166. A. Scaphoid fat
    B. Trapezoid
    C. Trapezium
    D. Second
    E. Ulnar styloid
    F. Carpal bones
167. A bony projection
168. A. 45
    B. Externally
169. Trapeziotrapezoidal
170. Trapezium
171. A. Third metacarpal
    B. Midforearm

172. The posterior margin will be projected distally to the anterior margin by 0.25 inch.
173. Posterior
174. A. In profile
    B. The elbow should be placed in a lateral projection and the humerus should be placed parallel with the IR.
175. Perpendicular
176. The carpal bones, one fourth of the distal forearm, and half of the proximal metacarpals
177. The patient's wrist was in less than a 45-degree externally rotated PA oblique projection.
178. The patient's wrist was in radial flexion deviation.
179. The patient's proximal forearm was depressed.
180. The trapezoid and trapezium are superimposed, the trapeziotrapezoidal joint space is obscured, and the trapezoid demonstrates minimal capitate superimposition. Increase the degree of obliquity until the wrist forms a 45-degree angle with the IR.
181. The scaphoid demonstrates foreshortening, and the long axis of the third metacarpal is not aligned with the midforearm and the second and third metacarpal joints are closed. Ulnar-deviate the wrist until the third metacarpal and midforearm are aligned and decrease hand flexion until metacarpals are at a 10- to 15-degree angle.
182. The trapezium demonstrates minimal trapezoidal superimposition, the capitate is superimposed by the trapezoid, and the trapeziotrapezoidal joint space is obscured. Decrease the degree of obliquity until the wrist forms a 45-degree angle with the IR.
183. The scaphoid is demonstrated with decreased foreshortening, the second carpometacarpal and scaphotrapezium joints are closed, and more than 0.25 inch (0.6 cm) of the radial articulating surface is demonstrated. Radial-deviate the wrist until the long axis of the third metacarpal and midforearm are aligned, decrease the amount of hand flexion until the metacarpals are at a 10- to 15-degree angle, and depress the proximal forearm until the forearm is parallel.
184. A. Capitate
    B. Lunate
    C. Ulnar styloid
    D. Radius
    E. Pisiform
    F. Distal scaphoid
    G. Trapezium
    H. First metacarpal
185. A. Pronator
    B. Anterior
    C. First metacarpal
    D. Posteriorly
    E. Trapezium
186. It is convex in shape and is located next to the anterior surface of the distal radius.
187. Changes in the shape and visualization of this stripe may indicate a fracture.
188. A. Distal scaphoid and pisiform
    B. Radius and ulna

189. A. Ulnar
    B. Lateromedial
    C. Pisiform
190. Align the long axes of the third metacarpal and the midforearm parallel with the IR.
191. A. Distal
    B. Proximal
192. Radial
193. Position the first metacarpal next to the second metacarpal and align it parallel with the forearm.
194. Position the humerus parallel with the IR and the elbow in a lateral projection.
195. Allow the humerus to hang without abduction, and position the elbow in an AP projection.
196. The position described in question 195, when the elbow is in an AP projection and the humerus is not abducted
197. Depress the distal first metacarpal until it is parallel with IR and at the same level as the second metacarpal.
198. Perpendicular
199. The carpal bones, one fourth of the distal ulna and radius, and half of the proximal metacarpals
200. Within 0.5 inch (1.25 cm) of skin line
201. A. AP projection
    B. Lateral projection
202. The patient's wrist was externally rotated (or supinated).
203. The patient's wrist was internally rotated (or pronated).
204. The wrist was in radial deviation.
205. The wrist was in ulnar deviation
206. The humerus was not abducted and the elbow was in an AP projection.
207. The first metacarpal was elevated.
208. The distal scaphoid is demonstrated anterior to the pisiform. Externally rotate the wrist until it is lateral. The ulnar styloid is in profile.
209. The distal scaphoid is demonstrated posterior to the pisiform. Internally rotate the wrist until it is lateral. The ulnar styloid is in profile.
210. The wrist is in extension. Place the wrist in a neutral position by positioning the first metacarpal adjacent to the second metacarpal and aligning the first metacarpal parallel with the forearm. The ulnar styloid is in profile.
211. The trapezium is superimposed by the proximal first metacarpal. Lower the first metacarpal until it is parallel with the IR and at the same level as the second metacarpal. The ulnar styloid is in profile.
212. The wrist is flexed and radial deviated. The pisiform is seen proximal to the scaphoid. Decrease wrist flexion by aligning the first metacarpal parallel with the forearm and ulnar deviate until the third metacarpal and mid-forearm are aligned. The ulnar styloid is in profile.
213. Angle the central ray posteriorly until it is parallel with the midcoronal plane.
214. A. Capitate
    B. Hamate
    C. Scaphocapitate joint
    D. Ulnar styloid

E. Radioulnar articulation
F. Scapholunate joint
G. Radioscaphoid joint
H. Scaphoid
I. Scaphotrapezoidal joint
J. Scaphotrapezium joint
K. Trapezium
L. Trapezoid
M. CM joint
N. First metacarpal

215. A. Scaphoid
     B. Scaphotrapezium
     C. Medially
     D. Scaphoid
216. Scaphoid fat stripe
217. A. First metacarpal
     B. Radius
     C. Radius
218. In ulnar deviation, the scaphoid has the space that it needs to move posteriorly and will demonstrate a decrease in foreshortening.
219. Position the patient's wrist in a 25-degree external PA oblique projection.
220. 15 degrees proximally
221. A. 20 degrees proximally
     B. Without ulnar deviation, the distal scaphoid is positioned anteriorly and the scaphoid demonstrates increased foreshortening.
222. Waist
223. A. Increase 5 to 10 degrees
     B. Decrease 5 to 10 degrees
224. No
225. Elevate the proximal forearm 5 to 6 degrees.
226. The carpal bones, radioulnar joint, and proximal first through fourth metacarpals
227. A. Distal fracture. The first metacarpal is not aligned with the ulna, so the starting central ray angulation should be 20 degrees. This should then be increased by 5 to 10 degrees to a maximum angle of 25 degrees. A 25-degree angle should be used.
     B. Proximal fracture. The first metacarpal and ulna are aligned, so the starting central ray angulation should be 15 degrees. This amount should then be decreased by 5 degrees because the fracture is close to the waist. A 10-degree angle should be used.
     C. Waist fracture. The first metacarpal is aligned with the ulna. A 15-degree central ray angulation should be used.
228. The wrist was externally rotated more than needed.
229. The patient's hand and fingers were flexed.
230. The scapholunate joint is closed and the capitate and hamate demonstrate a small degree of superimposition. Decrease the degree of external wrist rotation.
231. The scaphocapitate joint space is closed, the capitate and hamate are demonstrated without

superimposition, and the first metacarpal is not aligned with the radius. Increase the degree of medial obliquity until the wrist forms a 25-degree angle with the IR and, if the patient is capable, ulnar-deviate the wrist until the first metacarpal and radius are aligned.
232. The scaphotrapezium, scaphotrapezoid, and carpometacarpal joints are closed. Extend the fingers and place the hand flat against the IR.
233. A. First metacarpal
     B. Trapezium
     C. Scaphoid
     D. Capitate
     E. Carpal canal
     F. Hamulus of hamate
     G. Triquetrum
     H. Pisiform
234. A. Pisiform
     B. Carpal canal
235. A. Narrowing
     B. Fractures
236. The patient's hand is rotated 10 degrees internally until the fifth metacarpal is aligned perpendicular to the IR.
237. A. Vertically
     B. 25 degrees proximally
238. A. Increased
     B. 35 degrees
     C. Acute angle between the central ray and IR.
239. The patient's wrist and distal forearm were either in a PA projection or in slight external rotation.
240. The angle between the central ray and metacarpals was too great.
241. The angle between the central ray and metacarpals was too small.
242. The pisiform is superimposed over the hamulus of the hamate. Internally (toward the radius) rotate the hand until the fifth metacarpal is vertical.
243. The metacarpal bases obscure the bases of the hamate's hamulus process, pisiform, and scaphoid. Increase the central ray angle until it is 15 degrees from the palmar surface or increase the amount of wrist hyperextension by pulling the fingers posteriorly until the metacarpals are vertical.
244. The carpal canal is not demonstrated in its entirety, and the carpal bones are foreshortened. Decrease the central ray angle until it is within 15 degrees of the palmar surface.
245. A. Radioscaphoid joint
     B. Radial styloid
     C. Radius
     D. Radial tuberosity
     E. Radial head
     F. Capitulum-radial joint
     G. Lateral epicondyle
     H. Olecranon fossa
     I. Medial epicondyle
     J. Olecranon
     K. Ulnar midshaft

L. Radioulnar articulation
M. Ulnar head
N. Ulnar styloid
O. Fifth metacarpal base
246. Position the wrist at the anode end and the elbow at the cathode end of the tube.
247. So they will still be included on the image when they are projected by the diverged beams used to record them
248. It is located 0.75 inch (2 cm) distal to the medial epicondyle.
249. A. Forearm midshaft
    B. Perpendicular
    C. Midforearm
250. The radius, ulna, wrist and elbow joints, and forearm soft tissue
251. A. Medially
    B. Ulna
252. The joint that is closer to the area of interest or near the fracture site should be positioned into an AP projection, whereas the other joint is positioned as close to an AP projection as possible.
253. Humeral epicondyles
254. A. 0.25 inch (0.6 cm)
    B. Humeral epicondyles
255. Because the diverged x-ray beams used to record this joint do not align parallel with the joint
256. Parallel
257. Supinate the hand and wrist, placing them in an AP projection.
258. The elbow was accurately positioned, but the hand and wrist were internally rotated.
259. The wrist and hand were accurately positioned, but the elbow was externally rotated.
260. The elbow is accurately positioned, but the hand was pronated.
261. The wrist was internally rotated and the elbow was laterally rotated.
262. The lateral and PA projections of the forearm reflect accurate positioning. When forearm images are obtained on a patient with a fracture, and the patient is unable to position the distal and proximal forearm in a true position simultaneously, the joint closer to the fracture site should be placed in the true position. For these images, the wrist joint demonstrates accurate positioning.
263. The radial head is demonstrated without being superimposed over the ulna. Internally rotate the elbow until an imaginary line connecting the humeral epicondyles is aligned parallel with the IR while maintaining the same wrist positioning.
264. The radial head is demonstrated without superimposition over the ulna. Align the central ray perpendicular to an imaginary line connecting the humeral epicondyles; this will require the central ray to be adjusted medially. Prop the IR as needed to align it perpendicular to the central ray.
265. A. Ulnar styloid
    B. Ulna

C. Coronoid
D. Olecranon
E. Humerus
F. Elbow joint
G. Radial head
H. Radius
I. Pisiform
J. Distal scaphoid
266. Position the wrist at the anode end and the elbow at the cathode end of the tube.
267. Forearm midpoint
268. The radius, ulna, wrist and elbow joints, and forearm soft tissue
269. A. Distal
    B. Superimposed
270. Ulnar (medial)
271. The distal scaphoid will be anterior to the pisiform.
272. A. It will be demonstrated in profile posteriorly.
    B. Place the elbow in a lateral projection with the humeral epicondyles aligned parallel with the IR.
273. A. No
    B. Supinate the hand to place the tuberosity in profile anteriorly, and pronate the hand to place the tuberosity in profile posteriorly.
274. A. Thick or muscular proximal forearm
    B. Thick or muscular distal forearm
275. The radial head will be too posterior to the coronoid.
276. Place the elbow and proximal forearm in a lateral projection and allow the distal forearm to rotate as close to a lateral projection as the patient will allow.
277. The arm could have been externally rotated a slight amount to superimpose the distal radius and ulna; otherwise, the image is accurately positioned.
278. The patient's hand and wrist were externally rotated.
279. The patient's hand and wrist were internally rotated, and the proximal humerus was depressed more than the distal humerus.
280. The patient's elbow was not in a lateral projection, but was closer to an AP projection.
281. The patient's wrist and hand were in external rotation.
282. The proximal humerus was elevated.
283. The radial head is posterior to the coronoid and the distal scaphoid is anterior to the pisiform. Depress the proximal humerus until the humerus is parallel with the IR, and externally rotate the wrist until it is in a lateral projection.
284. Adjust the central ray angle posteriorly until it is aligned parallel with the midcoronal plane. Prop the IR as needed to align it perpendicular to the central ray.
285. A. Olecranon
    B. Lateral epicondyle
    C. Capitulum-radial joint
    D. Radial head
    E. Radial neck
    F. Radius

G. Ulna
H. Radial tuberosity
I. Coronoid
J. Medial trochlea
K. Medial epicondyle
L. Olecranon fossa
M. Humerus

286. A. Profile
B. 0.25 inch (0.6 cm)
C. Medially
D. Elbow joint

287. Medial and lateral humeral epicondyles

288. Lateral

289. The wrist and hand position

290. A. Central ray accurately centered to joint
B. Forearm aligned parallel with the IR

291. Find where the central ray was positioned by diagonally connecting the corners on the collimated elbow image. The two lines connect where the central ray was located. Determine if the olecranon is within the olecranon fossa.

292. Do two AP views—one with the humerus parallel with the IR and one with the forearm parallel with the IR.

293. A. Perpendicular
B. 0.75 inch (2 cm)
C. Distal
D. Because it protrudes more than the lateral epicondyle

294. The elbow joint, one fourth of the proximal forearm and distal humerus, and the lateral soft tissue

295. Dislocated elbow. Note that the radial head and capitulum do not articulate.

296. The patient's arm was internally (medially) rotated.

297. The patient's arm was externally (laterally) rotated.

298. The hand was pronated.

299. The distal forearm was elevated.

300. The humeral epicondyles are not in profile, and the radial head superimposes over the ulna by more than 0.25 inch (0.6 cm). Externally rotate the elbow until the humeral epicondyles are at equal distances to the IR.

301. The humeral epicondyles are not in profile, and the radial head demonstrates less than 0.25 inch (0.6 cm) of ulnar superimposition. Internally rotate the elbow until the humeral epicondyles are at equal distances from the IR.

302. The capitulum–radial joint is closed and the radial head articulating surface is demonstrated. If the patient's condition allows, fully extend the elbow. If the patient is unable to extend the elbow, take the AP exposure with the forearm parallel with the IR.

303. Angle the central ray laterally until it is aligned perpendicular to an imaginary line connecting the humeral epicondyles. Prop the IR as needed to align it perpendicular to the central ray and parallel with the humeral epicondyle line.

304. Angle the central ray medially until it is aligned perpendicular to an imaginary line connecting the humeral epicondyles, center the central ray to the elbow joint, and prop the IR as needed to align it perpendicular to the central ray and parallel with the humeral epicondyle line.

305. A. Medial epicondyle
B. Medial trochlea
C. Coronoid
D. Radial tuberosity
E. Radial head

306. A. Radial tuberosity
B. Ulna
C. Radial head
D. Capitulum

307. A. Capitulum
B. Radial tuberosity
C. Ulna
D. Coronoid process
E. Elbow joint

308. A. The forearm was not positioned parallel with the IR.
B. The central ray was not centered to the elbow joint.

309. The olecranon will move away from the olecranon fossa with elbow flexion.

310. A. Forearm
B. Forearm
C. Humerus
D. Humerus
E. Forearm

311. 45 degrees

312. Externally

313. A. Perpendicular
B. 0.75 inch (2 cm)
C. Medial epicondyle

314. The elbow joint, one fourth of the distal humerus and proximal forearm, and the lateral soft tissue

315. The distal forearm was elevated.

316. The patient's arm was rotated less than 45 degrees.

317. The patient's arm was rotated more than 45 degrees.

318. The patient's arm was rotated less than 45 degrees.

319. The patient's arm was rotated more than 45 degrees.

320. A small portion of the radial head and tuberosity is superimposed over the ulna. Increase the degree of external obliquity until the humeral epicondyles are at a 45-degree angle to the IR.

321. The capitulum–radial head joint is closed and a small portion of the radial head is superimposed over the ulna. If the patient's condition allows, fully extend the arm and, if the patient is unable to extend the arm fully, position the forearm parallel with the IR. Increase the degree of external obliquity until the humeral epicondyles are at a 45-degree angle to the IR.

322. The radial head is demonstrated lateral to the coronoid process without complete superimposition of the ulna and the capitulm-radial head joint is closed. Increase the degree of internal obliquity until the humeral epicondyles are at a 45-degree angle to the IR and position the forearm parallel with the IR.

323. The radial head is demonstrated lateral to the coronoid process without complete superimposition of the ulna, the capitulum–radial joint is closed, and the articulating surface of the radial head is demonstrated. Increase the degree of internal obliquity until the humeral epicondyles are at a 45-degree angle with the IR. If the patient's condition allows, fully extend the arm and, if the patient is unable to extend the arm fully, position the forearm parallel with the IR.

324. A. Medial trochlea
   B. Coronoid
   C. Radial head
   D. Radius
   E. Ulna
   F. Trochlear notch
   G. Olecranon process
   H. Capitulum
   I. Trochlear sulcus
   J. Humerus

325. A. Supinator
   B. Trochlear sulcus
   C. Anterior
   D. Profile
   E. Elbow joint

326. A. Anterior fat pad, anterior to the distal humerus
   B. Posterior fat pad, within the olecranon fossa
   C. Supinator fat stripe, seen parallel to the anterior aspect of the distal radius
   D. Joint effusion and elbow injury

327. The posterior fat pad can be used as a diagnosing tool only when the elbow is flexed 90 degrees and the olecranon is out of the fossa.

328. A. Capitulum
   B. Trochlear sulcus
   C. Medial aspect of the trochlea
   D. Trochlear sulcus
   E. Medial trochlea
   F. It will close it.

329. The capitulum would be distal to the medial trochlea.

330. The radial head would be distal to the coronoid, and the capitulum would be anterior to the medial trochlea.

331. The radial head will be proximal to the coronoid.

332. The radial head will be anterior to the coronoid, and the capitulum will be proximal to the medial trochlea.

333. A. Superimposed by the radius
   B. In profile, anteriorly
   C. In profile, posteriorly
   D. Superimposed by the radius

334. A. Perpendicular
   B. 0.75 inch (2 cm)
   C. Distal

335. The elbow joint, one fourth of the proximal forearm and distal humerus, and the surrounding soft tissue

336. The patient's arm was in extension.

337. The patient's hand and wrist were supinated.

338. The patient's proximal humerus was elevated.

339. The patient's proximal humerus was depressed.

340. The patient's distal forearm was not adequately elevated.

341. The patient's distal forearm was elevated more than needed.

342. The radial head is proximal to the coronoid (capitulum is posterior to the medial trochlea), and the radial tuberosity is seen anteriorly. Depress the distal forearm until the humeral epicondyles are aligned perpendicular to the IR, and internally rotate the distal forearm until the wrist is in a lateral projection.

343. The radial head is distal to the coronoid (capitulum is anterior to the medial trochlea). Elevate the distal forearm until the humeral epicondyles are aligned perpendicular to the IR.

344. The radial head is distal and posterior to the coronoid (capitulum is distal and anterior to the medial trochlea), the radial tuberosity is demonstrated anteriorly, and the elbow is not flexed to 90 degrees. Elevate the distal forearm and depress the proximal humerus until the humeral epicondyles are aligned perpendicular to the IR, externally rotate the distal forearm until the wrist is in a lateral projection, and flex the elbow to 90 degrees.

345. The radial head is proximal and anterior to the coronoid (capitulum is posterior and proximal to the medial trochlea) and the radial tuberosity is visible posteriorly. Depress the distal forearm and elevate the proximal humerus until the humeral epicondyles are aligned perpendicular to the IR, and externally rotate the distal forearm until the wrist is in a lateral projection.

346. The radial head is distal and anterior to the coronoid (capitulum is anterior and proximal to the medial trochlea). Elevate the distal forearm and proximal humerus until the humeral epicondyles are aligned perpendicular to the IR.

347. Adjust the central ray angle posteriorly with the humerus (proximally on the forearm) until it is aligned parallel with a line connecting the humeral epicondyles. Prop the IR as needed to align it perpendicular to the central ray and to a line connecting the humeral epicondyles.

348. Adjust the angle anteriorly on the humerus (distally on the forearm) until it is aligned parallel with the humeral epicondyles. Prop the IR as needed to align it perpendicular to the central ray and to a line connecting the humeral epicondyles.

349. A. Capitulum
   B. Capitulum–radial joint
   C. Radial head
   D. Radial tuberosity
   E. Coronoid
   F. Medial trochlea

350. A. Medial trochlea
   B. Open
   C. Radial head

351. Lateral projection

352. Radial head and coronoid and the capitulum and medial trochlea
353. The radial head will be proximal to the coronoid, and the capitulum will be posterior to the medial trochlea.
354. The capitulum will be anterior to the medial trochlea.
355. A. Perpendicular
    B. 45
    C. Proximally
    D. Radial head
    E. Capitulum
356. Radial tuberosity
357. A. The radial tuberosity will be in profile posteriorly, the lateral surface of the radial head will be in profile anteriorly, and the medial surface will be in profile posteriorly.
    B. The radial tuberosity will not be in profile but will be superimposed by the radius. The anterior surface of the radial head will appear in profile anteriorly, and the posterior surface will appear in profile posteriorly.
358. A. Lateral
    B. Medial
359. Radial head, located 0.75 inch (2 cm) distal to the lateral epicondyle
360. The proximal forearm, distal humerus, and surrounding soft tissue
361. The patient's distal forearm was positioned too close to the IR.
362. The patient's distal forearm was positioned too far away from the IR.
363. The capitulum–radial joint space is closed, the radial head is demonstrated distal to the coronoid process, and the capitulum is demonstrated too far anterior to the medial trochlea. Elevate the distal forearm until the humeral epicondyles are aligned perpendicular to the IR.
364. The capitulum–radial joint space is closed and the radial head is too distal to the coronoid process (capitulum is too anterior to the medial trochlea). The radial head is not anterior enough to the coronoid (capitulum is not proximal enough to the medial trochlea). Elevate the distal forearm and elevate the proximal humerus.
365. First, align the central ray parallel with an imaginary line connecting the humeral epicondyles, and then adjust the central ray 45 degrees proximally (toward the humerus). The resulting angle will be more than 45 degrees. Prop the IR as needed to align it perpendicular to the humeral epicondyles.
366. The central ray was aligned at an angle halfway between the humerus and forearm instead of toward the proximal humerus.
367. A. Greater tubercle
    B. Lesser tubercle
    C. Humeral midshaft
    D. Medial epicondyle
    E. Lateral epicondyle
    F. Radial head
    G. Ulna
368. A. 10
    B. 70
369. Position the elbow at the anode end of the x-ray tube and the shoulder at the cathode end.
370. A. 0.25 inch (0.6 cm)
    B. Humeral epicondyles
371. A. Greater
    B. Humeral head
    C. Lesser tubercle
372. A. Arm
    B. Humeral epicondyles
373. A. Forced external rotation may result in an increased risk of radial nerve damage.
    B. Rotate the patient 35 to 40 degrees toward the affected side for the proximal humerus, and rotate the patient toward the affected side until the humeral epicondyles are parallel with the IR when the distal humerus is of interest.
374. Abduct the humerus and place it diagonally on the IR.
375. To ensure that the joints will be included after the beam's divergence projects the elbow joint distally and the shoulder joint proximally
376. A. Located at the same level as the coracoid
    B. Located 0.75 inch (2 cm) distal to the epicondyles
377. Humeral midshaft
378. The humerus, shoulder and elbow joints, and lateral humeral soft tissue
379. The patient's arm was externally rotated.
380. The patient's arm was internally rotated.
381. The greater tubercle and the humeral epicondyles are not in profile, and the radial head is superimposed over more than 0.25 inch (0.6 cm) of the ulna. Externally rotate the arm until the humeral epicondyles are at equal distances to the IR.
382. The greater and lesser tubercles are almost superimposed and the ulna is demonstrated without radial head superimposition. Internally rotate the arm until the humeral epicondyles are at equal distances from the IR.
383. Lateromedial
384. A. Lesser tubercle
    B. Humeral shaft
    C. Medial trochlea
    D. Coronoid
    E. Radial tuberosity
    F. Radial head
    G. Capitulum
385. Mediolateral
386. A. Lesser tubercle
    B. Humeral shaft
    C. Capitulum
    D. Radial head
    E. Radial tuberosity
    F. Capitulum–radial joint
    G. Medial trochlea
387. Mediolateral

388. A. Lesser
    B. Medially
    C. Lateromedial
389. Mediolateral
390. The effect of the x-ray's divergence on the ana-
    tomic structure positioned farthest from the IR
391. A. Arm
    B. Humeral epicondyles
392. A. PA oblique (scapular Y) projection
    B. Transthoracic lateral projection
393. The lesser tubercle will be in profile medially.
394. They will be magnified and may be superimposed
    over the area of interest.
395. Humeral midshaft
396. The humerus, elbow and shoulder joints, and
    lateral soft tissue
397. The patient's torso was not in a PA projection but
    was rotated toward the affected humerus.
398. The lesser tubercle is not in profile and the
    capitulum is demonstrated posterior to the medial
    trochlea. Move the distal humerus away from the
    IR until the humeral epicondyles are perpendicular
    to the IR.
399. The image demonstrates a lateral projection, as
    indicated by the optimal distal humerus position-
    ing. The density is lighter at the proximal humerus
    than at the distal humerus, preventing proximal
    humerus visualization. Rotate the torso away from
    the proximal humerus into a PA projection.

CHAPTER 5   SHOULDER

1. A. With the anterior surface up and posterior surface
    down; marker is correct.
    B. As if the patient is standing in an upright posi-
    tion; marker is correct.
    C. As if the patient is standing in an upright posi-
    tion; marker is reversed.
2. Soft tissue and bony trabecular patterns and cortical
    outlines of the shoulder structures
3. A. 65-75
    B. 40 to 48 inches
4. Use a compensating filter over the acromion process
    and lateral clavicular end.
5. When the part thickness measurement is more than
    4 inches (10 cm)
6. A. Superior scapular angle
    B. Clavicle
    C. Acromion process
    D. Humeral head
    E. Greater tubercle
    F. Glenoid cavity
    G. Superolateral border of the scapula
    H. Thorax
    I. Coracoid process
7. A. Thorax
    B. Vertebral column
    C. Midclavicle

D. Greater
E. Medially
F. Laterally
G. Medially
H. Lesser
8. A. Describes an image that has too much density
    because the mAs was too high
    B. Backward movement of the shoulder
    C. Condition that results when the humeral head
    has been pulled away from the glenoid cavity
9. A. Position the arrow so it is pointing toward the
    torso.
    B. Position the arrow so it is pointing away from
    the torso.
10. Position the shoulders at equal distances from the
    imaging table or IR holder.
11. A. 35 to 45 degrees
    B. Lateral
12. Glenoid cavity
13. Anterior
14. The midcoronal plane should be positioned parallel
    with the IR.
15. Midclavicle
16. Angle the central ray cephalically until it is perpen-
    dicular to the scapular body.
17. A. Laterally
    B. Superiorly
18. A. Greater tubercle
    B. Head
19. A. Position the humeral epicondyles at a 45-degree
    angle with the IR.
    B. Position the humeral epicondyles perpendicular
    to the IR.
    C. Position the humeral epicondyles parallel with
    the IR.
    D. Position the humeral epicondyles parallel with
    the IR
20. Do not move the patient's arm. The image should be
    taken with the arm positioned as is.
21. A. Perpendicular
    B. Inferior to the coracoid process
22. The glenohumeral joint, lateral two thirds of the
    clavicle, proximal third of the humerus, and superior
    scapula
23. The coracoid process is located 1 inch (2.5 cm)
    inferior to the midpoint of the lateral half of the
    clavicle.
24. The patient was rotated toward the affected
    shoulder.
25. The patient was rotated toward the unaffected
    shoulder.
26. The patient's upper midcoronal plane was tilted
    away from the IR.
27. The patient's humerus was externally rotated until
    the humeral epicondyles were positioned parallel
    with the IR.
28. The patient's humerus was rotated internally until
    the humeral epicondyles were aligned perpendicular
    to the IR.

29. The superior scapular angle is demonstrated superior to the clavicle and the lesser tubercle is demonstrated in profile medially. Tilt the upper midcoronal plane posteriorly until it is aligned parallel with the IR and, if a neutral shoulder is indicated, externally rotate the arm until the humeral epicondyles are at a 45-degree angle to the IR.

30. The superior scapular angle is demonstrated inferior to the clavicle. Tilt the upper midcoronal plane anteriorly until it is aligned parallel with the IR.

31. The medial clavicular end is superimposed over the vertebral column, the superior scapular angle is demonstrated superior to the clavicle, and the lesser tubercle is demonstrated in profile medially. Rotate the patient toward the left shoulder until the shoulders are at equal distances from the IR, and tilt the upper midcoronal plane posteriorly until it is aligned parallel with the IR. If a neutral shoulder is indicated, externally rotate the arm until the humeral epicondyles are at a 45-degree angle to the IR.

32. A. Greater tubercle
    B. Acromion process
    C. Scapular spine
    D. Glenohumeral joint
    E. Clavicle
    F. Coracoid process
    G. Humeral head
    H. Lesser tubercle

33. A. Glenoid cavity
    B. Inferior
    C. Parallel
    D. 45-degree angle

34. A. Glenohumeral joint
    B. Scapula

35. 30- to 35-degree

36. Align the central ray at a 30- to 35-degree angle with the lateral body surface.

37. A. The angle should be decreased to approximately 20 degrees.
    B. Because the humerus has not been abducted enough to move the glenoid cavity superiorly

38. Position the IR vertically at the top of the affected shoulder so it is aligned perpendicular to the central ray.

39. When it is abducted less than 90 degrees

40. A. Lesser tubercle in partial profile anteriorly and posterolateral aspect of the humeral head in profile posteriorly
    B. Humeral head and neck in profile anteriorly and the greater tubercle in profile posteriorly
    C. Humeral head and neck in profile posteriorly and the lesser tubercle in profile anteriorly

41. A. Hill-Sachs defect
    B. Arm is externally rotated until humeral epicondyles are at a 45-degree angle with floor

42. A. Horizontal
    B. Coracoid process

43. The glenoid cavity, coracoid process, acromion process, scapular spine, and one third of the proximal humerus

44. Posterior

45. A. Coracoid process
    B. Glenoid cavity
    C. Proximal humerus

46. A. The humeral epicondyles were at a 45-degree angle with the floor.
    B. The humeral epicondyles were perpendicular to the floor.

47. The angle formed between the lateral body surface and the central ray was smaller than needed to align the central ray parallel with the glenohumeral joint space.

48. The angle formed between the lateral body surface and the central ray was larger than needed to align the central ray parallel with the glenohumeral joint.

49. The humerus was externally rotated enough to position the humeral epicondyles perpendicular to the floor.

50. The patient's shoulder was not adequately elevated with a sponge or washcloth.

51. The glenoid fossa is demonstrated lateral to the base of the coracoid process. Increase the angle formed by the lateral body and central ray.

52. The inferior margin of the glenoid fossa is demonstrated medial to the coracoid process base. Decrease the angle formed by the lateral body and the central ray.

53. The coracoid is not included in the image. Laterally flex the neck toward the right shoulder, and position the IR more medially.

54. A. Clavicle
    B. Scapular neck
    C. Coracoid process
    D. Humeral head
    E. Glenohumeral joint

55. A. Profile
    B. 0.25 inch (0.6 cm)
    C. Glenohumeral joint

56. Forward movement of the shoulder

57. A. Sternoclavicular
    B. Acromioclavicular

58. A. Coracoid process
    B. Acromion angle

59. A. The patient is kyphotic.
    B. The patient is imaged in a recumbent position.
    C. The patient leans against the IR while in an upright position.

60. A. The lateral coracoid process will be superimposed over the humeral head by approximately 0.25 inch (0.6 cm).
    B. On overrotation, the coracoid process is superimposed over more than 0.25 inch (0.6 cm) of the humeral head.
    C. On underrotation, the coracoid process is superimposed over less than 0.25 inch (0.6 cm) of the humeral head.

61. Vertically

62. A. Perpendicular
    B. Inferior
    C. Medial
    D. Coracoid process

63. The glenoid cavity, humeral head, coracoid process, acromion process, and lateral clavicle
64. The patient was rotated more than needed to obtain an open glenohumeral joint space.
65. The patient was rotated less than needed to obtain an open glenohumeral joint space.
66. The patient was rotated more than needed to obtain an open glenohumeral joint space.
67. The glenohumeral joint space is closed, more than 0.25 inch (0.6 cm) of the lateral tip of the coracoid process is superimposed over the humeral head, and the clavicle demonstrates excessive transverse foreshortening. Decrease the degree of patient obliquity.
68. The glenohumeral joint space is closed, the lateral tip of the coracoid process is not superimposed over the humeral head, and the clavicle demonstrates little foreshortening. Increase the degree of patient obliquity.
69. A. Humeral head
    B. Coracoid process
    C. Clavicle
    D. Superior scapular angle
    E. Acromion process
    F. Glenoid cavity
    G. Scapular body
70. A. Superimposed
    B. Acromion process
    C. Coracoid process
    D. Clavicle
    E. Midscapular body
71. A. Least scapular and proximal humerus magnification
    B. Greater scapular and proximal humerus detail sharpness
72. A. Acromion process
    B. Coracoid process
    C. Scapular body
    D. Glenoid cavity
73. Vertebral (medial) border
74. A. Acromion process angle
    B. Coracoid process
75. A. Shoulder dislocation
    B. Proximal humeral fracture
76. A. Affected
    B. Unaffected
77. The cortical outline of the lateral border is thicker than the cortical outline of the vertebral border.
78. Identify the scapular border positioned closest to the thoracic cavity.
79. The humeral head should be superimposed over the glenoid cavity and the humeral shaft should be superimposed over the scapular body.
80. Yes
81. A. Anteriorly and beneath the coracoid process
    B. Posteriorly and beneath the acromion process

82. Position the midcoronal plane vertically so it is parallel with the IR.
83. A. Kyphosis
    B. Angle the central ray caudally until it is perpendicular to the scapular body.
    C. Angle the central ray cephalically until it is perpendicular to the scapular body.
84. A. Perpendicular
    B. Vertebral (medial)
    C. Inferior scapular angle
    D. Acromion angle
85. The entire scapula and proximal humerus
86. The patient was rotated more than needed to superimpose the scapular body.
87. The patient was rotated less than needed to superimpose the scapular body.
88. The patient's upper midcoronal plane was leaning toward the IR.
89. The lateral and vertebral borders of the scapula are demonstrated without superimposition. The vertebral scapular border is demonstrated next to the ribs and the lateral border is demonstrated laterally. Increase the degree of patient obliquity.
90. The lateral and vertebral borders of the scapula are demonstrated without superimposition. The lateral border is demonstrated next to the ribs and the vertebral border is demonstrated laterally. Decrease the degree of patient rotation.
91. The superior scapular angle is demonstrated superior to the clavicle. Tilt the patient's upper midcoronal plane posteriorly until it is parallel with the IR.
92. The lateral and vertebral borders of the scapula are demonstrated without superimposition. The vertebral scapular border is demonstrated next to the ribs and the lateral border appears laterally. Increase the degree of patient obliquity.
93. A. Greater tubercle
    B. Posterolateral humeral head
    C. Conoid tubercle
    D. Coracoid process
    E. Clavicle
    F. Lesser tubercle
94. A. Conoid tubercle
    B. Posterolateral
    C. Coracoid process
    D. Coracoid process
95. A. Hill-Sachs
    B. Posterolateral
96. A. Vertical
    B. On top of the patient's head
97. Coracoid process
98. Humeral head, coracoid process, lateral clavicle, and glenoid cavity
99. The central ray was angled less than the required 10-degree cephalic angle.

100. The distal humerus is tilted laterally.
101. The humerus was elevated to less than a vertical position
102. The coracoid process is seen inferior to the clavicle and the humeral shaft demonstrates increased foreshortening. Place a 10-degree cephalic angulation on the central ray.
103. The posterolateral humeral head is obscured and the humeral shaft demonstrates increased foreshortening and a decrease in density. Elevate the humerus until it is placed at a 90-degree position with the patient's torso.
104. The posterolateral humeral head and lesser tubercle are obscured. The greater tubercle is in profile laterally. Tilt the distal humerus laterally until it is parallel with midsagittal plane.
105. A. Scapular body
    B. Glenoid cavity
    C. Humeral head
    D. Acromion process
    E. Clavicle
    F. Superior scapular angle
    G. Coracoid process
    H. Thorax
106. A Superimposed
    B. Scapular body
    C. Acromion
    D. Coracoid
    E. Coracoid process
    F. Clavicle
    G. AC joint
107. Anterior
108. A. Vertebral
    B. 45 degrees
109. The lateral border is thick, with two cortical outlines that are separated by approximately 0.25 inch (0.6 cm), whereas the cortical outline of the vertebral border demonstrates a single thin line.
110. Inferior
111. A. Midcoronal
    B. 10 to 15 degrees caudally
112. Acromion and coracoid processes, lateral clavicle, superior scapular spine, and half of the scapular body
113. The patient was rotated more than needed to superimpose the scapular body.
114. The upper midcoronal plane was tilted toward the IR and/or the central ray was not angled 10 to 15 degrees caudally.
115. The lateral and vertebral borders of the scapula are demonstrated without superimposition, and the glenoid cavity is not demonstrated on end but is seen medially. The lateral scapular border is demonstrated next to the ribs and the vertebral border is demonstrated laterally. Decrease patient obliquity until the scapular borders are superimposed.
116. The lateral clavicle and acromion process are demonstrated less than 0.5 inch (1.25 cm) superior to the humeral head and supraspinous fossa, and the superior scapular spine appears superior to the clavicle. Tilt the midcoronal plane posteriorly until it is vertical, and place a 10- to 15-degree caudal angle on the central ray.
117. A. Acromion process
    B. Lateral clavicle
    C. Coracoid process
    D. Superior scapular angle
    E. Vertebral border of scapula
    F. Medial clavicle
    G. Vertebral column
118. A. Lateral edge
    B. Superior scapular angle
    C. Midclavicle
119. Over or under the lateral clavicular end
120. A. PA
    B. It results in increased patient discomfort and difficulty in clavicle palpation.
121. Both shoulders should be placed at equal distances from the table or IR holder.
122. When the midcoronal plane is not positioned parallel with the IR
123. A. Perpendicular
    B. Medial
    C. Lateral
124. The lateral, middle, and medial thirds of the clavicle and acromion process
125. The patient was rotated away from the affected shoulder.
126. The patient was rotated toward the affected shoulder.
127. The patient's upper midcoronal plane was leaning away from the IR.
128. The superior scapular angle is demonstrated superior to the clavicle. Tilt the upper midcoronal plane posteriorly until it is aligned parallel with the IR.
129. The medial clavicular end is superimposed over the vertebral column and the vertebral border of the scapula is positioned away from the thoracic cavity. Rotate the patient toward the affected shoulder.
130. A. Acromion process
    B. Lateral clavicle
    C. Middle clavicle
    D. Superior scapular angle
    E. Medial clavicle
131. A. Medial
    B. First, second, or third
    C. Acromion process
    D. Midclavicle
132. A 15- to 30-degree cephalic angle
133. Middle third of the clavicle
134. A. Medial
    B. Lateral
135. The lateral, middle, and medial thirds of the clavicle and the acromion process
136. The patient was rotated toward the affected shoulder.
137. The central ray was not angled enough cephalically.

138. The lateral and medial thirds of the clavicle are superimposed over the scapula, and the medial clavicular end is superimposed over the vertebral column. Increase the degree of cephalic central ray angulation, and rotate the patient toward the right shoulder until the shoulders are at equal distances from the IR.
139. A. Superior scapular angle
    B. Scapular spine
    C. Lateral clavicle
    D. AC joint
    E. Acromial apex
140. A. Word or arrow
    B. Horizontal
    C. Acromion process
    D. Scapular spine
    E. AC joint
141. A. Act of holding weights or standing to place pressure on the structure
    B. Regarding only one side
    C. Regarding both sides
142. A. To identify the weight-bearing from the non–weight-bearing image
    B. Laterally within the collimated field and pointing downward if it is an arrow
143. Both shoulders should be positioned at equal distances from the upright IR holder.
144. To evaluate the AC joint for possible ligament injury
145. Separation between the acromion process and clavicle will be increased when one compares the weight-bearing with the non–weight-bearing images.
146. 5 to 8 lb
147. A. When the upper midcoronal plane is tilted away from the IR and is positioned parallel with the IR
    B. The middle and lateral clavicles are superimposed over the acromion process and scapular spine.
148. A. Inferior
    B. Lateral tip of the clavicle
149. The AC joint, lateral clavicle, and acromion process
150. To ensure that the same centering is obtained and the x-ray beam's divergence does not result in a false reading
151. The patient is rotated toward the affected AC joint.
152. The superior scapular angle is demonstrated superior to the clavicle. Tilt the upper midcoronal plane posteriorly until it is parallel with the IR.
153. A. Acromion process
    B. Lesser tubercle
    C. Glenoid cavity
    D. Glenoid neck
    E. Lateral border
    F. Inferior angle
    G. Vertebral border
    H. Scapular body

I. Supraspinous fossa
J. Scapular spine
K. Coracoid process
L. Superior angle
M. Clavicle
154. A. Glenoid cavity
    B. Clavicle
    C. Thoracic cavity
    D. Midscapular body
155. Because the thorax, which is filled with air, has less density than the shoulder soft tissue
156. Expiration
157. A. Longitudinal
    B. Transverse
158. A. 35 to 45 degrees
    B. Transverse
159. A. The arm is abducted to a 90-degree angle with the body, the elbow is flexed, and the hand is supinated by externally rotating the arm.
    B. It forces it to retract.
    C. When the arm is positioned to cause retraction, the glenoid cavity is positioned closer to profile.
160. Longitudinal
161. A. Perpendicular
    B. 2
    C. Inferior
162. The entire scapula, which includes the inferior and superior angles, coracoid and acromion processes, body, and glenoid cavity
163. Place the patient supine to maximize shoulder retraction. If the glenoid cavity area is of interest, roll the patient onto the affected shoulder.
164. Make sure that the arm is abducted to 90 degrees and externally rotate by flexing the elbow and supinating the hand.
165. A portion of the inferolateral border of the scapula is superimposed by the thoracic cavity and the superior angle is superimposed by the clavicle. Abduct the humerus to a full 90-degree angle with the body.
166. The inferolateral border of the scapula is superimposed by the thoracic cavity and the superior angle is superimposed by the clavicle. Abduct the humerus to a 90-degree angle with the body.
167. A. Clavicle
    B. Coracoid process
    C. Thorax
    D. Inferior angle
    E. Scapular body
    F. Acromion process
    G. Glenoid cavity
168. A. Superimposed
    B. Superior scapular angle
    C. Midscapular body
169. A. Away from
    B. Toward
170. The elevation of the humerus
171. Lateral

172. The borders of the scapula will not be superimposed.
173. A. Body
    B. Neck
174. Placing the humerus at a 90-degree angle with the body
175. Elevating the humerus higher than a 90-degree angle with the body
176. A. Less
    B. Because the scapula is drawn laterally around the thorax as the humerus is abducted
177. A. Perpendicular
    B. Anterior
    C. Inferior scapular
    D. Acromion process
178. The entire scapula, which includes the inferior and superior angles, coracoid and acromion processes, and scapular body
179. The patient was rotated more than needed to superimpose the scapular borders.
180. The patient was rotated less than needed to superimpose the scapular borders.
181. The lateral and vertebral borders of the scapula are demonstrated without superimposition. The vertebral border is visible next to the ribs. Increase the degree of patient rotation.
182. The lateral and vertebral borders of the scapula are demonstrated without superimposition. The lateral border is next to the ribs, and the vertebral border is demonstrated laterally. The patient's arm was not elevated, positioning the vertebral border of the scapula parallel with the IR. Decrease the degree of patient obliquity and elevate the arm to 90 degrees with the torso.

CHAPTER 6   LOWER EXTREMITY

1. A. As if the patient is hanging from the toes. The marker is correct.
   B. As if hung by the patient's hip or in an upright position. The marker is correct.
   C. As if hung by the patient's hip or in an upright position. The marker is correct.
   D. As if hung by the patient's hip or in an upright position. The marker is correct.
2. A. 55-65 kVp
   B. 65-75 kVp
   C. 70-80 kVp
3. A. 3
   B. 9
   C. 7
   D. 10
   E. 2
   F. 4
   G. 1
   H. 6
   I. 5
   J. 8

4. A. Distal phalanx
   B. Distal interphalangeal joint
   C. Middle phalanx
   D. Proximal interphalangeal joint
   E. Proximal phalanx
   F. Metatarsophalangeal joint
   G. Metatarsal
5. A. IP
   B. MTP
   C. MTP
   D. Third
6. A. Plantar
   B. Foot
   C. Ankle
   D. Lower leg
7. A. Lateral
   B. Lateral
8. Medially
9. A. Parallel
   B. Perpendicular
10. Collimated field
11. The toes are spread.
12. MTP joint
13. The distal and proximal phalanges and half of the metatarsal
14. The foot and toe were laterally rotated.
15. The foot and toe were medially rotated.
16. The patient's toe was flexed.
17. The proximal phalanx demonstrates greater soft tissue width and midshaft concavity on the medial surface. The toenail is facing laterally. Medially rotate the foot and toe until they are placed flat against the IR. The IP joint space is closed, and the distal phalanx is foreshortened. Angle the central ray proximally until it is aligned perpendicular to the distal phalanx or elevate the toe on a radiolucent sponge, bringing the distal phalanx parallel with the IR.
18. A. Distal phalanx
    B. Interphalangeal joint
    C. Proximal phalanx
    D. Metatarsophalangeal joint
    E. Metatarsal
    F. Tarsometatarsal joint
19. A. Twice
    B. Away from
    C. IP
    D. MTP
    E. MTP
20. A. 45 degrees
    B. Twice as much soft tissue width is present on the side of the digit rotated away from the IR when accurate.
21. A. Medially
    B. Laterally
    C. To obtain an oblique using the least amount of OID
22. Closed joint spaces and foreshortened phalanges
23. MTP joint

24. The distal and proximal phalanges and half of the metatarsal
25. Connecting tissue between the toes
26. The patient's toe and foot were close to an AP projection.
27. The patient's toe was close to a lateral projection.
28. The patient's toe was flexed and the central ray was not aligned perpendicular to the phalanges or parallel with the joint spaces.
29. Almost equal soft tissue width and midshaft concavity are demonstrated on each side of the phalanges. Increase the degree of toe and foot obliquity until the affected toe is at a 45-degree angle with the IR.
30. Soft tissue and bony overlap of the adjacent digit onto the affected digit is present. Draw the unaffected toes away from the affected toe.
31. The proximal phalanx demonstrates more concavity on the lateral aspect of the toe than the medial aspect, and more than twice as much soft tissue is shown on one side of the toe as on the other. Decrease the degree of toe and foot obliquity until the toe is at a 45-degree angle with the IR.
32. A. Distal phalanx
    B. Distal interphalangeal joint
    C. Middle phalanx
    D. Proximal interphalangeal joint
    E. Proximal phalanx
    F. Metatarsophalangeal joint
    G. Metatarsal
33. A. Posterior
    B. Anterior
    C. PIP
34. A. Medially
    B. Laterally
35. Anteriorly
36. A. Perpendicular
    B. PIP joint
37. The distal and proximal phalanges and the MTP joint space
38. The foot and toe were not rotated enough to place the toe in a lateral projection.
39. The foot and toe were rotated too much to place the toe in a lateral projection.
40. The adjacent unaffected digits were not drawn away from the affected digit.
41. The proximal and distal phalanges demonstrate almost equal midshaft concavity, the condyles of the proximal phalanx are demonstrated without superimposition, and the first and second metacarpal heads are not superimposed. Increase the patient's toe and foot obliquity until the affected toe is in a lateral projection.
42. The proximal phalange's condyles are not superimposed, and the metacarpal heads demonstrate slight superimposition. Decrease the patient's toe and foot obliquity until the affected toe is in a lateral projection.
43. A. Phalanges
    B. Metatarsals

C. Medial cuneiform
D. Medial-intermediate cuneiform joint
E. Intermediate cuneiform
F. Navicular-cuneiform joint
G. Navicular bone
H. Talus
I. Calcaneus
J. Cuboid
K. Lateral cuneiform
L. Fifth metatarsal tuberosity
M. Fourth tarsometatarsal joint
N. Fifth metatarsal base
44. A. Medial (first)
    B. Intermediate (second)
    C. 0.75
    D. TMT
    E. Third
45. A. Because of the anteroposterior thickness difference that exists between the distal and proximal foot
    B. Position a compensating filter over the phalanges and distal metatarsals.
46. A. 1
    B. Proximal
47. A. Plantar
    B. Lower leg
    C. Ankle
    D. Foot
48. No
49. Medial
50. Lateral
51. A. 10-15
    B. 1.0
    C. 15
52. A. 0.5
    B. Fifth metatarsal tuberosity
53. Proximal calcaneus, talar neck, tarsals, metatarsals, phalanges, and surrounding soft tissue
54. The foot was laterally rotated.
55. The foot was medially rotated.
56. The central ray was not angled enough proximally.
57. The joint space between the medial and intermediate cuneiforms is closed, the navicular bone is demonstrated in profile, and less than 0.75 inch (2 cm) of the calcaneus is demonstrated without talar superimposition. Rotate the foot medially until the pressure is equal over the entire plantar surface.
58. The joint space between the medial and intermediate cuneiforms is closed, the distal calcaneus is demonstrated without talar superimposition, and the metatarsal bases demonstrate decreased superimposition. Rotate the foot laterally until the pressure is equal over the entire plantar surface.
59. A. Phalanges
    B. Metatarsals
    C. Medial cuneiform
    D. Lateral cuneiform
    E. Intermediate cuneiform
    F. Navicular bone

598

G. Talus
H. Tarsal sinus
I. Calcaneus
J. Cuboid
K. Cuboid-cuneiform joint
L. Fifth metatarsal tuberosity
M. Intermetatarsal joint
N. Fifth metatarsal base
60. A. Cuboid-cuneiform
B. Second through fifth
C. Fifth
D. Third metatarsal
61. Cuboid-cuneiform
62. Medially
63. A. 60 degrees
B. 30 degrees
C. 45 degrees
64. A. High
B. Once repeated the first metatarsal base will superimpose the second and part of the third metatarsal bases.
65. A. Figure 6-15
B. More of the cuboid is demonstrated posterior to the navicular bone in Figure 6-15 than in Figure 6-17.
66. A. First
B. Second
C. Closer to
67. A. Fourth metatarsal tubercle
B. The fifth metatarsal will be superimposed over the fourth metatarsal tubercle.
68. A. Perpendicular
B. Midline
C. Fifth metatarsal tuberosity
69. The phalanges, metatarsals, tarsals, calcaneus, and surrounding soft tissue
70. The patient's foot was positioned too close to an AP projection.
71. The patient's foot was positioned too close to a lateral projection.
72. The lateral cuneiform-cuboid, navicular-cuboid, and third through fifth intermetatarsal joint spaces are closed. The fifth metatarsal is not superimposed over the fourth metatarsal tubercle. Increase the degree of medial foot obliquity.
73. A. Fibula
B. Calcaneus
C. Cuboid
D. Metatarsals
E. Phalanges
F. Cuneiforms
G. Navicular bone
H. Talus
I. Tibiotalar joint
J. Tibia
74. A. Anterior patellar
B. Posterior pericapsular
C. Tibiotalar
D. Proximal metatarsals

75. Lateral
76. A. Posterior pericapsular located within indention formed by the articulation of the posterior tibia and talar bone
B. Anterior pretalar located anterior to the ankle joint, next to the talus
77. Position the lower leg parallel with the imaging table.
78. A. Position the long axis of the foot at a 90-degree angle with the lower leg.
B. Position the lateral foot surface parallel with the IR.
79. A. The medial talar dome would be demonstrated distal to the lateral talar dome.
B. Elevate the distal lower leg and ankle until the lower leg is parallel with the imaging table.
80. A. Posterior
B. Navicular bone
81. 0.5 inch (1.25 cm)
82. A. Less
B. More
83. Talar domes
84. The most medial and lateral aspects of the talar's trochlear surface
85. A. Leg
B. Foot
86. This question can be answered in two different ways:
A. Medial
B. Proximal
C. Lateral
D. Higher
or
A. Lateral
B. Distal
C. Media
D. Higher
87. This question can be answered in two different ways:
A. Medial
B. Distal
C. Lateral
D. Lower
or
A. Lateral
B. Proximal
C. Medial
D. Lower
88. Lateral
89. This question can be answered in two different ways:
A. Medial
B. Posterior
C. Lateral
D. Anterior
or
A. Lateral
B. Anterior
C. Medial
D. Anterior

90. This question can be answered in two different ways:
    A. Medial
    B. Anterior
    C. Lateral
    D. Posterior
    or
    A. Lateral
    B. Posterior
    C. Medial
    D. Posterior
91. A. It demonstrates the anterior pretalar fat pad without forced flattening.
    B. It places the tibiotalar joint in a neutral position.
    C. It prevents anterior foot rotation.
92. A. Medial
    B. Lateral
93. Move the patient's heel away from the IR.
94. A. Perpendicular
    B. Heel
95. The phalanges, metatarsals, tarsals, talus, calcaneus, 1 inch (2.5 cm) of the distal lower leg, and the surrounding foot soft tissue
96. The proximal lower leg was elevated higher than the distal lower leg.
97. The distal lower leg was elevated higher than the proximal lower leg.
98. The heel was elevated and the forefoot was depressed.
99. The heel was depressed and the forefoot was elevated.
100. The lower leg and long axis of the foot do not form a 90-degree angle. The patient's foot was in plantar flexion. Dorsiflex the foot until the lower leg and long axis of the foot form a 90-degree angle.
101. The medial talar dome is positioned posterior to the lateral dome and the distal fibula is anterior on the tibia. Depress the patient's forefoot and elevate the heel (external leg rotation) until the lateral foot surface is parallel with the IR.
102. The lateral talar dome is proximal to the medial talar dome and less than half of the cuboid is seen posterior to the navicular. Depress the proximal lower leg or elevate the distal lower leg.
103. The lateral talar dome is posterior to the medial talar dome and the fibula is posterior to the tibia. Move the heel away from the IR (internal leg rotation).
104. A. Talus
     B. Talocalcaneal joint
     C. Sustentaculum tali
     D. Tuberosity
     E. Fifth metatarsal base
105. A. Talocalcaneal
     B. Medial
     C. Lateral
     D. Calcaneal tuberosity

106. A. Vertical
     B. 40
     C. Plantar
107. A. Parallel
     B. Perpendicular
108. A. Increase the degree of central ray angulation.
     B. Decrease the degree of central ray angulation.
109. Base of the fifth metatarsal and distal point of the fibula.
110. Along the lateral foot surface, approximately halfway between the ball of the foot and heel
111. A. Place the ankle in an AP projection without medial or lateral rotation.
     B. The first metatarsal will be demonstrated medially or the fourth and fifth metatarsals will be demonstrated laterally.
112. Fifth metatarsal base
113. The calcaneal tuberosity and talocalcaneal joint
114. The foot was dorsiflexed beyond the vertical position.
115. The foot was in plantar flexion.
116. The leg and ankle were internally rotated.
117. The leg and ankle were externally rotated.
118. The second through fifth metatarsals are demonstrated laterally. Internally rotate the leg until the ankle is in an AP projection.
119. The talocalcaneal joint space is obscured and the calcaneal tuberosity is foreshortened. If the patient's condition allows, dorsiflex the foot to a vertical neutral position. If the patient cannot dorsiflex the foot, increase the central ray angulation, aligning the central ray with the fifth metatarsal base and the distal point of the fibula.
120. The talocalcaneal joint space is obscured and the calcaneal tuberosity is elongated. The foot was dorsiflexed beyond the vertical position and a 40-degree central angulation was used. Plantar-flex the foot to a vertical position and use a 40-degree angulation.
121. A. Tibiotalar joint
     B. Talar domes
     C. Calcaneus
     D. Tuberosity
     E. Talocalcaneal joint
     F. Cuboid
     G. Navicular bone
     H. Talus
     I. Tibia
122. A. Posterior
     B. Lower leg
     C. Midcalcaneus
123. Parallel with the imaging table
124. A. Position the long axis of the foot at a 90-degree angle with the lower leg.
     B. Position the lateral foot surface parallel with the IR.
125. The medial talar dome would be demonstrated distal to the lateral talar dome.
126. A. Posterior
     B. Navicular bone

127. 0.5 inch (1.25 cm)
128. A. Less
    B. More
129. Talar domes
130. The most medial and lateral aspects of the talar's trochlear surface
131. A. Leg
    B. Foot
132. This question can be answered in two different ways:
    A. Medial
    B. Proximal
    C. Lateral
    D. Higher
    or
    A. Lateral
    B. Distal
    C. Medial
    D. Higher
133. This question can be answered in two different ways:
    A. Medial
    B. Distal
    C. Lateral
    D. Lower
    or
    A. Lateral
    B. Proximal
    C. Medial
    D. Lower
134. This question can be answered in two different ways:
    A. Medial
    B. Posterior
    C. Lateral
    D. Anterior
    or
    A. Lateral
    B. Anterior
    C. Medial
    D. Anterior
135. This question can be answered in two different ways:
    A. Medial
    B. Anterior
    C. Lateral
    D. Posterior
    or
    A. Lateral
    B. Posterior
    C. Medial
    D. Posterior
136. Anterior
137. A. Perpendicular
    B. Distal
    C. Medial malleolus
138. The tibiotalar joint, talus, calcaneus, and calcaneal articulating tarsal bones
139. A. Medial malleolus
    B. Medial malleolus
140. The proximal tibia was elevated.

141. The distal tibia was elevated.
142. The forefoot was depressed, and the heel was elevated (leg externally rotated).
143. The forefoot was elevated, and the heel was depressed (leg internally rotated).
144. The medial talar dome is anterior to the lateral talar dome, and the fibula is too posterior on the tibia. Elevate the forefoot and depress the heel until the lateral foot surface is parallel with the IR.
145. The foot is plantar-flexed, the medial talar dome is posterior and distal to the lateral talar dome, the fibula is too anterior on the tibia, and less than 0.5 inch (1.25 cm) of the cuboid is demonstrated posterior to the navicular bone. Dorsiflex the foot to a 90-degree angle with the lower leg, depress the forefoot and elevate the heel (externally rotate leg) until the lateral foot surface is parallel with the IR, and depress the proximal lower leg until it is parallel with the imaging table.
146. The lateral talar dome is posterior and proximal to the medial talar dome, the fibula is too far posterior on the tibia, and more than 0.5 inch (1.25 cm) of the cuboid is demonstrated posterior to the navicular bone. Internally rotate the leg until the lateral foot surface is parallel with the IR and elevate the proximal lower leg until it is parallel with the IR.
147. A. Tibia
    B. Medial malleolus
    C. Medial mortise
    D. Talus
    E. Lateral malleolus
    F. Tibiotalar joint
    G. Fibula
148. A. Distal fibula
    B. Lateral
    C. Tibiotalar
149. Medial malleolus
150. The tibia is superimposed over the fibula.
151. 15 to 20 degrees
152. The tibia and talus will demonstrate increased superimposition of the fibula and the medial mortise will be closed.
153. The lower leg should be positioned parallel with the IR.
154. The tibiotalar joint space will be closed or narrowed and the anterior tibial margin will be projected distally.
155. A. Perpendicular
    B. Medial malleolus
156. The distal fourth of the tibia and fibula, talus, and surrounding ankle soft tissue
157. The ankle was externally rotated.
158. The ankle was internally rotated.
159. The proximal tibia was elevated, or the central ray was centered too proximally.
160. The medial mortise is obscured, the tibia and talus demonstrate increased superimposition of the fibula, and the posterior aspect of the medial malleolus is situated medial to the anterior aspect. Rotate the leg internally, placing the long axis of the foot in a vertical position.

161. The talus is demonstrated without fibular super-imposition. Externally rotate the leg until the long axis of the foot is vertical.
162. A. Fibula
    B. Lateral malleolus
    C. Lateral mortise
    D. Calcaneus
    E. Talus
    F. Medial mortise
    G. Medial malleolus
    H. Tibiotalar joint
    I. Tibia
163. A. Talar
    B. Lateral
    C. Tibial
    D. Tibial
    E. Distal
    F. Tibiotalar joint
164. A. 15 to 20 degrees
    B. Medially (internally)
165. Position the lower leg parallel with the imaging table.
166. The anterior tibial margin will be projected too far superior to the posterior margin, expanding the tibiotalar joint space.
167. Dorsiflex the foot to a 90-degree angle with the lower leg.
168. A. Perpendicular
    B. Medial malleolus
169. The distal fourth of the fibula and tibia, talus, and surrounding ankle soft tissue
170. The patient's leg and ankle were underrotated.
171. The patient's leg and ankle were overrotated.
172. The patient's leg and ankle were internally rotated more than 45 degrees.
173. The distal tibia was elevated or the central ray was positioned distal to the joint space.
174. The foot was in plantar flexion.
175. The calcaneus is obscuring the distal aspect of the lateral mortise and the distal fibula. Dorsiflex the foot until its long axis forms a 90-degree angle with the lower leg.
176. The lateral mortise is closed, the medial mortise is open, and the tarsal sinus is not demonstrated. Increase the degree of internal (medial) leg rotation until the most prominent aspects of the malleoli are positioned at equal distances from the IR.
177. The medial mortise is partially closed, the fibula is demonstrated without tibial superimposition, and the tarsal sinus is partially shown. Decrease the degree of internal (medial) leg rotation until the malleoli are positioned at equal distances from the IR.
178. The lateral and medial mortises are closed and the tarsal sinus is demonstrated. Rotate the leg later-ally until the long axis of the foot is at a 45-degree angle with the IR.
179. The lateral and medial mortises are closed and the tarsal sinus is demonstrated. Rotate the leg later-ally until the long axis of the foot is at a 45-degree angle with the IR.

180. The tibia superimposes the fibula by 0.5 inch. Angle the central ray medially.
181. A. Fibula
    B. Tibiotalar joint
    C. Talar domes
    D. Calcaneus
    E. Talocancaneal joint
    F. Cuboid
    G. Fifth metatarsal tuberosity
    H. Navicular bone
    I. Talus
    J. Tibia
182. A. Open
    B. Distal tibia
    C. Lower leg
    D. Tibiotalar joint
183. Displacement of these pads may indicate underlying injuries and joint effusion.
184. A. Parallel
    B. Lateral
185. A. Posterior
    B. Navicular
    C. 0.5 inch (1.25 cm)
    D. 0.75 inch (2 cm)
    E. 0.25 inch (0.6 cm)
186. The most medial and lateral aspects of the talar's trochlear surface
187. Proximal-distal
188. This question can be answered in two different ways:
    A. Medial
    B. Proximal
    C. Lateral
    D. Higher
    or
    A. Lateral
    B. Distal
    C. Medial
    D. Higher
189. This question can be answered in two different ways:
    A. Medial
    B. Distal
    C. Lateral
    D. Lower
    or
    A. Lateral
    B. Proximal
    C. Medial
    D. Lower
190. Anteroposterior
191. This question can be answered in two different ways:
    A. Medial
    B. Posterior
    C. Lateral
    D. Anterior
    or
    A. Lateral
    B. Anterior
    C. Medial
    D. Anterior

192. This question can be answered in two different ways:
   A. Medial
   B. Anterior
   C. Lateral
   D. Posterior
   or
   A. Lateral
   B. Posterior
   C. Medial
   D. Posterior
193. A. It allows the anterior pretalar fat pad to be used to detect joint effusion.
   B. It places the ankle joint in a neutral position.
   C. It prevents the patient from rotating anteriorly.
194. A. Perpendicular
   B. Medial malleolus
195. The talus, 1 inch (2.5 cm) of the fifth metatarsal base, surrounding ankle soft tissue, and distal fourth of the fibula and tibia
196. A fracture of the fifth metatarsal base that results from inversion of the foot
197. So the fifth metatarsal base will be included on the projection to rule out a Jones fracture
198. The proximal lower leg was elevated.
199. The distal lower leg was elevated.
200. The heel was elevated, and the forefoot was depressed.
201. The heel was depressed, and the forefoot was elevated.
202. The foot is plantar-flexed. Dorsiflex the foot until the long axis of the foot forms a 90-degree angle with the lower leg.
203. The lateral talar dome is demonstrated distal to the medial dome, more than 0.5 inch (1.25 cm) of the cuboid is demonstrated posterior to the navicular bone, and the talocalcaneal joint is widened. Depress the distal lower leg until the lower leg is aligned parallel with the IR.
204. The lateral talar dome is proximal to the medial dome. Less than 0.5 inch (1.25 cm) of the cuboid is demonstrated posterior to the navicular bone and the talocalcaneal joint is narrowed. Elevate the distal lower leg until the lower leg is parallel with the IR.
205. The lateral talar dome is demonstrated anterior to the medial dome and the fibula is too far anterior on the tibia. Move the calcaneus toward the IR (internally rotate the leg) until the lateral surface of the foot is aligned parallel with the IR and depress the proximal tibia or adjust the central ray angle posteriorly.
206. The lateral talar dome is posterior to the medial dome and the fibula is posterior on the tibia. Adjust the central ray anteriorly until it is aligned perpendicular to the lateral aspect of the foot or 10 degrees; (the domes are physically approximately 1 inch (2.5 cm) apart and are off by 0.25 (0.6 cm) inch on projection, with a needed 5-degree angulation adjustment for every 0.125 inch (0.3 cm) that the domes are off.

207. The lateral talar dome is proximal and anterior to the medial talar dome.
   Patient: Adjust the distal lower leg 0.125 inch (0.3 cm) toward the IR (need to move half the distance the talar domes are off), and externally rotate the ankle and leg 0.125 inch (0.3 cm) or until the lateral foot surface is parallel with the IR.
   Central ray: Adjust the central ray distally and posteriorly 5 degrees for every 0.125 inch (0.3 cm) the domes are off anteriorly-posteriorly and proximally-distally, respectively (10 degrees proximally and anteriorly).
208. The foot is plantar-flexed, the fibula is too posterior on the tibia, and the lateral talar dome is posterior to the medial talar dome. Dorsiflex the foot if the patient is able and angle the central ray anteriorly.
209. A. Intercondylar fossa
   B. Lateral femoral condyle
   C. Fibular head
   D. Fibula
   E. Tibia
   F. Intercondylar eminence
   G. Medial femoral condyle
210. A. Tibial
   B. Closed
   C. Tibial midshaft
211. Position the ankle toward the anode end of the tube and the knee toward the cathode end.
212. A. Extending
   B. Internally
   C. Femoral epicondyles
213. Medial
214. A. The tibia is partially superimposed over the fibular head.
   B. The tibia and fibula are demonstrated without superimposition.
   C. The distal tibia and talus are partially superimposed over the fibula.
215. A. The fibula will be demonstrated with reduced or without tibial superimposition.
   B. The fibula will be demonstrated with reduced or without tibial and talar superimposition.
216. Place the knee in an AP projection and allow the ankle to be positioned as is.
217. A. Yes
   B. The proximal tibia slopes in the opposite direction as the diverged x-rays and the distal tibia does not slope at the same degree as the diverged x-rays. If the x-ray divergence and joints are not parallel, the joints will be closed.
218. To ensure that the diverged beams used to record the ankle and knee will be included on the projection
219. A. Medial malleolus
   B. Distal
   C. Medial epicondyle
220. Tibial midshaft
221. The tibia, fibula, ankle and knee joints, and surrounding lower leg soft tissue

222. The patient's leg was externally rotated.
223. The patient's leg was internally rotated.
224. The distal lower leg has been clipped, and the distal and proximal fibula are free of talar superimposition. Move the central ray and IR 1 inch (2.5 cm) distally and laterally rotate the patient's leg until the femoral epicondyles are positioned at equal distances from the IR.
225. A. Medial femoral condyle
    B. Fibula
    C. Talar domes
    D. Tibia
226. A. Posterior
    B. Midshaft
    C. Extended
    D. 30
    E. Tibial midshaft
227. Position the distal lower leg at the anode end of the tube and the proximal lower leg at the cathode end.
228. Lateral
229. A. The tibia is partially superimposed over the fibular head.
    B. The tibia and fibula midshafts are free of superimposition.
    C. The distal fibula is superimposed by the posterior half of the distal tibia.
230. A. The fibula will be demonstrated with reduced or without tibial superimposition.
    B. The fibula will be demonstrated with reduced or without tibial superimposition.
231. A. No
    B. Yes
232. Place the ankle in a lateral projection and allow the knee to be positioned as is.
233. At least 1 inch
234. Tibial midshaft
235. The tibia, fibula, ankle and knee joints, and surrounding lower leg soft tissue
236. The patient's leg was rotated too far anteriorly.
237. The patient's leg was rotated too far posteriorly.
238. The fibula is superimposed by the tibia. Rotate the patient's leg externally.
239. The fibular head is demonstrated without tibia superimposition and the fibula is demonstrated too posterior on the tibia. Rotate the patient's leg internally.
240. A. Patella
    B. Lateral epicondyle
    C. Lateral condyle
    D. Intercondylar eminence
    E. Fibular head
    F. Tibia
    G. Femorotibial joint
    H. Medial epicondyles
    I. Femur
241. A. Profile
    B. 0.25
    C. Tibial plateau
    D. Superior
    E. Lateral
    F. Knee joint

242. 10
243. A. Extended
    B. Internally
    C. Equal distances
244. The proximal tibia is superimposed over the proximal fibula.
245. Farther away
246. The medial condyle will appear larger than the lateral condyle, and the head, neck, and possibly the shaft of the fibula will be superimposed by the tibia.
247. Parallel with it
248. The tibial plateau slopes approximately 5 degrees anterior to posterior.
249. The thicker the upper thigh, the more the leg slopes down toward the IR and the more distally the anterior tibial margin and proximal the posterior tibial margin will move.
250. No
251. A. 5 degrees cephalic
    B. 5 degrees caudal
252. A. The fibular head will be foreshortened and demonstrated more than 0.5 inch (1.25 cm) distal to the tibial plateau.
    B. The fibular head will be elongated and demonstrated less than 0.5 inch (1.25 cm) distal to the tibial plateau.
253. A. Lateral compartment
    B. Medial compartment
254. Valgus
255. Decrease the angulation approximately 5 degrees to align it with the tibial plateau.
256. The patella lies just superior to the patellar surface of the femur and is situated slightly lateral to the knee midline.
257. A. Distally
    B. Medially
    C. Laterally
258. A. It is demonstrated superior to the patellar surface.
    B. It is demonstrated on the patellar surface.
    C. It is demonstrated between the patellar surface and intercondylar fossa.
259. A. It is demonstrated farther laterally than it would be demonstrated on a nonsubluxed knee projection.
    B. Lateral (external)
    C. When the patella is subluxed, the condyles will remain symmetrical and the tibia will be superimposed over the fibular head. Rotation will alter these two relationships.
260. A. 1 inch (2.5 cm)
    B. Distal
    C. Medial epicondyle
261. One fourth of the distal femur and proximal lower leg and surrounding knee soft tissue
262. The patient's leg was externally (laterally) rotated.
263. The patient's leg was internally (medially) rotated.
264. The central ray was angled too cephalically.

604

265. The central ray was angled too caudally.
266. The femorotibial joint space is obscured, the fibular head is more than 0.5 inch (1.25 cm) distal to the tibial plateau, and the fibular head is foreshortened. Adjust the central ray angulation 5 degrees caudally.
267. The femorotibial joint space is obscured, the fibular head is less than 0.5 inch (1.25 cm) distal to the tibial plateau, and the fibular head is elongated. Adjust the central ray angulation 5 degrees cephalically.
268. The medial femoral condyle appears larger than the lateral condyle and the head, neck, and shaft of the fibula are almost entirely superimposed by the tibia. Internally rotate the patient's leg until the femoral epicondyles are at equal distances from the IR. The femorotibial joint space is obscured and the fibular head is less than 0.5 inch (1.25 cm) distal to the tibial plateau. Adjust the central ray angulation 5 degrees cephalically.
269. The lateral femoral condyle appears larger than the medial condyle and the tibia demonstrates very little superimposition of the fibular head. Externally rotate the patient's leg until the femoral epicondyles are at equal distances from the IR.
270. Angle the central ray until it is perpendicular to the anterior surface of the lower leg, and then adjust the angle 5 degrees distally, aligning the central ray with the tibial plateau.
271. The medial femoral condyle appears larger than the lateral condyle and the head, neck, and shaft of the fibula are almost entirely superimposed by the tibia. Angle the central ray medially until it is perpendicular to a line connecting the femoral epicondyles.
272. The lateral femoral condyle appears larger than the medial condyle, the tibia demonstrates very little superimposition of the fibular head, the femorotibial joint space is obscured, and the fibular head is more than 0.5 inch (1.25 cm) distal to the tibial plateau. Angle the central ray laterally until it is perpendicular with an imaginary line connecting the femoral epicondyles and rotate the imaging tube until the central ray is aligned perpendicular to the anterior surface of the lower leg; then adjust the angle 5 degrees distally, aligning the central ray with the tibial plateau.
273. A. Femur
   B. Patella
   C. Medial condyle
   D. Tibia
   E. Fibular head
   F. Tibiofibular joint
   G. Femorotibial joint
   H. Lateral condyle
274. A. Femur
   B. Medial condyle
   C. Tibia
   D. Fibula

   E. Femorotibial joint
   F. Lateral condyle
   G. Patella
275. A. Distal
   B. Tibial plateau
   C. Tibial
   D. Anterior
   E. Knee joint
276. 45
277. A. The fibular head should be demonstrated without tibial superimposition.
   B. Lateral
278. The femoral condyles will be almost superimposed.
279. A. The fibula is superimposed by the tibia and the fibular head is aligned with the anterior edge of the tibia.
   B. Medial
280. The fibular head will be aligned with the anterior edge of the tibia but will be positioned posterior to this placement.
281. A. Angle 5 degrees caudally.
   B. The patient's hip is often elevated to accomplish the degree of needed internal obliquity.
   C. The patient's hip is placed closer to the imaging table to obtain the needed external obliquity.
282. A. Midline of the knee
   B. Knee joint
283. One fourth of the distal femur and proximal lower leg and surrounding knee soft tissue
284. The patient's knee was rotated less than 45 degrees.
285. The patient's knee was rotated more than 45 degrees.
286. The patient's knee was rotated less than 45 degrees.
287. The central ray was angled too cephalically.
288. The tibia is partially superimposed over the fibular head. Increase the degree of internal knee obliquity until an imaginary line connecting the femoral epicondyles is aligned at a 45-degree angle with the IR.
289. The fibular head, neck, and shaft are not entirely superimposed by the tibia. Increase the degree of external knee obliquity until an imaginary line connecting the femoral epicondyles is aligned at a 45-degree angle with the IR.
290. The fibular head is not aligned with the anterior edge of the tibia but is situated posterior to this placement. Decrease the degree of external knee rotation until the femoral epicondyles are aligned at a 45-degree angle with the IR.
291. A. Femur
   B. Femoral condyles
   C. Intercondylar eminence
   D. Fibular head
   E. Fibular neck
   F. Tibia
   G. Femorotibial joint
   H. Patellofemoral joint
   I. Patella

292. A. Suprapatellar
    B. Proximal
    C. Femoral condyles
    D. Fibular head
    E. Knee joint
293. A. Anterior suprapatellar fat pad
    B. Posterior suprapatellar fat pad
294. When the knee is flexed more than 20 degrees, the muscles and tendons tighten, forcing the patella to come into contact with the patellar surface of the femur and obscuring the fat pads.
295. A. Parallel
    B. Medially
    C. 10 to 15
    D. Wide
    E. Short
296. A. Medial
    B. Distal
    C. Lateral
297. A. 5 to 7
    B. Medial
    C. Reduced
298. A. Locate the adductor tubercle on the posterior aspect of the medial condyle.
    B. Locate the distal articulating surface that is the flattest. It is the lateral condyle.
299. When the leg is laterally abducted
300. A. The tibia will be partially superimposed over the fibular head.
    B. The fibula will be demonstrated free of tibial superimposition.
301. Because it is situated farthest from the IR
302. Adjust the angle approximately 5 degrees for every 0.25 inch (0.6 cm) of distance demonstrated between the distal surfaces of the condyles.
303. A. Posteriorly
    B. Medial
304. The proximal tibia is superimposed over the proximal fibula.
305. The fibula will be demonstrated with decreased or without tibial superimposition.
306. The fibula will be demonstrated with increased or complete tibial superimposition.
307. A. 1 (2.5 cm)
    B. Distal
    C. Medial epicondyle
308. One fourth of the distal femur and proximal lower leg and surrounding knee soft tissue
309. The patient's knee was overflexed.
310. The central ray was not angled cephalically enough.
311. The central ray was angled too cephalically.
312. The patient's patella was situated too far away from the IR (leg internally rotated).
313. The patient's patella was situated too close to the IR (leg externally rotated).
314. The patient's knee is overflexed; the patella is in contact with the patellar surface of the femur. The marker is superimposed over the soft tissue structures. Decrease the degree of knee flexion to meet

your facility's requirements. Move the marker off the soft tissue structures.
315. The medial femoral condyle is anterior to the lateral condyle. Rotate the patella farther away from the IR (internal leg rotation).
316. The medial femoral condyle is posterior to the lateral condyle. Rotate the patella closer to the IR (external leg rotation).
317. The medial femoral condyle is proximal to the lateral condyle and the tibiofibular joint is visualized. Adjust the central ray angle 5 to 7 degrees caudally.
318. The knee is overflexed; the patella demonstrates a fracture. If a patellar or other knee fracture is suspected, the knee should remain extended to prevent displacement of bony fragments or vascular injury.
319. The medial femoral condyle is anterior to the lateral condyle. Rotate the knee internally until the femoral epicondyles are parallel with the imaging table or the cart on which the patient is lying or adjust the central ray anteriorly until it is aligned parallel with the femoral epicondyles.
320. The medial femoral condyle is distal to the lateral condyle. Adduct the patient's leg until the epicondyles are perpendicular to the IR or rotate the x-ray tube toward the patient's feet, adjusting the central ray caudally (this moves the lateral condyle toward the medial condyle).
321. The lateral femoral condyle is proximal and posterior to the medial condyle. Rotate the imaging tube to direct central ray distally and angle the central ray anteriorly.
322. A. Lateral fossa surfaces
    B. Lateral epicondyle
    C. Lateral condyle
    D. Tibial condylar margin
    E. Fibular head
    F. Intercondylar eminence
    G. Femorotibial joint
    H. Medial condyle
    I. Medial epicondyle
    J. Medial fossa surfaces
    K. Intercondylar fossa
    L. Proximal fossa surfaces
323. A. Fibular head
    B. Superimposed
    C. Proximal
    D. Open
    E. Distal
    F. Intercondylar fossa
324. A. Allow the femur to incline medially approximately 10 to 15 degrees.
    B. Position the long axis of the foot perpendicular to the imaging table.
325. A. The patella rotates laterally.
    B. The patella rotates medially.
326. A. 20 to 30
    B. 60 to 70

327. Distally
328. Distally
329. A. The posterior tibial margin is distal to the anterior tibial margin.
    B. Dorsiflex the foot until its long axis is aligned perpendicular to the imaging table.
    C. Femorotibial
    D. Intercondylar eminence
    E. Tubercles
330. A. Perpendicular
    B. 1
    C. Medial femoral epicondyle
331. The distal femur, proximal tibia and intercondylar fossa, eminence, and tubercles
332. The femur was too vertical or the heel was rotated medially.
333. The patient's heel was laterally rotated.
334. The patient's knee was overflexed; the femur was too close to vertical.
335. The patient's knee was underflexed; the femur was more than 20 to 30 degrees from vertical.
336. The foot was in plantar flexion.
337. The proximal surfaces of the intercondylar fossa are demonstrated without superimposition, and the patellar apex is positioned too far above the inter-condylar fossa. Increase knee flexion, positioning the proximal femur farther from the imaging table. The femorotibial joint is closed and the fibular head is slightly less than 0.5 inch (1.25 cm) from the tibial plateau. Decrease the degree of foot dorsiflexion, elevating the distal lower leg.
338. The femorotibial joint is obscured, the tibial pla-teau is demonstrated, and the fibular head is less than 0.5 inch (1.25 cm) from the tibial plateau. Plantar-flex the foot, lowering the distal lower leg.
339. The proximal surfaces of the intercondylar fossa are demonstrated without superimposition, and the patellar apex is positioned too far above the intercondylar fossa. Increase the degree of knee flexion. The femorotibial joint is closed, and the fibular head is more than 0.5 (1.25 cm) from the tibial plateau. Increase the degree of foot dorsiflexion.
340. A. Medial epicondyle
    B. Proximal intercondylar fossa surfaces
    C. Intercondylar fossa
    D. Medial intercondylar fossa surfaces
    E. Medial femoral condyle
    F. Femorotibial joint space
    G. Intercondylar eminence
    H. Fibular head
    I. Lateral condyle
    J. Lateral intercondylar fossa surfaces
    K. Lateral epicondyle
341. A. Femoral epicondyles
    B. Fibular head
    C. Proximal
    D. Superimposed

E. 0.5 inch
    F. Intercondylar fossa
342. Internally rotated to AP projection, with femoral epicondyles parallel with the imaging table
343. A. Central ray aligned parallel with tibial plateau
    B. Femur position at a 60-degree angle with the imaging table
344. A. Distally
    B. Intercondylar fossa
345. A. Central ray
    B. Tibial plateau
346. A. Perpendicular
    B. Decreasing
    C. Medial femoral condyle
347. Distal femur, proximal tibia, and intercondylar fossa, eminences, and tubercles
348. The patient's leg was internally rotated.
349. The patient's leg was externally rotated.
350. The femur was angled more than 60 degrees with the imaging table, resulting in over-flexion.
351. The femur was angled less than 60 degrees with the imaging table, resulting in under-flexion.
352. The distal lower leg was depressed or the central ray was angled too caudally.
353. The distal lower leg was elevated too high or the central ray was angled too cephalically.
354. The medial and the lateral aspects of the inter-condylar fossa are not superimposed, the medial femoral condyle is wider than the lateral condyle, and the fibular head demonstrates increased tibial superimposition. Internally rotate the leg until an imaginary line connecting the femoral epicondyles is aligned parallel with the imaging table.
355. The proximal surfaces of the intercondylar fossa are not superimposed, and the patellar apex is demonstrated within the intercondylar fossa. Decrease the degree of hip and knee flexion until the long axis of the femur is aligned 60 degrees with the imaging table. The femorotibial joint is closed and the fibular head is demonstrated less than 0.5 inch (1.25 cm) distal to the tibial plateau. Elevate the distal lower leg until the knee is flexed 45 degrees or adjust the central ray cephalically.
356. A. Patella
    B. Patellofemoral joint
    C. Anterolateral femoral condyle
    D. Intercondylar sulcus
    E. Anteromedial femoral condyle
357. A. Lateral
    B. Medial
    C. Open
    D. Patellofemoral joint space
358. Because a long OID is used
359. Patellofemoral joint spaces
360. Internally rotate the legs and secure them by wrap-ping the Velcro straps of the axial viewer around the patient's calves.

361. A. They will be situated laterally.
    B. The condyles will demonstrate equal heights or the medial condyle will demonstrate more height than the lateral condyle.
362. A. Patellar subluxation
    B. The patella will be demonstrated laterally.
    C. The intercondylar sulci will remain facing superiorly on a subluxed patella but not on a rotated one.
363. Because tightening of the quadriceps muscles will prevent patella subluxation from being demonstrated
364. Parallel with the imaging table
365. Directly above the bend of the axial viewer until the knees are flexed 45 degrees
366. A. Decrease the angulation set on the axial viewer, or increase the central ray angulation 5 to 10 degrees.
    B. The tibial tuberosities will be demonstrated within the patellofemoral joint spaces.
367. 60 degrees caudally
368. 105 degrees
369. To offset the magnification caused by the large OID
370. Patellofemoral joints
371. The patellae, anterior femoral condyles, and inter-condylar sulci
372. The patient's legs were externally rotated.
373. The height of the axial viewer was not set high enough to position the long axes of the femurs parallel with the imaging table.
374. The posterior knee curve was positioned at or below the bend of the axial viewer.
375. The posterior knee curve was positioned too far above the bend of the axial viewer.
376. The patellae are demonstrated directly above the intercondylar sulci and rotated laterally, and the heights of the lateral and medial condyles are almost equal. Internally rotate the patient's legs until the patellae are situated superiorly and restrain the legs with the Velcro straps of the axial viewer.
377. The patellae are resting against the intercondylar sulci, obscuring the patellofemoral joint spaces. Slide the patient's knees away from the axial viewer until the patient's posterior knee curvatures are positioned just superior to the bend of the axial viewer.
378. The tibial tuberosities are demonstrated within the patellofemoral joint spaces. Slide the patient's knees toward the axial viewer until the posterior knee curvatures are just superior to the bend of the axial viewer.
379. The patellae, anterior femoral condyles, and intercondylar sulci are demonstrated superiorly, the lateral femoral condyle demonstrates more height than the medial condyle, the patellofemoral joint space is open, and the patellae are laterally located. Positioning is accurate; the patient's patellae are subluxed.

380. A. Femoral shaft
    B. Lateral epicondyle
    C. Lateral condyle
    D. Femorotibial joint
    E. Fibular head
    F. Medial condyle
    G. Medial epicondyle
381. A. Pelvic brim
    B. Obturator foramen
    C. Lesser trochanter
    D. Femoral shaft
    E. Greater trochanter
    F. Femoral neck
    G. Femoral head
    H. Acetabulum
382. A. Profile
    B. Fibular head
    C. Distal femoral shaft
383. A. Pelvic brim
    B. Greater
    C. Lesser
    D. Proximal femoral shaft
384. Position the knee toward the anode end of the tube and the hip toward the cathode end.
385. It can be used to detect subcutaneous air or hematomas.
386. A. Supine
    B. Extended
    C. Internally
387. A. No
    B. Forced internal rotation of a fractured femur may cause injury to the blood supply and nerves that surround the injured area.
388. The diverged x-rays used to record the femorotibial joint are angled against the joint.
389. A. 2
    B. Femorotibial
390. The distal femoral shaft, surrounding femoral soft tissue, femorotibial joint, and 1 inch (2.5 cm) of the lower leg
391. Position the anterior superior iliac spines at equal distances from the imaging table.
392. A. Parallel with the imaging table
    B. It will demonstrate the femoral neck without foreshortening and the greater trochanter in profile.
393. A. Proximal femoral shaft
    B. ASIS
394. To allow the reviewer to detect subcutaneous air or hematomas
395. The proximal femoral shaft, hip joint, and surrounding femoral soft tissue
396. The patient's leg was externally rotated.
397. The patient's leg was internally rotated.
398. The patient's pelvis was rotated toward the affected femur.
399. The patient was rotated away from the affected femur.
400. The patient's leg was externally rotated.

401. The femoral epicondyles are not in profile, the medial condyle appears larger than the lateral condyle, and the tibia superimposes the fibular head. Internally rotate the leg until the femoral epicondyles are at equal distances from the IR.

402. The femoral epicondyles are not in profile, the lateral condyle appears larger than the medial condyle, the fibular head is demonstrated without tibial superimposition, and not enough of the femur has been included. Externally rotate the leg until the femoral epicondyles are at equal distances from the IR, increase the IR size, and enter the central ray proximally, including more of the proximal femurs.

403. The femoral neck is partially foreshortened and the lesser trochanter is demonstrated in profile medially. Internally rotate the patient's leg until the femoral epicondyles are positioned at equal distances from the imaging table.

404. A. Femoral shaft
     B. Fibula
     C. Tibia
     D. Medial femoral condyle
     E. Patella
     F. Lateral femoral condyle

405. A. Femoral head
     B. Femoral neck
     C. Femoral shaft
     D. Lesser trochanter
     E. Greater trochanter

406. A. Femoral shaft
     B. Femoral neck
     C. Femoral head
     D. Lesser trochanter
     E. Greater trochanter

407. A. Femoral
     B. Fibular head
     C. Medial
     D. Lateral
     E. Distal femoral shaft

408. A. Medially
     B. Greater trochanter
     C. Greater
     D. Proximal femoral shaft

409. Position the knee toward the anode end of the tube and the hip toward the cathode end.

410. A. Lateral
     B. Perpendicular

411. A. Medial
     B. The reduction in medial femoral inclination that results when the patient is in a recumbent lateral projection
     C. The x-rays used to record the condyles are caudally diverged and project the medial condyle, which is situated farther from the IR distally.

412. The femur should not be moved or the patient rotated. The projection is obtained using a cross-table (horizontal) beam.

413. It allows the technologist to collimate tightly.

414. A. 2
     B. Femorotibial joint

415. The distal femoral shaft, surrounding femoral soft tissue, femorotibial joint, and 1 inch (2.5 cm) of the lower leg

416. The pelvis is rotated until the femoral epicondyles are aligned perpendicular to the imaging table.

417. The lateral surface of femur is placed next to the imaging table.

418. The patient's leg should not be moved, nor the body rotated. Take the projection with the patient in an axiolateral projection.

419. A. Proximal femoral shaft
     B. ASIS

420. The proximal femoral shaft, hip joint, and surrounding femoral soft tissue

421. The patient's patella was positioned too far away from the IR.

422. The patient's patella was positioned too close to the IR.

423. The pelvis is overrotated and the femoral epicondyles are not aligned perpendicular to the imaging table; the medial epicondyle is anterior to the lateral epicondyle.

424. The pelvis is underrotated and the femoral epicondyles are not aligned perpendicular to the imaging table; the medial epicondyle is posterior to the lateral epicondyle.

425. The medial femoral condyle is anterior to the lateral epicondyle. Internally rotate the leg (moving the patella away from the IR).

426. The medial femoral condyle is anterior to the lateral epicondyle. Internally rotate the femur until the femoral epicondyles are aligned perpendicular to the IR, or angle the central ray anteriorly until it is aligned parallel with the femoral epicondyles.

427. The greater trochanter is positioned laterally, the femoral neck is demonstrated with only partial foreshortening, and the femoral shaft is foreshortened. Rotate the pelvis, increase the degree of external leg rotation, and abduct the leg as needed to place the femur against the imaging table, with the femoral epicondyles aligned perpendicular to the IR.

428. The soft tissue from the unaffected thigh is superimposed over the acetabulum and femoral head of the affected femur. Flex and abduct the unaffected leg, drawing it away from the affected acetabulum and femoral head.

429. The greater trochanter is demonstrated posteriorly and the lesser trochanter is superimposed over the femoral shaft. A proximal femoral shaft fracture is present. The patient's affected leg was in external rotation. Do not attempt to adjust the patient's leg position if a fracture of the proximal femur is suspected. No corrective movement is needed.

1. A. With the anterior surface upward and the posterior downward. The marker should be correct.
   B. As if the patient is standing in an upright position. The marker should be correct.
   C. As if the patient is standing in an upright position. The marker should be correct. The side positioned farther from the IR is marked.
2. Patient's hand

3. A. The obturator internus fat plane lies within the pelvic inlet next to the pelvic brim.
   B. The iliopsoas fat plane lies medial to the lesser trochanter.
   C. The pericapsular fat plane is found superior to the femoral neck.
   D. The gluteal fat plane lies superior to the pericapsular fat plane.
   E. They will aid in the detection of intra-articular and periarticular disease.

4.

Hip and Pelvis Technical Data				
Projection	kVp	Grid	AEC Chamber(s)	SID
AP, hip	70 – 85	Grid	Center	40 – 48 inches (100 –120 cm)
AP oblique, hip	70 – 85	Grid	Center	40 – 48 inches (100 –120 cm)
Axiolateral, hip	75 – 85	Grid		40 – 48 inches (100 –120 cm)
AP, pelvis	65 – 85	Grid	Both outside	40 – 48 inches (100 –120 cm)
AP oblique, pelvis	65 – 85	Grid	Both outside	40 – 48 inches (100 –120 cm)
AP axial, sacroiliac joints	80 – 85	Grid	Center	40 – 48 inches (100 –120 cm)
AP oblique, sacroiliac joints	75 – 85	Grid	Center	40 – 48 inches (100 –120 cm)

5. A. ASIS
   B. Iliac ala
   C. Acetabulum
   D. Femoral head
   E. Femoral neck
   F. Greater trochanter
   G. Lesser trochanter
   H. Ischial tuberosity
   I. Inferior ramus of pubis
   J. Symphysis pubis
   K. Obturator foramen
   L. Superior ramus of pubis
   M. Pelvis brim
   N. Coccyx
   O. Ischial spine
   P. Sacrum
6. A. Pelvic brim
   B. Symphysis pubis
   C. Laterally
   D. Femoral neck
7. Make sure that the ASISs are at equal distances from the imaging table.
8. A. The sacrum would not be aligned with the symphysis pubis but would be rotated toward the affected hip.

   B. The iliac spine would be closer to the acetabulum than the pelvic brim.
9. It will be narrower.
10. A. The femoral neck will be demonstrated on end, and the lesser trochanter will be demonstrated in profile medially.
    B. The lesser trochanter is in partial profile medially, and the femoral neck is only partially foreshortened.
    C. The femoral neck is demonstrated without foreshortening, the greater trochanter is demonstrated in profile laterally, and the lesser trochanter is obscured.
11. The foot should be tilted internally 15 to 20 degrees from vertical and an imaginary line connecting the epicondyles should be positioned parallel with the imaging table.
12. A. No
    B. Forced internal rotation of a fractured or dislocated hip may result in injury to the blood supply and nerves that surround the injured area.
13. A. Perpendicular
    B. Distal
    C. Symphysis pubis

14. The acetabulum, greater and lesser trochanters, femoral head and neck, and half of the sacrum, coccyx, and symphysis pubis
15. A larger IR and lower central ray centering may be required.
16. A. Yes, no anatomic structures will be covered.
    B. Yes, but use a shield that is small enough and is shaped for the female pelvis to avoid covering any pelvic structures.
17. The patient was rotated toward the affected hip.
18. The patient was rotated away from the affected hip.
19. The patient's leg was in external rotation, with the foot and femoral epicondyles positioned at a 45-degree angle with the imaging table.
20. The ischial spine is demonstrated without pelvic brim superimposition, the sacrum and coccyx are not aligned with the symphysis pubis but are rotated away from the affected hip, and the obturator foramen is narrowed. Rotate the patient away from the affected hip. The lesser trochanter is demonstrated in profile. Internally rotate the leg until the femoral epicondyles are aligned parallel with the imaging table.
21. The ischial spine is not aligned with the pelvic brim but is demonstrated closer to the acetabulum, the sacrum and coccyx are not aligned with the symphysis pubis but are rotated toward the affected hip, and the iliac ala is narrowed. Rotate the patient toward the affected hip. The lesser trochanter is demonstrated in profile. Internally rotate the leg until femoral epicondyles are aligned parallel with the imaging table.
22. The femoral neck is partially foreshortened and the lesser trochanter is demonstrated in profile. The patient's leg was externally rotated, bringing the foot vertical and the femoral epicondyles positioned at approximately a 15- to 20-degree angle with the imaging table. Internally rotate the patient's leg until the foot is angled 15 to 20 degrees from vertical and the femoral epicondyles are positioned parallel with the imaging table.
23. The lesser trochanter is in profile and there is a proximal femur fracture. The leg should not be internally rotated when a femoral or hip fracture is suspected. Adequate positioning is demonstrated.
24. A. Iliac ala
    B. Acetabulum
    C. Femoral head
    D. Femoral neck
    E. Greater trochanter
    F. Femoral shaft
    G. Lesser trochanter
    H. Ischial tuberosity
    I. Obturator foramen
    J. Superior ramus
    K. Inferior ramus

L. Symphysis pubis
M. Coccyx
N. Pelvic brim
O. Ischial spine
P. Sacrum
25. A. Ischial spine
    B. Lesser trochanter
    C. Femoral neck
    D. Femoral neck
    E. Greater trochanter
26. Position the ASISs at equal distances from the imaging table.
27. A. Toward
    B. Against the imaging table
28. Profile
29. 60 to 70 degrees
30. A. The amount of femoral neck foreshortening
    B. The transverse level at which the greater trochanter will be demonstrated between the femoral head and lesser trochanter
31. A. Demonstrates the femoral neck on end and the greater trochanter at the same transverse level as the femoral head
    B. Demonstrates the femoral neck with only partial foreshortening and positions the greater trochanter at a transverse level halfway between the femoral neck and lesser trochanter
    C. Demonstrates the femoral neck without foreshortening and the greater trochanter at the same transverse level as the lesser trochanter
32. A. Perpendicular
    B. 2.5 (6.25 cm)
    C. ASIS
33. The acetabulum, greater and lesser trochanters, femoral head and neck, and half of the sacrum, coccyx, and symphysis pubis
34. The patient was rotated toward the affected hip.
35. The patient's knee was flexed more than needed, placing the femur at an angle greater than 60 to 70 degrees with the imaging table.
36. The patient's knee was not flexed enough to align the femur at a 60- to 70-degree angle with the imaging table or the affected leg's foot and ankle were resting on top of the unaffected leg, elevating it off the imaging table.
37. The patient's femur was abducted until it was positioned next to the imaging table.
38. The ischial spine is demonstrated without pelvic brim superimposition, the sacrum and coccyx are rotated toward the right hip, and the left obturator foramen is narrowed. Rotate the patient away from the affected hip until the ASISs are at equal distances from the imaging table.
39. The ischial spine is not aligned with the pelvic brim but is demonstrated closer to the acetabulum, the sacrum and coccyx are not aligned with the symphysis pubis but are rotated toward the affected

hip, the iliac ala is narrowed, and the obturator foramen is widened. Rotate the patient toward the affected hip.

40. The femoral neck is foreshortened and the greater trochanter is demonstrated at the same transverse level as the femoral head. Adduct the patient's femur until it is aligned at a 45-degree angle with the imaging table.

41. The greater trochanter is positioned laterally. The patient's knee was not flexed enough to align the femur at a 60- to 70-degree angle with the imaging table (20 to 30 degrees from vertical). Increase the knee flexion until the femur is aligned at a 60- to 70-degree angle with the imaging table.

42. The greater trochanter is positioned medially. Decrease knee flexion until the femur is at a 60- to 70-degree angle with the imaging table (20 to 30 degrees from vertical).

43. A. Acetabulum
    B. Femoral head
    C. Femoral neck
    D. Greater trochanter
    E. Lesser trochanter
    F. Femoral shaft
    G. Ischial tuberosity

44. A. Proximal greater
    B. Posteriorly
    C. Femoral shaft

45. A. Use tight collimation.
    B. Place a flat lead contact strip over the top of the unused half of the IR.
    C. Use a grid.

46. Align the thin end of the filter with the femoral neck and the thicker end with the proximal femur.

47. Place the unaffected leg in maximum flexion and abduction.

48. A. Against the patient's affected side at the level of the iliac crest
    B. Parallel
    C. It should be positioned superior to the iliac crest.
    D. Perpendicular to both

49. Find the center of an imaginary line drawn between the superior symphysis pubis and the ASIS. Bisect that line and draw a perpendicular line distally. This imaginary line parallels the long axis of the femoral neck.

50. A. Femoral neck will be foreshortened
    B. The greater trochanter will be demonstrated proximal or distal to the lesser trochanter depending on the angle.

51. Injury to the blood supply and nerves that surround the injured area

52. Internally rotate the leg until an imaginary line connecting the femoral epicondyles is positioned parallel with the imaging table.

53. Femoral neck

54. The acetabulum, femoral head and neck, greater and lesser trochanters, and ischial tuberosity

55. The unaffected leg was not adequately flexed and abducted.

56. The angle of the central ray to the femur was too great.

57. The patient's leg was in external rotation.

58. Soft tissue from the unaffected thigh is superimposed over the acetabulum and femoral head of the affected hip. Flex and abduct the unaffected leg, drawing it away from the affected acetabulum and femoral head. If the patient is unable to adjust the unaffected leg further, the kVp and mAs can be increased to demonstrate this area. A wedge-type compensating filter may also be added to prevent overexposure of the femoral neck and shaft.

59. The greater trochanter is demonstrated at a transverse level proximal to the lesser trochanter, and the femoral neck is partially foreshortened. Localize the femoral neck. Position the IR parallel with the femoral neck and the central ray perpendicular to the IR and femoral neck.

60. The greater trochanter is demonstrated posteriorly, the lesser trochanter is superimposed over the femoral shaft, the greater trochanter is demonstrated at a transverse level proximal to the lesser trochanter, and the femoral neck is foreshortened. Internally rotate the patient's leg and decrease the angle of the central ray to the femur.

61. A fracture of the femoral neck is present. The greater trochanter is demonstrated posteriorly, and the lesser trochanter is superimposed over the femoral shaft. Do not attempt to adjust the patient's leg position if a fracture of the proximal femur is suspected. No corrective movement is needed.

62. A. Iliac crest
    B. Iliac ala
    C. ASIS
    D. Acetabulum
    E. Femoral head
    F. Femoral neck
    G. Greater trochanter
    H. Lesser trochanter
    I. Ischial tuberosity
    J. Obturator foramen
    K. Inferior ramus of ischium
    L. Symphysis pubis
    M. Superior ramus of pubis
    N. Coccyx
    O. Superior ramus of ischium
    P. Pelvic brim
    Q. Ischial spine
    R. Sacrum

63.

Male and Female Pelvic Differences		
Parameter	Male	Female
Overall shape	Bulkier, deeper, narrower	Smaller, shallower, and wider
Ala	Narrower, nonflared	Wider, flared
Pubic arch angle	Acute angle	Obtuse angle
Inlet shape	Smaller, heart shaped	Larger, rounded shape
Obturator foramen	Larger	Smaller

64. A. Pelvic brim
    B. Greater
    C. Lesser
65. A. Female
    B. Male
66. Make sure that the ASISs are positioned at equal distances from the IR.
67. The sacrum and coccyx would not be aligned with the symphysis pubis but would be rotated toward the left hip; the right iliac spine would be demonstrated within the inlet pelvis without pelvic brim superimposition; and the left iliac spine would be demonstrated next to the left acetabulum.
68. A. The patient's legs were internally rotated with the feet at 15 to 20 degrees from vertical and the femoral epicondyles placed parallel with the imaging table.
    B. The patient's legs were externally rotated with the feet at a 45-degree angle from vertical and the femoral epicondyles positioned at a 60- to 65-degree angle with the imaging table.
    C. The patient's legs were externally rotated with the feet vertical and the femoral epicondyles at a 15- to 20-degree angle with the imaging table.
69. The feet are tilted internally 15 to 20 degrees from vertical and the line connecting the femoral epicondyles is aligned parallel with the imaging table.
70. A. Perpendicular
    B. Symphysis pubis
    C. ASISs
71. The ilia, pubis, ischia, acetabula, femoral necks and heads, and greater and lesser trochanters
72. The pelvis was rotated onto the right side (RPO position).
73. The patient's legs were externally rotated, with the feet and an imaginary line connecting the femoral epicondyles positioned at a 45-degree angle with the table.
74. The femoral necks are completely foreshortened, and the lesser trochanters are demonstrated in profile. The patient's legs were externally rotated, with the patient's feet at a 45-degree angle and the femoral epicondyles positioned at a 60- to 65-degree angle with the imaging table. Internally rotate the patient's legs until the feet are angled 15 to 20 degrees from vertical and the femoral epicondyles are positioned parallel with the imaging table.

75. The left obturator foramen is narrower than the right foramen, the left ischial spine is demonstrated without pelvic brim superimposition, and the sacrum and coccyx are rotated toward the right hip. Rotate the patient toward the right hip until the ASISs are positioned at equal distances from the imaging table.
76. The femoral necks are foreshortened and the lesser trochanters are demonstrated in profile. The right obturator foramen is narrower, the right ischial spine is demonstrated without pelvic brim superimposition, and the sacrum and coccyx are rotated toward the left hip. Internally rotate the legs until the femoral epicondyles are positioned parallel with the imaging table and rotate the patient toward the left hip until the ASISs are positioned at equal distances from the imaging table.
77. A. Ischial spine
    B. Pelvic brim
    C. Coccyx
    D. Symphysis pubis
    E. Ischial tuberosity
    F. Obturator foramen
    G. Lesser trochanter
    H. Greater trochanter
    I. Femoral neck
    J. Femoral head
    K. Sacrum
    L. Acetabulum
    M. Iliac ala
    N. ASIS
    O. Iliac crest
78. A. Medially
    B. Femoral necks
    C. Proximal greater trochanters
79. Place the anterior iliac spines at equal distances from the IR.
80. The sacrum and coccyx would not be aligned with the symphysis pubis but would be rotated toward the right hip, the left iliac spine would be demonstrated within the inlet pelvis without pelvic brim superimposition, and the right iliac spine would be demonstrated next to the right acetabulum.
81. Profile
82. 60 to 70 degrees
83. The greater trochanters will be demonstrated lateral to the proximal femur.

84. A. The amount of femoral neck foreshortening
    B. The transverse level at which the greater trochanters will be demonstrated between the femoral heads and lesser trochanters
85. A. The femoral necks would be demonstrated on end and the greater trochanters would be demonstrated at the same transverse level as the femoral heads.
    B. The femoral necks would be partially foreshortened and the greater trochanters would be positioned at a transverse level halfway between the femoral heads and lesser trochanters.
    C. The femoral necks would be demonstrated without foreshortening and the greater trochanters would be positioned at the same transverse level as the lesser trochanters.
86. A. Perpendicular
    B. Midsagittal
    C. 1 inch (2.5 cm)
    D. Symphysis pubis
87. The ilea, pubis, ischia, acetabula, femoral necks and heads, and greater and lesser trochanters
88. The left side of the patient's pelvis was rotated closer to the IR than the right (LPO).
89. The patient's femurs were abducted beyond 45 degrees.
90. The femoral necks are demonstrated on end. The greater trochanters are demonstrated on the same transverse level as the femoral heads. Consult with reviewers in your facility to determine whether this is an acceptable image. Because the femoral necks cannot be evaluated because of foreshortening, it may be necessary to position the femurs at a 45-degree angle with the imaging table. The iliac crest has been clipped. The central ray and IR were positioned too inferiorly.
91. The femoral necks are demonstrated on end. The greater trochanters are demonstrated on the same transverse level as the femoral heads. Consult with reviewers in your facility to determine whether this is an acceptable image. Because the femoral necks cannot be evaluated because of foreshortening, it may be necessary to position the femurs at a 45-degree angle with the imaging table.
92. The greater trochanters are partially demonstrated laterally. Increase the degree of knee and hip flexion until the femurs are placed at a 60- to 70-degree angle with the imaging table.
93. The sacrum is rotated toward the right hip, the patient's hands are demonstrated within the collimated field, the right femur is abducted more than the left, and the inferior sacrum is not in the center of the image. Rotate the patient toward the right hip, move the patient's hands away from the collimated field, and abduct both femurs equally and accurately center the central ray.
94. A. Median sacral crest
    B. Symphysis pubis
    C. Pelvic brim
    D. Second sacral segment
    E. Ilium
    F. Sacroiliac joint
    G. Sacral ala
95. A. Symphysis pubis
    B. Symphysis pubis
96. Position the ASISs at equal distances from the imaging table.
97. A. Opposite
    B. Farther
98. A. 30 degrees cephalic
    B. 35 degrees cephalic
    C. Increase the angle over the routine amount used until the central ray and sacroiliac joints are aligned.
    D. Decrease the angle over the routine amount used until the central ray and sacroiliac joints are aligned.
99. A. To obtain tight collimation
    B. To ensure that the central ray is accurately aligned with the sacroiliac joints
100. A. Midsagittal
    B. ASISs
    C. Symphysis pubis
101. The sacroiliac joints and first through fourth sacral segments
102. The right side of the patient's pelvis was situated farther away from the IR than the left side (LPO position).
103. The central ray was inadequately angled.
104. The sacroiliac joints are foreshortened, and the inferior sacrum is demonstrated without symphysis pubis superimposition. Increase the degree of cephalic central ray angulation.
105. The central ray is centered to the L5-S1 joint disk space, causing less diverged beams to record the sacroiliac joints than required to demonstrate them without foreshortening. Move the central ray inferiorly, centering to the second sacral segment (1.5 inches superior to the symphysis pubis).
106. The sacroiliac joints and sacrum are elongated and the symphysis pubis is superimposed over the inferior aspects of the sacrum and sacroiliac joints. Angle the central ray 30 to 35 degrees cephalad.
107. A. Ilium
    B. Iliac tuberosity
    C. Inferior sacral ala
    D. Sacrum
    E. Superior sacral ala
    F. Sacroiliac joint
108. A. Sacrum
    B. Long axis
109. A. Ilium
    B. Sacrum
110. A. Ilium
    B. Sacrum
111. A. Midcoronal
    B. 25 to 30
112. A. Right
    B. Right
113. A. Medial
    B. ASIS

614

114. The sacroiliac joint, sacral ala, and ilium
115. The patient was underrotated.
116. The patient was overrotated.
117. The sacroiliac joint is closed. The superior and inferior sacral alae are demonstrated without iliac superimposition, and the lateral sacral ala is superimposed over the iliac tuberosity. Increase the pelvic obliquity.
118. The sacroiliac joint is closed and the ilium is superimposed over the lateral sacral ala and the inferior sacrum. Decrease the degree of pelvic obliquity.

CHAPTER 8   CERVICAL AND THORACIC VERTEBRAE

1. A. As if the patient is standing in an upright position. The marker is correct.
   B. As if the patient is standing in an upright position. The marker is reversed.
   C. As if the patient is standing in an upright position. The marker is correct.
   D. As if the patient is standing in an upright position. The marker is correct.

2.

Cervical and Thoracic Vertebrae Technical Data				
Projection	kVp	Grid	AEC Chamber(s)	SID
AP axial, cervical vertebrae	70 – 80	Grid	Center	40 – 48 inches (100 –120 cm)
AP, open-mouth, C1 and C2	70 – 80	Grid	Center	40 – 48 inches (100 –120 cm)
Lateral, cervical vertebrae	70 – 80	Air-gap technique		72 inches (150 – 180 cm)
AP axial oblique, cervical vertebrae	70 – 80	Air-gap technique		72 inches (150 – 180 cm)
Lateral (Twining method), cervicothoracic vertebrae	65 – 85	Grid	Center	40 – 48 inches (100 –120 cm)
AP, thoracic vertebrae	75 – 85	Grid	Center	40 – 48 inches (100 –120 cm)
Lateral, thoracic vertebrae	80 – 90	Grid	Center	40 – 48 inches (100 –120 cm)

3. A. Imaginary line connecting the point where the upper lip and nose meet with the external ear opening.
   B. Slow shallow breathing; used with a long exposure time to blur chest details
   C. External auditory meatus
   D. Imaginary line connecting the inferior orbital margin and the external acoustic opening
   E. Chewing surface of maxillary teeth
4. A. Articular pillar
   B. Pedicle
   C. Sixth to seventh intervertebral disk space
   D. Fourth spinous process
   E. Fifth vertebral body
   F. Seventh uncinate process
   G. Air-filled trachea
5. A. Spinous processes
   B. Lateral
   C. Inferior
   D. Superimposed
6. No more than 3 inches (7.5 cm) from the IR center
7. A. Position the mastoid tips and mandibular angles at equal distances from the imaging table.
   B. Position the shoulders at equal distances from the imaging table.

8. A. Closer to
   B. Farther from
9. A. No
   B. The upper and lower cervical vertebrae can move independently of each other.
10. A. No
    B. No
    C. Spinal cord injury may be caused by moving the patient when a fracture is suspected.
11. Lordotic
12. A. Upwardly, anteriorly to posteriorly
    B. Higher when upright
    C. 15 degrees cephalad
    D. 20 degrees cephalad
    E. The gravitational pull on the vertebrae that results when the patient is supine
13. A. Closed
    B. Its vertebral body
14. Within the inferior adjoining vertebral body
15. Too much
16. The patient's chin was adjusted until an imaginary line connecting the upper occlusal plane and the posterior occiput's inferior edge was aligned perpendicular to the imaging table or until the acanthiomeatal line was aligned perpendicular to the imaging table.

17. A. Midsagittal
    B. External auditory meatus (EAM)
    C. Jugular notch
18. The second through seventh cervical vertebrae, first thoracic vertebra, and surrounding soft tissue
19. The patient's head was turned and the torso was rotated toward the right side.
20. The central ray was not angled cephalically enough.
21. The central ray was angled too cephalically.
22. The chin was not adequately tucked, positioning the upper occlusal plane superior to the posterior occiput's inferior edge.
23. The chin was overtucked, positioning the upper occlusal plane inferior to the base of the occiput.
24. The patient's head and upper cervical vertebrae's midsagittal plane were not aligned with the lower cervical vertebrae.
25. The spinous processes are not aligned with the midline of the cervical bodies but are closer to the right side, the medial end of the right clavicle is superimposed over the vertebral column, the antero-inferior aspects of the cervical bodies are obscuring the intervertebral disk spaces, and each vertebra's spinous process is demonstrated within its vertebral body. Rotate the patient toward the right side until the shoulders are at equal distances from the imaging table or upright grid holder and increase the amount of cephalic central ray angulation.
26. The spinous processes are closer to the left side, the medial end of the left clavicle superimposes the vertebral column, and the patient's face is turned toward the right side. Rotate the patient's body and face toward the left side until the shoulders are at equal distances from the IR and the face is looking forward.
27. The anteroinferior aspects of the cervical bodies are obscuring the intervertebral disk spaces and each vertebra's spinous process is demonstrated within its vertebral body. Increase the amount of cephalic central ray angulation.
28. The anteroinferior aspects of the cervical bodies are obscuring the intervertebral disk spaces, and each vertebra's spinous process is demonstrated within its vertebral body. The head and upper cervical vertebrae are tilting toward the right side. Increase the amount of cephalic central ray angulation and align the midsagittal planes of the head and cervical vertebrae.
29. The posteroinferior aspects of the cervical bodies are obscuring the intervertebral disk spaces, the uncinate processes are elongated, and each vertebra's spinous process is demonstrated within the inferior adjoining vertebral body. Decrease the amount of cephalic central ray angulation.
30. A portion of the third cervical vertebra is superimposed over the posterior occipital bone, preventing clear visualization of the third cervical vertebra. Tuck the chin half the distance demonstrated between the base of the skull and the mandibular mentum or until an imaginary line connecting

the upper occlusal plane and the base of the skull is aligned perpendicular to the imaging table or upright grid holder.
31. The mandible is superimposed over a portion of the third cervical vertebra, the anteroinferior aspects of the cervical bodies are obscuring the intervertebral disk spaces, and each vertebra's spinous process is demonstrated within its vertebra body. Raise the chin half the distance demonstrated between the base of the skull and mandibular mentum, or until an imaginary line connecting the upper occlusal plane and the inferior base of the posterior occiput is aligned perpendicular to the imaging table or upright grid holder, and increase the degree of cephalic central ray angulation.
32. A. Upper incisors
    B. Posterior occipital bone
    C. Dens
    D. C1 lateral mass
    E. Transverse process
    F. Atlantoaxial joint
    G. Mandibular ramus
    H. C2 spinous process
    I. C2 body
    J. Occipitoatlantal joint
33. A. Axis
    B. Dens
    C. Axis's
    D. Lateral masses
    E. Superior
    F. Midline
34. Position the patient's shoulders, mandibular angles, and mastoid tips at equal distances from the imaging table.
35. A. Posteriorly
    B. Anteriorly
36. A. Tuck the patient's chin until an imaginary line connecting the upper occlusal plane and the posterior occiput's inferior edge is aligned perpendicular to the imaging table, or until the acanthiomeatal line is perpendicular to the imaging table, and have the patient open the mouth.
    B. Imagine where the occlusal plane would be if the patient had teeth, and position the patient using this imaginary plane.
37. To offset the magnification of the upper incisors caused by the long object–image receptor distance (OID)
38. Angle the central ray until it is aligned parallel with the infraorbitomeatal line (IOML).
39. A. The atlantoaxial joint will be closed and the axis's spinous process will demonstrate an increased superior location to the dens.
    B. The atlantoaxial joint will be closed and the axis's spinous process will demonstrate an increased inferior location to the dens.
40. Midsagittal plane
41. The atlantoaxial and occipitoatlantal joints, atlas's lateral masses and transverse processes, and axis's dens and body

42. The patient's face was rotated toward the left side.
43. The central ray was not angled 5 degrees cephalad.
44. A. The patient's chin was tucked more than needed to position the acanthiomeatal line perpendicular to the imaging table.
    B. The central ray was angled too caudally.
45. A. The patient's chin was not tucked enough to position the acanthiomeatal line perpendicular to the imaging table.
    B. The central ray was angled too cephalically.
46. The distances from the atlas's lateral masses to the dens and from the mandibular rami to the dens are narrower on the left side than on the right side, and the dens is superimposed over the posterior occiput. Rotate the face toward the left side until the mandibular angles and mastoid tips are positioned at equal distances from the imaging table or upright grid holder and tuck the chin toward the chest until an imaginary line connecting the upper occlusal plane with the base of the skull is aligned perpendicular to the IR.
47. The dens is superimposed over the posterior occiput. The upper incisors are demonstrated directly superior to the dens. Tuck the chin toward the chest until an imaginary line connecting the upper occlusal plane with the base of the skull is aligned perpendicular to the IR. A 5-degree cephalad angulation should be used.
48. The upper incisors are demonstrated inferior to the base of the skull, superimposing the dens and atlantoaxial articulation. The base of the skull is demonstrated directly superior to the dens. If the upper occlusal plane and base of the skull were aligned perpendicular to the imaging table, and a perpendicular central ray was used for this image, do not adjust patient positioning; simply direct the central ray 5 degrees cephalad. If a 5 degree cephalad angulation was used for this image, do not adjust patient positioning; simply increase the cephalad angulation by 5 degrees.
49. The atlantoaxial joint space is closed and the axis's spinous process is demonstrated too inferior to the dens. The neck was in extension. Place a small sponge under the patient's head to reduce neck extension and then realign the upper occlusal plane and the base of the skull.
50. The upper incisors are demonstrated superior to the dens and the base of the skull, and the dens is superimposed over the posterior occiput. Adjust the central ray angulation caudally until it is aligned parallel with the IOML.
51. A. Sella turcica
    B. Clivus
    C. Posterior occipital bone
    D. Inferior cranial cortices
    E. Posterior arch
    F. Dens
    G. Third spinous process
    H. Fifth through sixth zygapophyseal joints
    I. Articular pillars
    J. Sixth lamina
    K. First thoracic vertebra
    L. Seventh cervical vertebra
    M. Intervertebral disk space
    N. Mandibular rami
52. A. Prevertebral
    B. Superimposed
    C. Profile
    D. Posterior occiput
    E. Superimposed
    F. Zygapophyseal joints
53. Prevertebral fat stripe
54. Using a long SID will decrease the cervical magnification that results from the long OID created between the cervical vertebrae and IR.
55. Midcoronal
56. Align the shoulders, mastoid tips, and mandibular rami.
57. The articular right or left pillars and zygapophyseal joints will be demonstrated one anterior to the other.
58. Position the head's midsagittal plane parallel with the IR and the acanthomeatal line parallel with the floor.
59. Position the midsagittal plane parallel with the IR and the interpupillary line perpendicular to the IR.
60. A. Places the cervical vertebrae in a neutral position
    B. Allows for tight transverse collimation
61. To demonstrate AP vertebral mobility
62. Instruct the patient to tuck the chin against the chest as tightly as possible.
63. Instruct the patient to extend the chin up and backward as far as possible.
64. A. Midcoronal
    B. EAM
    C. Jugular notch
65. The sella turcica, clivus, first through seventh cervical vertebrae, superior half of the first thoracic vertebra, and surrounding soft tissue
66. The clivus with the dens can be used to evaluate cervical injury.
67. A. Take the image with the patient in an upright position.
    B. Have the patient hold weights on each arm to depress the shoulders.
    C. Take the exposure on suspended expiration.
68. Lateral cervicothoracic (Twining method)
69. The midsagittal plane was not parallel with IR.
70. The patient's head was rotated.
71. The patient's head and upper cervical vertebrae were tilted toward the IR.
72. The articular pillars and zygapophyseal joints on one side of the patient are situated anterior to those on the other side. Rotate the patient until the midcoronal plane is aligned perpendicular to the IR.
73. Neither the inferior nor posterior cortices of the cranium or mandible are superimposed, the posterior arch of C1 is demonstrated in profile, and the right and left articular pillars and zygapophyseal joints

617

demonstrate a superoinferior separation. Rotate the head until the midsagittal plane is aligned parallel with the IR, and then tilt the head toward the IR until the interpupillary line is perpendicular to the IR.

74. The vertebral body of C7 is not demonstrated in its entirety, and the superior body of T1 is not demonstrated. Have the patient hold 5- to 10-lb weights on each arm to depress the shoulders. If the patient cannot hold weights or if the weights do not drop the shoulders sufficiently, a special image known as the cervicothoracic lateral (Twining method) should be taken to demonstrate this area.

75. The posterior cortices of the mandible are not superimposed, causing C1 and C2 to superimpose the left mandibular ramus, the left articular pillars and zygapophyseal joints demonstrate a superoinferior separation, and the long axis of the cervical vertebral column is not aligned with the long axis of the collimated field. Rotate the face away from the IR until the midsagittal plane is parallel with the IR, tilt the head toward the IR until the interpupillary line is perpendicular to the IR, and elevate the chin until the eyes are facing forward and the long axis of the neck is aligned with the long axis of the collimated field.

76. A. Inferior mandibular cortices
    B. Pedicle
    C. Sixth vertebral body
    D. Intervertebral foramen
    E. Intervertebral disk space
    F. Pedicle
    G. Fourth uncinate process
    H. Posterior arch
    I. Inferior cranial cortices

77. A. Seventh
    B. Profile
    C. Anterior
    D. Vertebral foramen

78. To offset the magnification that would result because of the long OID used for the examination

79. When a long OID is used, causing scatter radiation to be diverged away from the IR and decreasing the amount of scatter radiation that reaches the IR

80. A. Right
    B. Right
    C. Left
    D. Left

81. 45 degrees

82. Midcoronal

83. A. Align the left mastoid tip with the longitudinal axis of the IR and the right gonion with the transverse axis of the IR.
    B. Direct it 45 degrees medially and 15 degrees cephalically. Center it to the right side of the patient's neck halfway between the AP surfaces of the neck at the level of the thyroid cartilage.

84. A. 15 to 20 degrees caudally
    B. 15 to 20 degrees cephalically
    C. To open the intervertebral disk spaces and demonstrate undistorted vertebral bodies

85. Position the skull's midsagittal plane parallel with the IR and the acanthiomeatal line parallel with the floor.

86. Increase the degree of central ray angulation.

87. A. Left
    B. Left
    C. The angulation of the central ray projects the mandible situated farther from the IR inferiorly on PA oblique projections and superiorly on AP oblique projections.

88. A. Midsagittal plane
    B. EAM
    C. Jugular notch

89. The first through seventh cervical vertebrae, first thoracic vertebra, and surrounding soft tissue

90. The patient was rotated less than 45 degrees.

91. The patient was rotated more than 45 degrees.

92. The central ray was not angled enough caudally.

93. The patient's head was not turned to a lateral projection.

94. The head and upper cervical vertebrae were tilted away from the IR.

95. This patient was in a right PA axial oblique projection (RAO position), with the head in a PA oblique projection. The right pedicles and intervertebral foramina are obscured. Increase patient obliquity until the midcoronal plane is placed at a 45-degree angle with the IR.

96. This patient was in a left PA axial oblique projection (LAO position), with the head in a lateral projection. The intervertebral foramina are demonstrated, the left pedicles are visible (although they are not in true profile), the right pedicles are demonstrated in the midline of the vertebral bodies, and the left zygapophyseal joints are demonstrated. Decrease patient rotation until the midcoronal plane is placed at a 45-degree angle with the IR.

97. This patient was in a right PA axial oblique projection (RAO position), with the head in a lateral projection. The atlas and its posterior arch are obscured. The inferior cranial cortices demonstrate more than 0.25 inch (0.6 cm) between them, and the inferior cortices of the mandibular rami demonstrate more than 0.5 inch (1.25 cm) between them. The first thoracic vertebra is not included in its entirety. Tilt the patient's head toward the IR until the interpupillary line is aligned perpendicular to the IR and move the central ray and IR inferiorly.

98. This patient was in a right PA axial oblique projection (RAO position), with the head in a lateral projection. The intervertebral disk spaces are closed, the cervical bodies are distorted, the posterior tubercles are demonstrated within the intervertebral foramina, the C1 vertebral foramen is not demonstrated, and the inferior mandibular rami and cranial cortices are demonstrated with superimposition. The central ray was directed perpendicular to the IR. Angle the central ray 15 to 20 degrees caudally for PA oblique projections.

99. This patient was in a right PA axial oblique projection (RAO position), with the head in a lateral projection. The intervertebral foramina are demonstrated, the left pedicles are shown although they are not in true profile, the right pedicles are demonstrated in the midline of the vertebral bodies, and the left zygapophyseal joints are demonstrated. Decrease the degree of patient rotation to 45 degrees with the IR.

100. A. Humeral head
 B. Zygapophyseal joints
 C. C7 spinous process
 D. Intervertebral foramen
 E. Humeral head
 F. Clavicle
 G. T1 vertebra
 H. C7 vertebral body
 I. Intervertebral disk space
 J. Pedicles
 K. Articular pillars

101. A. Vertebral column
 B. Superimposed

102. A. When the routine lateral cervical projection demonstrates the seventh vertebra
 B. When the routine lateral thoracic projection does not demonstrate the first through third thoracic vertebrae

103. A. Use tight collimation.
 B. Use a high-ratio grid.
 C. Align a lead contact shield or apron along the posterior edge of the collimated field.

104. Expiration

105. A. The arm is elevated above the patient's head as high as possible.
 B. The arm is against the patient's side and should be depressed.

106. A. Position the patient's head in a lateral projection.
 B. Position the patient to superimpose the shoulders and inferior posterior ribs.

107. The right and left articular pillars, posterior ribs, and zygapophyseal joints will be demonstrated without superimposition.

108. The cervical and vertebral column should be positioned parallel with the IR.

109. A. Midcoronal
 B. Jugular notch
 C. Vertebral prominens

110. When the patient is unable to depress the shoulder positioned farther from the IR

111. The fifth through seventh cervical vertebrae and first through fourth thoracic vertebrae

112. The shoulder that was depressed and positioned farther from the IR was rotated anteriorly.

113. The shoulder that was depressed and positioned farther from the IR was rotated posteriorly.

114. The patient's vertebral column was not positioned parallel with the IR.

115. The intervertebral disk spaces are closed and the vertebral bodies are distorted. The patient's cervical vertebral column was not positioned parallel with the IR. Position the midsagittal plane of the head and cervical vertebral column parallel with the IR. It may be necessary to prop the head on a sponge to help the patient maintain the position.

116. The right and left articular pillars, zygapophyseal joints, and posterior ribs are demonstrated without superimposition. The patient's thorax was rotated. The humerus that was raised and situated closer to the IR is demonstrated anterior to the vertebral column. Rotate the shoulder positioned farther from the IR anteriorly until your flat palms placed against the shoulders and the posterior ribs, respectively, are aligned perpendicular to the imaging table and upright IR.

117. A. Medial clavicular end
 B. Spinous process
 C. Posterior rib
 D. Pedicle
 E. Vertebral body
 F. Intervertebral disk space

118. A. Vertebral bodies
 B. Spinous processes
 C. Open

119. To an 8-inch (20-cm) transverse field size

120. A. Use the anode heel effect.
 B. Use a wedge-compensating filter.

121. Position the thin edge of the filter at the inferior sternum, where it begins to decline. The thick end will be directed toward the cervical vertebrae.

122. Position the patient's head and upper thoracic vertebrae at the anode end of the tube and the lower thoracic vertebrae at the cathode end of the tube.

123. Suspended expiration

124. Position the shoulders and anterior superior iliac spines at equal distances from the imaging table.

125. Closer to

126. A. Scoliosis
 B. A rotated thoracic image will demonstrate rotation of the thoracolumbar vertebrae and either the upper thoracic or lower lumbar vertebrae, whereas scoliosis will demonstrate rotation of the thoracolumbar vertebrae without corresponding rotation of the upper thoracic or lower lumbar vertebrae.

127. A. Kyphotic
 B. Position the patient's head on a thin pillow and bend his or her knees, placing the feet flat against the imaging table.

128. A. Midsagittal
 B. Jugular notch

129. The seventh cervical vertebra, first through twelfth thoracic vertebrae, first lumbar vertebra, and 2.5 inches (6.25 cm) of the posterior ribs and mediastinum on each side of the vertebral column

130. The patient's legs were extended.

131. The left side of the patient was positioned closer to the IR than was the right side (LPO).

132. The patient's head was positioned at the cathode end of the tube, and a compensating filter was not positioned over the upper thoracic vertebrae.

133. The upper thoracic vertebrae demonstrate more distance from the left pedicle to the spinous process than from the right pedicle to the spinous process, and the left medial clavicle is demonstrated away from the vertebral column. Rotate the patient toward the right side until the shoulders are at equal distances from the imaging table.

134. The eighth through twelfth intervertebral disk spaces are obscured and the vertebral bodies are distorted. Flex the patient's hips and knees, placing the feet and back firmly against the imaging table.

135. A. First thoracic vertebra
     B. Posterior ribs
     C. Pedicles
     D. Intervertebral foramen
     E. Intervertebral disk space

136. A. Profile
     B. 0.5
     C. Open

137. It will blur the ribs and lung markings.

138. Suspended expiration

139. A. To prevent the humeri or their soft tissue from obscuring the thoracic vertebrae
     B. So the inferior scapular angle can be used to locate the seventh thoracic vertebra

140. Align the shoulders, posterior ribs, and posterior pelvic wings on top of each other.

141. By evaluating the superimposition of the right and left posterior surfaces of the vertebral bodies and the degree of posterior rib superimposition

142. The posterior ribs demonstrate differing degrees of rotation.

143. X-ray divergence will cause the posterior ribs situated farther from the IR to demonstrate more magnification than those situated closer to the IR.

144. The vertebral column should be positioned parallel with the IR.

145. A. A patient who has wide hips and a narrow waist
     B. Between the patient's lateral body surface and the imaging table, just superior to the iliac crest
     C. Angle the central ray 10 to 15 degrees cephalically.

146. Inferior scapular angle

147. The seventh cervical vertebra, first through twelfth thoracic vertebrae, and first lumbar vertebra

148. A. The vertebra that has the last rib attached to it is the twelfth.
     B. Follow the posterior vertebral bodies of the lower thoracic and upper lumbar vertebrae, locating the subtle change from kyphotic to lordotic that takes place between T12 and L1.

149. A. Counting up from the twelfth thoracic vertebra
     B. Locate the first vertebral prominens.

150. Cervicothoracic lateral (Twining method) projection

151. The elevated side of the thorax was rotated posteriorly.

152. The elevated side of the thorax was rotated anteriorly.

153. The thoracic vertebral column was not aligned parallel with the imaging table.

154. The posterior surfaces of the vertebral bodies are demonstrated without superimposition and the posterior ribs are superimposed. Rotate the elevated thorax posteriorly until a flat palm placed against the shoulder, posterior ribs, and posterior pelvic wings is aligned perpendicular to the imaging table.

155. The posterior surfaces of the vertebral bodies are demonstrated without superimposition, and more than 0.5 inch (1.25 cm) of space is demonstrated between the posterior ribs. Rotate the elevated thorax anteriorly until a flat palm placed against the shoulders and the posterior ribs is perpendicular to the imaging table. The T8 to T12 intervertebral disk spaces are obscured and the vertebral bodies are distorted. Position a radiolucent sponge between the lateral body surface and the imaging table just superior to the patient's iliac crest, aligning the thoracic and lumbar vertebral column parallel with the imaging table.

156. The T8 to T12 intervertebral disk spaces are obscured and the vertebral bodies are distorted. The vertebral column was not positioned parallel with the IR. The inferior posterior ribs situated farther from the IR are projected superior to the posterior ribs situated closer to the IR, indicating that the lower vertebral column was situated farther from the IR than the upper. Shift the lower half of the patient's body toward the IR until the vertebral column is parallel with the imaging table.

CHAPTER 9   LUMBAR VERTEBRAE, SACRUM, AND COCCYX

1. A. As if the patient is standing in an upright position. The marker is correct.
   B. As if the patient is standing in an upright position. The marker is correct.
   C. As if the patient is standing in an upright position. The marker is correct.

2.

Lumbar Vertebrae, Sacrum, and Coccyx Technical Data				
Projection	kVp	Grid	AEC Chamber(s)	SID
AP, lumbar vertebrae	75 – 80	Grid	Center	40 – 48 inches (100 –120 cm)
AP oblique, lumbar vertebrae	75 – 85	Grid		40 – 48 inches (100 –120 cm)
Lateral, lumbar vertebrae	85 – 95	Grid	Center	40 – 48 inches (100 –120 cm)
Lateral, L5-S1 lumbosacral junction	95 – 100	Grid	Center	40 – 48 inches (100 –120 cm)
AP axial, sacrum	75 – 80	Grid	Center	40 – 48 Inches (100 –120 cm)
Lateral, sacrum	85 – 95	Grid	Center	40 – 48 inches (100 –120 cm)
AP axial, coccyx	75 – 80	Grid	Center	40 – 48 inches (100 –120 cm)
Lateral, coccyx	80 – 85	Grid		40 – 48 inches (100 –120 cm)

3. A. First lumbar vertebra
   B. Intervertebral disk space
   C. Sacrum
   D. Coccyx
   E. Sacroiliac (SI) joint
   F. Ilium
   G. Lateral edge of psoas major muscle
   H. Zygapophyseal joint
   I. Lamina
   J. Pars interarticularis
   K. Inferior articular process
   L. Superior articular process
   M. Spinous process
   N. Pedicle
   O. Transverse process
4. A. Psoas
   B. Spinous processes
   C. Equal
   D. Open
   E. Spinous processes
5. A. Psoas major muscles
   B. Lateral to the lumbar vertebrae, originating at the first lumbar vertebra on each side and extending to the corresponding side's lesser trochanter
6. Position the shoulders and anterior superior iliac spines (ASISs) at equal distances from the imaging table.
7. By comparing the distance between each pedicle with the spinous process on the same vertebra and comparing the distance between each SI joint with the spinous processes
8. Rotated lumbar vertebrae will demonstrate corresponding upper or lower lumbar rotation as well as middle lumbar rotation, whereas a scoliotic patient

may demonstrate a rotated appearance in the middle of the vertebral column without corresponding upper or lower vertebrae rotation.
9. Flex the patient's knees and hips until the lower back rests firmly against the imaging table.
10. Lordotic
11. The iliac spines will be demonstrated without pelvic brim superimposition.
12. A. Use the xiphoid and a point halfway between the ASISs.
    B. It is often shifted to one side and not located directly above the lumbar vertebrae.
13. The patient has scoliosis.
14. A. Midsagittal
    B. Superior
    C. Iliac crest
15. The twelfth thoracic vertebra, first through fifth lumbar vertebrae, sacroiliac joints, and psoas major muscles
16. A. Midsagittal
    B. Iliac crest
17. The twelfth thoracic vertebra, first through fifth lumbar vertebrae, sacroiliac joints, sacrum, coccyx, and psoas major muscles
18. 8 inches (20 cm)
19. When the sacrum and coccyx are not of interest
20. The patient was rotated onto the left side (LPO position).
21. The upper torso was accurately positioned and the pelvis was rotated toward the right side.
22. The patient's legs were extended.
23. The distances from the left pedicles to the spinous processes of L1-4 are less than the distances from the right pedicles to the spinous processes, and the intervertebral disk spaces between T12 and L3 are closed. Rotate the patient toward the left side and

flex the hips and knee until the lower back rests firmly against the imaging table.

24. The distances from the right pedicles to the spinous processes are less than the distances from the left pedicles to the spinous processes and the right sacroiliac joint is clipped. Rotate the patient toward the right side until the ASISs are at equal distances to the IR and shift the patient slightly to the left and open the transverse collimation enough to include both sacroiliac joints.

25. The intervertebral disk spaces between T12 and L3 are closed. Flex the patient's hips and knees until the lower back rests firmly against the imaging table.

26. A. Second lumbar vertebra
    B. Zygapophyseal joint
    C. Transverse process
    D. Superior articular process
    E. Inferior articular process
    F. Pedicle
    G. Lamina
    H. Pars interarticularis

27. A. Articular processes
    B. Zygapophyseal
    C. Pedicles

28. A. Left
    B. Left
    C. Right
    D. Right

29. A. Midcoronal
    B. 45 degrees

30. A. Superior articular process
    B. Transverse process
    C. Lamina
    D. Pedicle
    E. Inferior articular process

31. A. Medial
    B. ASIS
    C. Iliac crest

32. The twelfth thoracic vertebra, first through fifth lumbar vertebrae, first and second sacral segments, and SI joints

33. The patient's lumbar vertebrae were rotated less than 45 degrees.

34. The patient's upper lumbar vertebrae were rotated more than 45 degrees.

35. The first and second lumbar vertebrae are accurately positioned, but the third through fifth lumbar vertebrae's superior and inferior articular processes are not demonstrated in profile, their corresponding zygapophyseal joint spaces are closed, and their pedicles are demonstrated adjacent to the vertebrae's lateral vertebral body border. While maintaining the degree of thoracic and upper lumbar vertebral obliquity, increase the lower lumbar vertebral and pelvic rotation.

36. The lumbar vertebrae's superior and inferior articular processes are not demonstrated in profile, their corresponding zygapophyseal joint spaces are

closed, their laminae are obscured, and their pedicles are aligned with the midline of the vertebral bodies. Decrease the degree of lumbar vertebrae rotation to 45 degrees.

37. The lumbar vertebrae's superior and inferior articular processes are not demonstrated in profile, their corresponding zygapophyseal joint spaces are closed, their laminae are obscured, and their pedicles are aligned with the midline of the vertebral bodies. Decrease the degree of lumbar vertebrae rotation to 45 degrees.

38. A. Pars interarticularis
    B. Intervertebral foramen
    C. Pedicle
    D. Zygapophyseal joint
    E. Sacrum
    F. Fifth lumbar vertebra
    G. Intervertebral disk space
    H. Third lumbar vertebra
    I. First lumbar vertebra

39. A. Spinous processes
    B. Superimposed
    C. Neutral

40. A. Use tight collimation.
    B. Use a high-ratio grid.
    C. Place a flat contact shield on the imaging table along the posterior edge of the collimated field.

41. A. Higher
    B. Increase

42. Align the shoulders, posterior ribs, and posterior pelvic wings perpendicular to the imaging table.

43. A. Scoliosis
    B. The patient should be positioned on the table so that the central ray is directed into the spinal curve.

44. It prevents the side of the patient positioned farther from the IR from rotating anteriorly.

45. By evaluating the superimposition of the right and left posterior surfaces of the vertebral bodies

46. A. No
    B. The upper and lower lumbar vertebrae can rotate independently or simultaneously.

47. Because the right and left sides are mirror images of each other

48. Align the lumbar column parallel with the imaging table.

49. A. Wide hips and a narrow waist
    B. Between the patient's lateral body surface and the imaging table just superior to the iliac crest
    C. Angle the central ray 5 to 8 degrees caudally.

50. To demonstrate AP vertebral mobility

51. A. Flex the shoulders, upper thorax, and knees anteriorly, rolling into a tight ball.
    B. Arch the back by extending the shoulders, upper thorax, and legs as far posteriorly as possible.

52. A. Decreased
    B. Increased

53. It is located halfway between the ASIS and posterior wing of the patient's side situated farther from the IR.

54. A. Coronal
    B. ASIS
    C. Posterior wing
    D. Iliac crest
55. The twelfth thoracic vertebra, first through fifth lumbar vertebrae, and L5-S1 intervertebral disk space
56. A. Coronal
    B. ASIS
    C. Posterior wing
    D. Iliac crest
57. The eleventh and twelfth thoracic vertebrae, first through fifth lumbar vertebrae, and sacrum
58. A. The L5-S1 area on a lateral lumbar projection is too light.
    B. The L5-S1 intervertebral disk spaces are closed on a lateral lumbar projection.
59. Position the edge of a flat contact shield against an imaginary line drawn between the coccyx and a point 1 inch (2.5 cm) posterior to the elevated ASIS.
60. The side of the patient situated farther from the IR was rotated anteriorly.
61. The lumbar vertebral column was not aligned parallel with the imaging table.
62. The patient has scoliosis and was not positioned so that the central ray was directed into the spinal curvature. A right lateral instead of a left lateral should be taken.
63. The posterior surfaces of the first through fourth vertebral bodies and the posterior ribs are demonstrated one anterior to the other. The posterior ribs demonstrating the greater magnification were positioned posteriorly. Rotate the side positioned farther from the IR anteriorly until the posterior ribs are superimposed while maintaining posterior pelvic wing superimposition.
64. The posterior surfaces of L1 through L3 are not superimposed. The posterior ribs demonstrating the greatest magnification are positioned posteriorly. Rotate the right side of the upper torso anteriorly until the posterior ribs are superimposed and position a radiolucent sponge between the patient's lateral body surface and imaging table just superior to the iliac crest. The sponge should be only thick enough to align the lumbar column parallel to the imaging table and IR.
65. The L4-L5 and L5-S1 intervertebral disk spaces are closed and the third through fifth vertebral bodies are distorted. Position a radiolucent sponge between the patient's lateral body surface and imaging table just superior to the iliac crest. The sponge should be only thick enough to align the lumbar column parallel with the imaging table and IR.
66. The lumbar vertebral column demonstrates excess lordotic curvature. The patient was in an extended position. If a neutral lateral projection is desired, flex the shoulders, upper thorax, and legs anteriorly until the posterior thorax and pelvic wings are aligned with the long axis of the imaging table.

67. A. Pedicles
    B. Intervertebral foramen
    C. Sacrum
    D. Greater sciatic notches
    E. L5-S1 disk space
    F. Fifth lumbar vertebra
    G. Pelvic wing
68. A. Pedicles
    B. Pelvic wings
    C. Open
69. 8 inches (10 cm)
70. A. Use tight collimation.
    B. Use a high-ratio grid.
    C. Place a flat contact shield on the imaging table along the posterior edge of the collimated field.
71. Align the shoulders, posterior ribs, and posterior pelvic wings perpendicular to the imaging table.
72. It prevents the side positioned farther from the IR from rotating anteriorly.
73. By evaluating the openness of the intervertebral foramen and superimposition of the greater sciatic notches and the femoral heads, when demonstrated.
74. Position the vertebral column parallel with the imaging table.
75. A. Wide hips and a narrow waist
    B. Between the patient's lateral body surface and imaging table just superior to the iliac crest
    C. The central ray can be angled until it is parallel with the interiliac line.
76. Angle the central ray cephalically until it parallels the interiliac line.
77. A. Posterior
    B. ASIS
    C. Inferior
    D. Iliac crest
78. The fifth lumbar vertebra and the first and second sacral segments
79. Position the edge of a flat contact shield against an imaginary line drawn between the coccyx and a point 1 inch (2.5 cm) posterior to the elevated ASIS.
80. The patient was rotated.
81. The vertebral column was not aligned parallel with the IR.
82. The L5-S1 intervertebral foramen is obscured and the greater sciatic notches and the femoral heads are demonstrated without superimposition. The femoral head positioned closer to the IR was rotated anteriorly. Rotate the patient's hip that was positioned farther from the IR toward the opposite hip until the posterior ribs and the posterior pelvic wings are superimposed.
83. The L5-S1 intervertebral disk space is closed, and the pelvic alae are not superimposed. Neither the long axis of the lumbar vertebral column nor the sacrum was aligned parallel with the imaging table, and the iliac crests were not positioned at different transverse levels. Position a radiolucent sponge

623

between the patient's lateral body surface and imaging table just superior to the patient's iliac crest. The sponge should be just thick enough to align the long axis of the vertebral column and sacrum parallel with the imaging table and place the iliac crests at the same transverse levels.

84. A. Ilium
    B. Sacral ala
    C. SI joint
    D. Second sacral segment
    E. Third sacral segment
    F. Fourth sacral segment
    G. Fifth sacral segment
    H. Ischial spine
    I. Coccyx
    J. Symphysis pubis
    K. Pelvic brim
    L. Sacral foramen
    M. Median sacral crest
    N. Sacral body
    O. Fifth lumbar vertebra
85. A. Pelvic brim
    B. Coccyx
    C. Fifth
    D. Symphysis pubis
86. It prevents urine, gas, and fecal material from obscuring the sacrum.
87. Position the ASISs and shoulder at equal distances from the IR.
88. A. Opposite
    B. Farther
89. Kyphotic
90. Position the patient supine with the legs extended and angle the central ray 15 degrees cephalically.
91. It will allow for tight collimation and ensure that the central ray is aligned correctly with the sacrum.
92. A. Midsagittal
    B. An imaginary line drawn between the ASISs
    C. Superior symphysis pubis
93. The fifth lumbar vertebra, first through fifth sacral segments, first coccygeal vertebra, symphysis pubis, and SI joints
94. A. No
    B. Using gonadal shielding on female patients will cover sacral information.
95. The patient's left side was positioned closer to the IR than was the right side.
96. The central ray was not angled enough cephalically.
97. The central ray was angled too cephalically.
98. The sacrum is elongated and the symphysis pubis is superimposed over the fifth sacral segment. Either the central ray was angled too cephalically or the patient's legs were not fully extended and a 15-degree central ray angle was used. If the patient's legs were extended, decrease the central ray. If the patient's legs were flexed and a 15-degree central ray angle was used, fully extend the patient's legs and use the same angulation.

99. The right ischial spine is demonstrated without pelvic brim superimposition and the median sacral crest and coccyx are rotated toward the left hip. The patient was rotated onto the right side (RPO position). Rotate the patient toward the left hip until the ASISs are positioned at equal distances from the imaging table.
100. The right ischial spine is demonstrated without pelvic brim superimposition and the first, second, and third sacral segments are foreshortened. Rotate the patient toward the left hip until the ASISs are positioned at equal distances from the imaging table and the patient's legs are fully extended, and then angle the central ray 15 degrees cephalad.
101. The first, second, and third sacral segments are foreshortened and fecal material superimposes the third through fifth sacral segments. Angle the central ray 15 degrees cephalad and ask the patient to empty the colon of gas and fecal material.
102. A. Median sacral crest
     B. Sacral canal
     C. First sacral segment
     D. Second sacral segment
     E. Third sacral segment
     F. Fourth sacral segment
     G. Fifth sacral segment
     H. Coccyx
     I. Greater sciatic notches
     J. Transverse ridges
     K. Sacral promontory
     L. L5-S1 disk space
     M. Fifth lumbar vertebra
     N. Femoral heads
103. A. Profile
     B. Pelvis wings
     C. Superimposed
104. Align the shoulders, posterior ribs, and posterior pelvic wings perpendicular to the imaging table.
105. It prevents the side of the patient positioned farther from the IR from rotating anteriorly.
106. By evaluating the superimposition of the greater sciatic notches and pelvic wings
107. Farther away from
108. Position the long axis of the vertebral column parallel with the imaging table.
109. A. Wide hips and a narrow waist
     B. Between the patient's lateral body surface and the imaging table just superior to the iliac crest
     C. Angle the central ray until it is parallel with the interiliac line.
110. Angle the central ray cephalically until it is parallel with the interiliac line.
111. A. Coronal
     B. ASIS
112. The fifth lumbar vertebra, first through fifth sacral segments, promontory, and first coccygeal vertebra
113. Position the edge of a flat contact shield against an imaginary line drawn between the coccyx and a point 1 inch (2.5 cm) posterior to the elevated ASIS.

114. The patient was not in a lateral projection. The side of the patient that was situated farther from the IR (right) was rotated posteriorly.

115. The long axis of the lumbar vertebral column was not positioned parallel with the imaging table.

116. The L5-S1 intervertebral disk space is closed, the sacrum is foreshortened, and the greater sciatic notches are demonstrated without superoinferior superimposition. The patient's long axis was not aligned parallel with the imaging table. Position the long axis of the lumbar vertebral column and sacrum parallel with the IR. It may be necessary to place a radiolucent sponge between the patient's lateral body surface and the imaging table just superior to the iliac crest. The sponge should be just thick enough to align the lumbar column parallel with the imaging table.

117. The L5-S1 intervertebral foramen is obscured, and the greater sciatic notches and the femoral heads are demonstrated without superimposition. The femoral head positioned closer to the IR was rotated anteriorly. Rotate the patient's hip that was positioned farther from the IR (right) toward the opposite hip until the posterior pelvic wings are superimposed.

118. The greater sciatic notches are demonstrated without superimposition. The superiorly positioned femoral head, which is the one situated closest to the IR, is rotated anteriorly. Rotate the patient's hip that was positioned farther from the IR (right) toward the opposite hip until the posterior pelvic wings are superimposed.

119. A. Sacrum
B. First coccygeal segment
C. Second coccygeal segment
D. Third coccygeal segment
E. Symphysis pubis

120. A. Symphysis pubis
B. Inlet pubis
C. Third

121. 6 inches (15 cm)

122. No more than 3 inches (7.5 cm) from the center of the IR

123. It will prevent urine, gas, and fecal material from obscuring the coccyx.

124. Position the ASISs at equal distances from the imaging table.

125. A. Opposite
B. Farther

126. The patient should be supine with the legs extended and the central ray should be angled 10 degrees caudally.

127. Kyphotic

128. A. Midsagittal
B. Symphysis pubis

129. The fifth sacral segment, three coccygeal vertebrae, symphysis pubis, and pelvic brim.

130. A. No
B. Shielding a female patient will obscure the coccyx.

131. The patient did not empty the bladder.

132. The patient was rotated toward the right side.

133. The central ray was not angled enough caudally.

134. The urinary bladder is dense and creating a shadow over the coccyx. The coccyx is not aligned with the symphysis pubis but is situated closer to the left lateral wall of the inlet pelvis. Have the patient empty the urinary bladder and rotate the patient toward the left side until the ASISs are positioned at equal distances from the imaging table and IR.

135. The symphysis pubis is superimposed over the inferior coccyx and the coccyx is foreshortened. Angle the central ray 10 degrees caudally.

136. A. Sacrum
B. Coccyx
C. Greater sciatic notches

137. A. Profile
B. Foreshortening

138. A. Use tight collimation.
B. Use a high-ratio grid.
C. Place a flat contact shield on the imaging table along the posterior edge of the collimated field.

139. Align the shoulders, posterior ribs, and posterior pelvic wings perpendicular to the imaging table.

140. It prevents the side of the patient positioned farther from the imaging table from rotating anteriorly.

141. By evaluating the superimposition of the greater sciatic notches

142. Position the vertebral column parallel with and the iliac line perpendicular to the imaging table.

143. A. Posteriorly
B. Inferiorly
C. ASIS

144. 4 inches (10 cm)

145. The fifth sacral segment, first through third coccygeal vertebrae, and inferior medial sacral crest

146. The patient was rotated.

147. The greater sciatic notches are demonstrated one anterior to the other and the ischium is almost superimposed over the third coccygeal segment. When rotation has occurred, it is most common for the elevated side of the patient to have been rotated anteriorly. Rotate the elevated pelvic wing posteriorly until the posterior pelvic wings are aligned perpendicular to the IR. It may be necessary to position a sponge or pillow between the patient's knees to help maintain this positioning.

1. A. As if the patient is in an upright position; the marker is reversed.
   B. As if the patient is in an upright position; the marker is correct.
   C. As if the patient is in an upright position; the marker is correct.

3. A. Thoracic vertebral column
   B. Jugular notch
   C. SC joint
   D. Manubrium
   E. Posterior rib
   F. Sternal body
   G. Inferior scapular angle
   H. Xiphoid process

2.

Sternum and Rib Technical Data			
Projection	kVp	Grid	SID
PA oblique (RAO position), sternum	60 – 70	Grid	30 – 40 inches (75 –100 cm)
Lateral, sternum	70 – 75	Grid	72 inches (180 cm)
AP or PA, upper ribs	65 – 70	Grid	40 – 48 inches (100 – 120 cm)
AP or PA, lower ribs	70 – 75	Grid	40 – 48 inches (100 – 120 cm)
AP oblique, upper ribs	70 – 80	Grid	40 – 48 inches (100 – 120 cm)
AP oblique, lower ribs	75 – 85	Grid	40 – 48 inches (100 – 120 cm)

4. A. Uniform in quality
   B. Shallow breathing
5. A. Blurred
   B. Left scapula
   C. Vertebral
6. Because it superimposes the heart shadow over the sternum
7. Homogeneous
8. A. Posterior ribs
   B. Lung markings
   C. Heart shadow
   D. Left inferior scapula
9. Higher
10. A. Costal
    B. Blur
    C. Posterior ribs
11. Blurred
12. A. Midcoronal
    B. 15 to 20
13. More
14. Midsternum
15. A. 3 inches (7.5 cm)
    B. Thoracic spinous processes
    C. Jugular notch
16. A. Superior
    B. Inferior
17. A. Thoracic spinous processes
    B. Left inferior angle of the scapula
18. A. Sternum
    B. Thoracic vertebrae
19. The patient was rotated less than 15 to 20 degrees.

20. The sternum and lung markings are blurry and unidentifiable. Instruct the patient to breathe shallowly instead of deeply. If the patient is unable to breathe costally, take the exposure on expiration.
21. The sternum is positioned to the left of the heart shadow. Decrease the degree of patient obliquity.
22. A. Anterior rib
    B. Sternal body
    C. Xiphoid process
23. A. Jugular notch
    B. Manubrium
    C. Sternal body
24. A. Profile
    B. Humeral
25. Because the pectoral muscles and female breast tissue are superimposed over the inferior sternum but not the superior sternum
26. A. Use a grid.
    B. Collimate tightly.
    C. Position a flat contact strip anterior to the sternum close to the shadow of the anterior skin line.
27. Align the shoulders, posterior ribs, and posterior pelvic wings perpendicular to the IR.
28. By evaluating the degree of anterior rib and sternal superimposition
29. The superior heart shadow will not continue into the anteriorly situated lung but will end at the sternum.
30. Anterior ribs
31. Extend the patient's arms behind the back and have the patient clasp the hands.

32. A. 1.5
    B. Jugular notch
    C. Perpendicular
33. To reduce the magnification that would result from the long OID
34. The jugular notch, sternal body, and xiphoid process
35. The patient's left side is positioned anterior to the right side.
36. The patient's right side is positioned anterior to the left side.
37. The anterior ribs are demonstrated without superimposition, the sternum is not in profile, the superior heart shadow does not extend beyond the sternum and into the anteriorly situated lung, and the humeri soft tissue is superimposed over the manubrium. Position the left thorax slightly anteriorly, extend the patient's arms behind the back, and have the patient clasp the hands.
38. A. Seventh posterior rib
    B. Eighth posterior rib
    C. Diaphragm
    D. Ninth posterior rib
    E. Eighth anterior rib
39. A. Vertebral column
    B. Vertebral column
    C. Superior ribs
    D. Nine
    E. Eighth
40. To aid the reviewer in pinpointing the exact location of the potential injury
41. A. Full suspended inspiration
    B. Full suspended expiration
42. Higher kVp is needed to penetrate the denser abdominal structures and demonstrate the ribs.
43. A. Upper thorax, axillary and neck soft tissues, and vascular lung markings.
    B. Upper abdominal tissue
44. A. Posteroanterior
    B. Anteroposterior
    C. The ribs of interest would demonstrate increased magnification.
45. In a rotated patient, the distances from the vertebral column to the lateral edge will be uniform down the length of the lung field and, in a patient with scoliosis, the distances from the vertebral column to the lateral lung edge will vary.
46. A. Flex the patient's knees, placing the feet flat against the imaging table and positioning the shoulders at equal distances from the IR.
    B. Place the patient's chin on a sponge so the patient can look straight ahead and position the patient's shoulders and anterior superior iliac spines (ASISs) at equal distances from the imaging table.
47. A. Place the back of the patient's hands on the hips, and rotate the elbows and shoulders anteriorly.
    B. Internally rotate the patient's arms, forcing the shoulders to rotate anteriorly.
48. Nine
49. Eight through twelfth

50. A. Midsagittal plane
    B. Jugular notch
    C. Xiphoid process
    D. Midsagittal plane
    E. Inferior scapular angle
51. The first through ninth ribs and vertebral column
52. A. Iliac crest
    B. Midsagittal plane
    C. Place the lower IR border 2 inches (5 cm) above the iliac crest.
53. The vertebral column and eighth through twelfth ribs
54. The patient's right side was positioned farther away from the IR than the left side.
55. The patient's left arm was not adequately internally rotated.
56. The projection was taken on inspiration.
57. The sternum is demonstrated to the right of the patient's vertebral column. Flex the patient's knees and rotate the thorax toward the left side until the shoulders are at equal distances from the IR. Seven posterior ribs are demonstrated above the diaphragm. Obtain the projection after full suspended inspiration.
58. Eight posterior ribs are demonstrated above the diaphragm. Obtain the projection after full suspended inspiration.
59. The distance from the spinous process to the pedicles on the right side is narrower than that on the left side. Rotate the patient toward the right side until the shoulders and ASISs are at equal distances from the IR.
60. A. Third axillary rib
    B. Inferior scapular angle
    C. Fifth anterior rib
    D. Sternum
61. A. Sixth anterior rib
    B. Ninth axillary rib
    C. Twelfth rib
62. A. Inferior sternal body
    B. Axillary ribs
    C. Ten
    D. Ninth
63. A. AP
    B. When posterior oblique ribs are taken, the axillary ribs are positioned closer to the IR, resulting in less magnification.
64. A. 45 degrees
    B. Midcoronal
65. A. Toward the affected side
    B. Away from the affected side
66. The inferior sternal body will be located halfway between the lateral body surface and vertebral column.
67. Full suspended inspiration
68. Full suspended expiration
69. A. Perpendicular
    B. Affected lateral rib surface
    C. Jugular notch
    D. Xiphoid process

70. The first through tenth axillary ribs of the affected side and thoracic vertebral column
71. A. Iliac crest
    B. Midsagittal plane
72. The vertebral column and tenth through twelfth axillary ribs of the affected side
73. The patient was rotated the wrong direction (toward the left side).
74. The patient was rotated less than 45 degrees.
75. The projection was not taken on full inspiration.
76. The sternum is situated next to the vertebral column. Increase the degree of patient obliquity to 45 degrees.
77. The axillary ribs demonstrate increased foreshortening. The patient was rotated the wrong direction. The patient should be rotated away from the affected ribs when a PA oblique projection is obtained. The ribs demonstrate increased magnification. Obtain the projection in an AP projection to decrease rib magnification.

CHAPTER 11   CRANIUM

1. A. As if the patient was in an upright position, with the marker correct
   B. As if the patient was in an upright position, with the marker reversed
   C. With the anterior mandible facing upward, with the marker correct
   D. As if the patient was in an upright position, with the marker correct

2.

Cranium, Facial Bones, Sinuses, and Mandible Technical Data					
Projection	Structure	kVp	Grid	AEC Chamber(s)	SID
AP or PA	Cranium	70 – 80	Grid	Center	40 – 48 inches (100 – 120 cm)
	Mandible	70 – 80	Grid		
PA axial (Caldwell method)	Cranium	70 – 80	Grid	Center	40 – 48 inches (100 – 120 cm)
	Facial bones	70 – 80	Grid	Center	
	Sinuses	70 – 80	Grid	Center	
AP axial (Towne method)	Cranium	70 – 80	Grid	Center	40 – 48 inches (100 – 120 cm)
	Mandible	70 – 80	Grid		
Lateral	Cranium	70 – 80	Grid	Center	40 – 48 inches (100 – 120 cm)
	Facial bones	70 – 80	Grid	Center	
	Sinuses	50 – 60	Grid		
	Nasal bones	70 – 80	Grid		
Submentovertex (Schueller method)	Cranium	70 – 80	Grid	Center	40 – 48 inches (100 – 120 cm)
	Mandible	70 – 80	Grid	Center	
	Sinuses	70 – 80	Grid	Center	
	Zygomatic arches	60 – 70	Nongrid		
Parietoacanthial (Waters method)	Facial bones	70 – 80	Grid	Center	40 – 48 inches (100 – 120 cm)
	Sinuses	70 – 80	Grid	Center	
Tangential (Superoinferior)	Nasal bones	50 – 60	Nongrid		40 – 48 inches (100 – 120 cm)

3. A. Frontal bone
   B. Anterior clinoid process
   C. Petrous ridge
   D. Oblique orbital line
   E. Nasal septum
   F. Internal auditory canal
   G. Supraorbital margin
   H. Lateral cranial cortex
   I. Dorsum sellae
   J. Crista galli
   K. Frontal sinus
4. A. Imaginary line connecting the outer eye canthus and external auditory opening
   B. Area located on the midsagittal plane at the level of the eyebrows
5. A. Cortices
   B. Ethmoid sinuses
   C. Supraorbital margins
   D. Nasal septum
6. A. Perpendicular
   B. Place an extended flat palm next to each parietal bone and adjust the head rotation until your hands are positioned perpendicular to the IR.
7. When the distance from the lateral orbital margin to the lateral cranial cortex or from the crista galli to the lateral cranial cortex on one side is greater than the opposite side
8. The patient's head should not be adjusted. The image should be taken with the head positioned as is.
9. A. AP projection
   B. PA projection
10. A. OML
    B. Perpendicular
11. Angle the central ray parallel with the OML.
12. Inferiorly
13. Angle the central ray parallel with the OML.
14. They would be demonstrated within the ethmoid sinuses.
15. Increase
16. A. Crista galli
    B. Nasal septum
17. A. Dorsum sellae
    B. Glabella
18. The outer cranial cortex and maxillary sinus
19. A. Midpoint between the mandibular rami
    B. Exit the acanthion
20. Entire mandible
21. The patient's face was rotated toward the right side.
22. A. The patient's chin was not tucked enough.
    B. The central ray was angled too cephalically.
23. A. The patient's chin was tucked too much.
    B. The central ray was angled too caudally.
24. The distances from the lateral orbital margins to the lateral cranial borders and from the crista galli to the lateral cranial cortex on the left side are greater than the same distances on the right side. Rotate the patient's face to the left until the midsagittal plane is aligned perpendicular to the IR.

25. The petrous ridges are demonstrated inferior to the supraorbital margins and the dorsum sellae and anterior clinoids are demonstrated within the ethmoid sinuses. Tuck the chin until the OML is aligned perpendicular to the IR or move the chin downward half the distance demonstrated between the petrous ridges and supraorbital margins.
26. The petrous ridges are demonstrated superior to the supraorbital margins and the internal auditory canals are distorted. Extend the chin, moving it away from the thorax until the OML is aligned perpendicular to the IR, or move the chin upward half the distance demonstrated between the petrous ridges and supraorbital margin.
27. The petrous ridges are demonstrated inferior to the supraorbital margins and the dorsum sellae and anterior clinoids are demonstrated within the ethmoid sinuses. The supraorbital margins need to be moved toward the petrous ridges. Tuck the chin until the OML is aligned perpendicular to the IR or adjust the central ray angulation caudally. The distance from the right lateral orbital margin to the lateral cranial cortex is less than the distance from the left lateral orbital margin to the lateral cranial cortex. If a cervical injury is not suspected and the patient allows, rotate the face toward the left side.
28. A. Lateral cranial cortex
    B. Greater sphenoidal wing
    C. Inferior orbital margin
    D. Nasal septum
    E. Ethmoid sinus
    F. Petrous pyramid
    G. Petrous ridge
    H. Oblique orbital line
    I. Superior orbital fissure
    J. Lesser sphenoidal wing
    K. Crista galli
29. A. Orbits
    B. Infraorbital margins
    C. Crista galli
30. Place an extended flat palm next to each parietal bone, and adjust the head rotation until your hands are positioned perpendicular to the IR.
31. Midsagittal
32. A. Away from
    B. Away from
33. A. Because the orbits are placed at a longer object–image receptor distance (OID) in the AP than in the PA projection
    B. AP projection
34. 15 degrees caudal
35. 15 degrees cephalic
36. Orbitomeatal
37. Position the OML as close as possible to perpendicular to the IR. Angle the central ray parallel with the patient's OML and adjust it 15 degrees caudally from this angle.
38. 5 degrees caudal
39. 10 degrees cephalic

40. Align the midsagittal plane with the long axis of the IR.
41. A. Ethmoid sinuses
    B. Exit at the nasion
42. Depression at the bridge of the nose.
43. A. The outer cranial cortex and ethmoid sinuses
    B. The frontal and ethmoid sinuses and lateral cranial cortices
44. A. Right
    B. The patient's head was turned toward the right side.
45. A. The patient's chin was not tucked enough.
    B. The central ray was angled too caudally.
46. A. The patient's chin was tucked more than needed.
    B. The central ray was angled too cephalically.
47. The distances from the lateral orbital margin to the lateral cranial cortex and from the crista galli to the lateral cranial cortex on the right side are greater than the distances on the left side. Rotate the patient's face toward the right side.
48. The petrous ridges and pyramids are demonstrated in the superior half of the orbits. Elevate the patient's chin until the OML is aligned perpendicular to the IR, or angle the central ray caudally.
49. The petrous ridges are demonstrated inferior to the inferior orbital margins and the patient's face is rotated toward the right side. Tuck the chin until the OML is aligned perpendicular to the IR, or adjust the central ray angulation cephalically and rotate the face toward the left side.
50. The petrous ridges are demonstrated too inferior in the orbits. Tuck the chin until the OML is perpendicular to the IR, or adjust the central ray angulation caudally.
51. A. Sagittal suture
    B. Parietal bone
    C. Lateral cranial cortex
    D. Posterior clinoid process
    E. Dorsum sellae
    F. Foramen magnum
    G. Occipital bone
    H. Petrous ridge
    I. Petrous pyramid
    J. Nasal septum
52. A. Mastoid process
    B. Condyle
    C. Coronoid process
    D. Ramus
    E. Body
    F. Symphysis
53. A. Foramen magnum
    B. Foramen magnum
    C. Posterior clinoids
    D. Superior
    E. Sagittal suture
54. Imaginary line connecting the lower orbital outline and external auditory meatus
55. Place an extended flat palm next to each lateral parietal bone, and adjust the patient's head rotation until your hands are positioned perpendicular to the IR.

56. A. By determining that the distance from the posterior clinoid process to the lateral border of the foramen magnum on one side is greater than the distance on the opposite side
    B. By determining that the dorsum sella is demonstrated closer to one side of the foramen magnum than the opposite side
57. A. Midsagittal
    B. Perpendicular
58. Toward
59. A. Dorsum sellae
    B. Foramen magnum
60. 35-40 degrees caudal
61. OML
62. Angle the central ray until it is parallel with the OML and adjust it 30 degrees caudally.
63. A. Sagittal suture
    B. Nasal septum
64. The outer cranial cortex, petrous ridges, dorsum sellae, and foramen magnum
65. The patient's face was rotated toward the left side.
66. A. The patient's chin was not tucked enough.
    B. The central ray was angled too cephalically.
67. A. The patient's chin was tucked more than needed.
    B. The central ray was angled too caudally.
68. The distance from the posterior clinoid process to the lateral foramen magnum on the patient's left side is less than the distance on the patient's right side. Rotate the patient's face toward the right side until the midsagittal plane is perpendicular to the IR.
69. The dorsum sellae and anterior clinoids are demonstrated superior to the foramen magnum. Tuck the patient's chin until the OML is perpendicular to the IR or adjust the central ray caudally. The symphysis is clipped. Lower the central ray and IR by 0.5 inch (1.25 cm).
70. The dorsum sella is foreshortened and superimposed over the atlas's posterior arch. Elevate the patient's chin or adjust the central ray angulation cephalically.
71. A. Inion
    B. Occipital bone
    C. Mastoid air cells
    D. External auditory meatus
    E. Posterior arch
    F. Clivus
    G. Dorsum sellae
    H. Posterior clinoid processes
    I. Sella turcica
    J. Anterior clinoid processes
    K. Sphenoidal sinuses
    L. Greater sphenoidal wings
    M. Orbital roofs
    N. Frontal sinuses
    O. Anterior cranial cortex
    P. Frontal bone
    Q. Parietal bone
    R. Superior cranial cortex

72. A. Frontal sinus
    B. Sella turcica
    C. Sphenoid sinuses
    D. Ethmoid air cells
    E. Maxillary sinuses
73. A. Nasofrontal suture
    B. Nasal bone
74. A. Profile
    B. Posterior arch
75. A. Imaginary line connecting the outer corners of each eyelid
    B. Outer corner where eyelids meet
    C. External auditory meatus
76. The sphenoid, ethmoid, frontal, and maxillary sinuses
77. To demonstrate air-fluid levels within the sinus cavities
78. A. Midsagittal
    B. Parallel
    C. Perpendicular
79. A. Elevate the occiput on a radiolucent sponge.
    B. Position the cassette 1 inch (2.5 cm) below the occipital bone.
80. When the patient's cranium is tilted, the inferior cortical outlines of superimposed structures are demonstrated without superimposition. When the cranium is rotated, the posterior and anterior cortices are demonstrated without superimposition.
81. Position the IOML perpendicular to the front edge of the IR.
82. A. Superior
    B. EAM
83. The outer cranial cortex
84. A. Zygoma and greater wings of the sphenoid
    B. Outer canthus
    C. EAM
85. The frontal, ethmoid, sphenoid, and maxillary sinuses and mandible
86. A. Nasal bones
    B. Inferior
87. Nasal bones, surrounding nasal soft tissue, anterior nasal spine of maxilla, anterior cranial cortices, orbital roofs, and zygomatic bones
88. The patient's head was rotated.
89. The patient's head was tilted toward the IR.
90. The greater wings of the sphenoid and the anterior cranial cortices are demonstrated without superimposition. One of each corresponding structure is demonstrated anterior to the other and the posterior arch is in profile. Rotate the patient's head until the midsagittal plane is parallel with the IR. The orbital roofs and inferior cranial cortices are demonstrated without superimposition. One of each corresponding structure is demonstrated superior to the other. Tilt the patient's head away from the IR until the midsagittal plane is parallel and the IP line is perpendicular to the IR.

91. The orbital roofs and inferior cranial cortices are demonstrated without superimposition. One of each corresponding structure is demonstrated superior to the other and the atlas's vertebral foramen is visualized. Tilt the patient's head toward the IR until the midsagittal plane is parallel and the IP line is perpendicular to the IR.
92. A. Mandibular mentum
    B. Maxillary sinus
    C. Posterior palatine bone
    D. Sphenoid sinus
    E. Mandibular condyle
    F. Dens
    G. Foramen magnum
    H. Petrous pyramid
    I. Cranial cortex
    J. Mastoid air cells
    K. Foramen spinosum
    L. Foramen ovale
    M. Mandibular ramus
    N. Mandibular coronoid
    O. Mandibular body
    P. Ethmoid sinus
    Q. Vomer and bony nasal septum
    R. Nasal fossae
93. A. Ethmoid sinuses
    B. Dens
94. A. IOML
    B. Parallel
95. A. Nasal fossae
    B. Ethmoid sinuses
    C. Foramen ovale
    D. Foramen spinosum
96. Angle the central ray until it is aligned perpendicular to the IOML.
97. A. By comparing the distance from the right mandibular ramus and body to its corresponding lateral cranial cortex with the distance from the left mandibular ramus and body to its corresponding lateral cranial cortex
    B. Align the midsagittal plane perpendicular to the IR.
98. A. Turn the patient's face until the midsagittal plane is aligned with the long axis of the collimator's longitudinal light.
    B. No
99. A. Dens
    B. Midsagittal
    C. 0.75 (2 cm)
    D. EAM
100. The mandible and outer cranial cortices
101. A. Sphenoid sinuses
    B. Midsagittal
    C. 1.5 (4 cm)
    D. Mandibular symphysis
102. The mandible, lateral cranial cortices, and mastoid air cells
103. The patient's neck was overextended, preventing the IOML from being positioned parallel with the IR.

104. A. The patient's neck was underextended, preventing the IOML from being positioned parallel with the IR.
    B. The central ray was angled too caudally.
105. The patient's vertex was tilted toward the left side.
106. The mandibular mentum is demonstrated too far anterior to the ethmoid sinuses. Depress the patient's chin until the IOML is aligned parallel with the IR or adjust the central ray angulation caudally.
107. The mandibular mentum is demonstrated posterior to the ethmoid sinuses. Elevate the patient's chin or adjust the central ray angulation cephalically. The distance from the right mandibular ramus and body to its corresponding lateral cranial cortex is greater than the distance from the left mandibular ramus and body to its corresponding lateral cranial cortex. Tilt the patient's cranial vertex toward the left side.
108. The distance from the right mandibular ramus and body to its corresponding lateral cranial cortex is greater than the distance from the left mandibular ramus and body to its corresponding lateral cranial cortex. Tilt the patient's cranial vertex toward the left side.
109. A. Supraorbital margin
    B. Lateral orbital margin
    C. Inferior orbital margin
    D. Zygomatic bone
    E. Zygomatic arch
    F. Coronoid process
    G. Petrous ridge
    H. Posterior maxillary process
    I. Sphenoid sinus
    J. Maxillary sinus
    K. Lateral cranial cortex
    L. Nasal septum
110. A. Inferior
    B. Laterally
111. Imaginary line connecting the chin with the external ear opening
112. Sphenoid sinuses
113. Position an extended flat palm next to each lateral parietal bone and adjust the head rotation until your hands are positioned perpendicular to the IR.
114. A. Away from
    B. Away from
115. A. Because they are placed at a longer OID for the acanthioparietal projection
    B. Acanthioparietal
116. Align the mentomeatal line perpendicular to the IR.
117. Align the cranium's midsagittal plane with the collimator's longitudinal light line.
118. A. It prevents tight collimation.
    B. It makes viewing the image more awkward.
119. A. Anterior nasal spine
    B. Acanthion
120. The frontal and maxillary (and sphenoidal with the open-mouth position) sinuses and lateral cranial cortices.

121. The patient's face was rotated toward the right side.
122. The patient's chin was not elevated enough to position the mentomeatal line perpendicular to the IR.
123. The patient's chin was elevated more than needed to align the mentomeatal line perpendicular to the IR.
124. The petrous ridges are inferior to the maxillary sinuses and posterior maxillary alveolar process, and the distance from the lateral orbital margin to the lateral cranial cortex on the left side is greater than on the right side. Tuck the patient's chin until the mentomeatal line (MML) is perpendicular to the IR and rotate the face toward the left side until the midsagittal plane is perpendicular to the IR.
125. The petrous ridges are demonstrated within the maxillary sinuses and superior to the posterior maxillary alveolar process. Elevate the patient's chin until the MML is perpendicular to the IR or adjust the central ray angulation caudally if air-fluid levels are not being evaluated.
126. The petrous ridges are inferior to the maxillary sinuses and posterior maxillary alveolar process. Depress the patient's chin until the MML is perpendicular to the IR or adjust the central ray angulation cephalically if air-fluid levels are not being evaluated.
127. A. Septal cartilage
    B. Nasal bone
128. Maxillary sinuses
129. Imaginary line connecting the glabella and maxillary alveolar
130. A. Perpendicular
    B. Midsagittal
131. Glabelloalveolar line (GAL)
132. A. Nasal bones
    B. Nasion
133. Nasal bones and surrounding nasal soft tissue.
134. The patient's chin was rotated toward the right side and cranium toward the left side.
135. The patient's chin was not elevated enough to position the GAL perpendicular to the IR.

CHAPTER 12 DIGESTIVE SYSTEM

1. The patient is instructed to remove the outer clothing and any underclothes containing artifacts, and then to change into a snapless hospital gown.
2. A. No preparation procedure is required
    B. Nothing by mouth (NPO) after midnight or at least 8 hours before the examination; avoid gum and tobacco products before procedure.
    C. Low-residue diet for 1 to 2 days before the examination, NPO after midnight or at least 8 hours before the examination; avoid gum and tobacco products before the examination.
    D. Low-residue diet for 2 to 3 days before the examination, followed by a clear liquid diet 1 day before the examination, laxatives the afternoon before the examination, and a suppository or cleaning enema the morning of the examination

3. Short exposure times are needed to control the image blur that may result from peristaltic activity within the system.
4. Peristalsis is the contraction and relaxation movements of the smooth muscles in the walls of the digestive system that mix food and secretions and move the materials through the system. Peristalsis is identified on an image by sharp bony cortices and blurry gastric and intestinal gases or barium.

5.

Digestive System Technical Data				
Projection	kVp	Grid	AEC	SID
UPPER GASTROINTESTINAL SYSTEM				
PA oblique (RAO position), esophagus	SC = 100 – 110	Grid	Center	40 – 48 inches (100 – 120 cm)
Lateral, esophagus	SC = 100 – 110	Grid	Center	40 – 48 inches (100 – 120 cm)
AP or PA, esophagus	SC = 100 – 110	Grid	Center	40 – 48 inches (100 – 120 cm)
PA oblique (RAO position), stomach	SC = 100 – 110 DC = 80 – 90	Grid	Center	40 – 48 inches (100 – 120 cm)
PA, stomach	SC = 100 – 110 DC = 80 – 90	Grid	Center	40 – 48 inches (100 – 120 cm)
Right lateral, stomach	SC = 100 – 110 DC = 80 – 90	Grid	Center	40 – 48 inches (100 – 120 cm)
AP oblique (LPO position), stomach	SC = 100 – 110 DC = 80 – 90	Grid	Center	40 – 48 inches (100 – 120 cm)
AP projection, stomach	SC = 100 – 110 DC = 80 – 90	Grid	Center	40 – 48 inches (100 – 120 cm)
SMALL INTESTINE				
PA or AP	SC = 100 – 125	Grid	All three	40 – 48 inches (100 – 120 cm)
Large intestine				
AP or AP	SC = 100 – 125 DC = 80 – 90	Grid	All three	40 – 48 inches (100 – 120 cm)
Lateral (rectum)	SC = 100 – 125 DC = 80 – 90	Grid	Center	40 – 48 inches (100 – 120 cm)
AP or PA (lateral decubitus position)	SC = 100 – 125 DC = 80 – 90	Grid	All three	40 – 48 inches (100 – 120 cm)
PA oblique (RAO position)	SC = 100 – 125 DC = 80 – 90	Grid	All three	40 – 48 inches (100 – 120 cm)
PA oblique (LAO position)	SC = 100 – 125 DC = 80 – 90	Grid	All three	40 – 48 inches (100 – 120 cm)
PA axial or PA axial oblique (RAO position)	SC = 100 – 125 DC = 80 – 90	Grid	All three	40 – 48 inches (100 – 120 cm)

AEC, Automatic exposure control; *AP*, anteroposterior; *DC*, double contrast; *kVp*, kilovoltage-peak; *LPO*, left posterior oblique; *PA*, posteroanterior; *RAO*, right anterior oblique; *SC*, single contrast; *SID*, source–image receptor distance.

6. A. Hypersthenic: The abdomen is broad and deep from anterior to posterior, the stomach is positioned high in the abdomen and lies transversely at the level of T9 to T12, and the duodenal bulb is demonstrated at the level of T11 to T12.
   B. Asthenic: The abdomen is narrow; the stomach is positioned low in the abdomen and runs vertically along the left side of the vertebral column, typically extending from T11 to L5, with the duodenal bulb at the level of L3 to L4.
   C. Sthenic: The abdomen is less broad than in the hypersthenic habitus and less narrow than in the asthenic habitus. The stomach also rests at a position between that in the hypersthenic and asthenic habitus and typically extends from T10 to L2, with the duodenal bulb at the level of L1 to L2.
7. A. Hypersthenic: The colic flexures and transverse colon tend to be high in the abdomen.
   B. Asthenic: The small and large intestinal structures tend to be positioned low in the abdomen.
   C. Sthenic: The small and large intestinal structures tend to be centered within the abdomen.
8. Ninth posterior rib. Full expiration allows increased abdominal space for the structures to be visualized without segment overlapping or foreshortening.
9. 30% to 50%
10. When foreign bodies and strictures of the esophagus are suspected
11. A. Left sternoclavicular end
    B. Vertebrae
    C. Esophagus
    D. Heart
12. A. Vertebrae
    B. Heart shadow
    C. 0.5
    D. 35 to 40
13. A. Midesophagus
    B. Spinous process
    C. 2 to 3
14. Entire esophagus

15. The patient did not swallow enough barium before and/or during the examination.
16. The patient was rotated less than the required 35 to 40 degrees.
17. The superior and inferior ends of the esophagus are not filled with barium. The patient should drink barium continuously during the exposure or should swallow two spoonfuls of thick barium and then given a third spoonful that is swallowed immediately before the exposure is taken.
18. The vertebrae are superimposed over the right sternoclavicular end and a portion of the esophagus. Increase the degree of patient obliquity until the midcoronal plane is at a 35- to 40-degree angle with the imaging table.
19. A. Vertebrae
    B. Left hemidiaphragm
    C. Esophagus
    D. Stomach
20. A. Posterior
    B. 0.5
    C. Posterior ribs
21. Align the posterior shoulders, ribs, and pelvis perpendicular to the imaging table.
22. Place the humeri at a 90-degree angle with the torso or separate the shoulders by positioning the arm and shoulder placed closer to the imaging table forward while maintaining a lateral thorax.
23. A. Midesophagus
    B. T5 to T6
    C. Jugular notch
24. Entire esophagus
25. The patient's elevated side was rotated posteriorly.
26. A. Vertebrae
    B. Left sternoclavicular end

C. Aortic arch
D. Esophagus
E. Heart
F. Left hemidiaphragm
G. Stomach
27. A. Vertebral column
    B. Sternal ends
28. Position the shoulders and anterosuperior iliac spines (ASISs) at equal distances from the imaging table.
29. Position the side of the patient with the breast removed at a greater OID than the opposite side.
30. A. Midesophagus
    B. T5 to T6
    C. Inferior scapular angle
31. Entire esophagus
32. The patient was rotated toward the left side.
33. The esophagus is to the left of the vertebrac and the left sternoclavicular end is demonstrated without vertebral column superimposition. Position the left shoulder toward the imaging table until the shoulders are at equal distances from the IR.
34. A. To demonstrate abnormalities of the stomach and lumen contour
    B. To visualize abnormalities in the mucosal details, and contour and lumen of stomach and duodenum
35. A. 30% to 50%
    B. 250%
36. A. Carbon dioxide
    B. Gastric distention and a smoothing of the rugae.
37. A. Mucosal surface
    B. Barium is washed over the gastric surface by having the patient turn 360 degrees and then positioning the patient so that the barium pool will be positioned away from the area of interest.

38.

Stomach	Barium-Filled Structures	Air-Filled Structures
PA oblique projection (RAO position)	Pylorus, duodenum	Fundus
PA projection	Pylorus, duodenum	Fundus
Right lateral projection	Pylorus, duodenum, body	Fundus
AP oblique projection (LPO position)	Fundus	Pylorus, duodenum
AP projection	Fundus	Pylorus, duodenum, body

39. A. Properties of the barium suspension
    B. Volume of barium and gas
    C. Frequency of washing
    D. Amount of fluid or secretions and viscosity of mucus in the stomach
40. A. Descending duodenum
    B. Duodenal bulb
    C. Pylorus
    D. Fundus
    E. Zygapophyseal joint
41. A. Hypersthenic; 70 degrees
    B. Sthenic; 45 degrees
    C. Asthenic; 40 degrees

42. A. Posterior third
    B. Descending
    C. Closed
43. A. Midline
    B. Descending
    C. Lesser curvature
44. A. Anterior third
    B. Descending
    C. Lesser curvature
45. Because of the difference in the amount of superimposition of the pylorus and duodenal bulb that exists among patients with a different habitus

46. A. Pylorus
    B. Vertebrae
    C. Lateral rib margin
    D. Superior
47. A. Center the central ray at a level 2 inches superior to the sthenic centering.
    B. Center the central ray at a level 2 inches inferior to the sthenic centering.
48. Stomach and duodenal loop
49. A. Pedicle
    B. Spinous process
    C. Pylorus
    D. Descending duodenum
    E. Small intestine
    F. Body
    G. Fundus
    H. Tenth thoracic vertebrae
50. A. Hypersthenic
    B. Asthenic
    C. Sthenic
51. A. Midline
    B. Spinous processes
52. A. Horizontally
    B. Eleventh to twelfth
    C. Anteriorly
    D. Esophagogastric junction
53. A. Vertically
    B. First or second
    C. Partial profile
54. A. Vertically
    B. Third to fourth
    C. J
    D. Lesser and greater curvatures, esophagogastric junction, pylorus, and duodenal bulb
55. A. Pylorus
    B. Vertebrae
    C. Left lateral rib border
    D. Superior
56. A. Direct the central ray just to the left of the vertebrae at a level 2 inches superior to the sthenic centering point.
    B. Direct the central ray 2 inches inferior to the sthenic habitus centering point.
57. Stomach and descending duodenum
58. The patient did not follow adequate preparation procedures.
59. The patient was rotated toward the left side.
60. A. Esophagus
    B. Fundus
    C. Duodenal bulb
    D. Descending duodenum
    E. Lumbar vertebra
    F. Pylorus
    G. Body
61. A. Sthenic
    B. Hypersthenic
    C. Asthenic
62. A. Posterior
    B. Retrogastric

63. A. Duodenal bulb
    B. Descending duodenum
    C. Closed
64. A. Duodenal bulb
    B. Descending duodenum
    C. Partially
    D. Partially closed
65. A. Duodenal bulb
    B. Descending duodenum
    C. Without
    D. Open
66. A. Pylorus
    B. Midcoronal plane
    C. Anterior abdomen
    D. Inferior rib margin
67. A. Direct the central ray at a level 2 inches superior to the sthenic habitus centering point.
    B. Direct the central ray at a level 2 inches inferior to the sthenic habitus centering point.
68. Stomach and duodenal loop.
69. The patient was not in a lateral projection but was rotated.
70. A. Esophagus
    B. Fundus
    C. Body
    D. Pylorus
    E. Duodenal bulb
    F. Descending duodenum
    G. Zygapophyseal joint
    H. Twelfth thoracic vertebra
71. A. Asthenic; 30 degrees
    B. Sthenic; 45 degrees
    C. Hypersthenic; 60 degrees
72. A. Posterior third
    B. Descending
    C. Vertebrae
73. A. Midline
    B. Descending
    C. Little if any
74. A. Anterior third
    B. Descending
    C. Little if any
75. A. Pylorus
    B. Vertebrae
    C. Left abdominal margin
    D. Midway
76. A. Center the central ray at a level 2 inches superior to the sthenic habitus central ray centering.
    B. Center the central ray at a level 2 inches inferior to the sthenic habitus central ray centering.
77. Stomach and duodenal loop
78. A. Fundus
    B. Body
    C. Small intestine
    D. Pylorus
    E. Descending duodenum
    F. Duodenal bulb
    G. Pedicle
    H. Spinous process

79. A. Sthenic
    B. Asthenic
    C. Hypersthenic
80. A. Midline
    B. Spinous processes
81. A. Horizontally
    B. Eleventh to twelfth
    C. Anteriorly
    D. Esophagogastric junction
82. A. Vertically
    B. First to second
    C. Partial profile
83. A. Vertically
    B. Third to fourth
    C. J
    D. Lesser and greater curvatures, esophagogastric junction, pylorus, duodenal bulb
84. A. Pylorus
    B. Vertebrae
    C. Left abdominal margin
    D. Midway
85. A. Center just to the left side of the vertebrae at a level 2 inches superior to the sthenic central ray centering.
    B. Center at a level 2 inches inferior to the sthenic central ray centering.
86. Stomach and duodenal loop
87. The patient was rotated with the left side positioned closest to the IR.
88. A. Stomach
    B. Left iliac ala
    C. Small intestine
    D. Spinous process
    E. Pedicle

89. With a right or left marker positioned laterally on the correct side and a time marker indicating the amount of time that has elapsed since the patient ingested the contrast
90. The first overhead is taken at 15 minutes, then 30 minutes, and then hourly until barium is demonstrated in the cecum.
91. A. Midline of the vertebral bodies
    B. Iliac ala
92. It will cause compression of the abdominal structures, increasing image quality.
93. The image in Figure 12-23 was taken earlier in the series than Figure 12-24. Figure 12-23 demonstrates more barium in the stomach, the central ray was centered above crest, and the barium has not reached as far into the colon when compared with Figure 12-24.
94. Barium is demonstrated in the cecum, which typically indicates the series is complete.
95. A. Small intestine
    B. Midsagittal plane
    C. Superior
    D. Iliac crest
96. The barium is in the stomach and upper small intestine directly after ingestion but moves to the lower small intestine later.
97. The stomach and proximal aspects of the small intestine on images taken early in the series, and the small intestine and cecum on images taken late in the series
98. A. Mucosal folds
    B. One third of the intestinal diameter
99. To wash away residual fecal material from the dependent surface, coat the mucosal surface, and fill any depressed lesions as the patient is rotated

100.

Double-Contrast Filling of Large Intestinal Structures		
Large Intestine	AP Projection (Supine Position)	PA Projection (Prone Position)
Cecum	Air	Barium
Ascending colon	Barium	Air
Ascending limb right colic (hepatic) flexure	Barium	Air
Descending limb right colic (hepatic) flexure	Barium	Air
Transverse colon	Air	Barium
Ascending limb left colic (splenic) flexure	Air	Barium
Descending limb left colic (splenic) flexure	Barium	Air
Descending colon	Barium	Air
Sigmoid colon	Air	Barium
Rectum	Barium	Air

101. Poor gaseous distention results in pockets of large barium pools and compacted intestinal segments, with tight mucosal folds.
102. Poor mucosal coating is demonstrated by thin, irregular, or interrupted barium coating or excessive barium pooling.
103. A. Pedicle
    B. Spinous process
    C. Transverse colon
    D. Left colic flexion
    E. Descending colon
    F. Iliac ala
    G. Sigmoid colon
    H. Rectum
    I. Cecum
    J. Ascending colon
    K. Right colic flexure

104. A. Midline
    B. Spinous processes
    C. Symmetrical
    D. Colic flexures
105. A. Shoulders
    B. ASISs
106. Farther
107. Wider
108. A. Fourth lumbar vertebra
    B. Midsagittal
    C. Iliac crest
109. A. Midsagittal plane
    B. Symphysis pubis
    C. ASIS
110. Entire large intestine, to include left colic (splenic) flexure and rectum
111. Figure 12-27 is an AP projection, and Figure 12-28 is a PA projection. The iliac alae are wider in Figure 12-27 than in Figure 12-28.
112. The patient was rotated toward the left side.
113. The central ray and IR were centered too low, or two crosswise IRs should have been used to include all of the structures.
114. The right iliac ala is narrow, the left iliac ala is wide, the distance from the right pedicles to the spinous processes is narrower than the corresponding distance on the left side, and the left colic (splenic) flexure demonstrates more ascending and descending limb superimposition. Rotate the patient toward the left side until the shoulders and iliac alae are equal distances to the imaging table.
115. The left colic (splenic) flexure and part of the transverse colon are not included on the image. Use two crosswise IRs with 2 to 3 inches of overlap.
116. A. Sigmoid
    B. Femoral heads
    C. Coccyx
    D. Rectum
    E. Sacrum
117. A lead sheet is placed on the imaging table at the edge of the posterior collimation field, and a grid is used.
118. A. Profile
    B. Femoral heads
119. A. Rectosigmoid region
    B. Midcoronal plane
    C. ASIS
120. Rectum, distal sigmoid, sacrum, and femoral heads
121. The patient's right side was rotated anteriorly.
122. The femoral heads are not superimposed; the right femoral head is rotated anterior to the left femoral head. Rotate the right side of the patient posteriorly until the posterior pelvic wings are superimposed and aligned perpendicular to the imaging table.
123. The femoral heads are not superimposed; the right femoral head is rotated posterior to the left femoral head. Rotate the right side of the patient anteriorly until the posterior pelvic wings are superimposed and aligned perpendicular to the imaging table.

124. A. Descending colon
    B. Iliac ala
    C. Sigmoid
    D. Rectum
    E. Cecum
    F. Ascending colon
    G. Right colic flexure
    H. Transverse colon
    I. Left colic flexure
125. Attach a wedge-compensating filter to the x-ray collimator head with the thick end positioned toward the patient's "up" side (thinnest part of abdomen) and the thin end toward the patient's "down" side (thickest part of abdomen).
126. A. Vertebral bodies
    B. Spinous processes
    C. Iliac ala
127. Farther
128. Narrower
129. To prevent the lateral abdomen, adjacent to the cart or imaging table, from being clipped or covered with artifact lines
130. A. Fourth lumbar vertebra
    B. Midsagittal
    C. Iliac crest
131. A. Midsagittal
    B. Symphysis pubis
    C. ASIS
132. Entire large intestine, including the left colic (splenic) flexure and rectum
133. The patient was not elevated on a cardiac board or radiolucent sponge.
134. The patient's right side was positioned farther from the IR than the left side.
135. A decrease in density is present across the entire image, and grid artifact lines are demonstrated longitudinally. Align the grid so it is perpendicular to the central ray.
136. This is an AP projection (the marker is correct). The distances from the right pedicles to the spinous processes are less than the distances from the left pedicles to the spinous processes, the left iliac ala is wider than the right, and the left colic (splenic) flexure demonstrates increased superimposition. Rotate the left side of the patient away from the IR until the shoulders and ASISs are at equal distances from the IR.
137. This is a PA projection (the marker is reversed). The distance from the right iliac ala is narrower than the left. Rotate the right side of the patient away from the IR until the shoulders and ASISs are at equal distances from the IR.
138. A. Left colic flexure
    B. Right colic flexure
    C. Descending colon
    D. Ascending colon
    E. Sigmoid
139. A. Right colic (hepatic) flexure
    B. Left colic (splenic) flexure
    C. Right

140. A. 35 to 45
    B. Ascending
    C. Descending
    D. Rectum
141. A. Midabdomen
    B. Left
    C. Iliac crest
142. Entire large intestine
143. The patient was insufficiently rotated.
144. A. Left colic flexure
    B. Right colic flexure
    C. Transverse colon
    D. Descending colon
    E. Ascending colon
    F. Sigmoid
145. A. Left
    B. Left
146. A. 35 to 45
    B. Descending
    C. Ascending
147. A. Midabdomen
    B. Right
    C. Iliac crest
148. Entire large intestine
149. A. Femoral head
    B. Inferior acetabulum
    C. Rectum
    D. Right superior acetabulum
    E. Sigmoid colon
    F. Anterior inferior iliac spine

150. A. Rectosigmoid segment
    B. Medial
    C. Left
151. A. Right
    B. Midcoronal
152. Symmetrical
153. A. Inferosuperior
    B. Distal rectum
    C. 30 to 40
    D. Caudally
154. A. Rectosigmoid segment
    B. ASIS
    C. ASIS
    D. Left
155. Rectum, sigmoid, and pelvic structures
156. The pelvis was rotated more than 45 degrees.
157. The central ray was insufficient.
158. The right SI joint is obscured and the left obturator foramen is closed. The inferior aspect of the left acetabulum is demonstrated superior to the distal rectum. Decrease pelvic rotation until the midcoronal plane is at a 30- to 45-degree angle with the imaging table and increase the degree of central ray angulation.
159. The right SI joint is obscured and the left obturator foramen is closed. The inferior aspect of the left acetabulum is demonstrated inferior to the distal rectum. Decrease pelvic rotation until the midcoronal plane is at a 30- to 45-degree angle with the imaging table and decrease the degree of central ray angulation.